HARRIET ROTH'S
CHOLESTEROL CONTROL COOKBOOK

D1469168

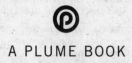

A PLUME BOOK

NOTE TO THE READER

The information contained in this book is not intended as a substitute for consulting with your physician. All matters regarding your health require medical supervision. Please note also that many of the products mentioned in this book are registered trademarks.

PLUME
Published by Penguin Group
Penguin Group (USA) Inc., 375 Hudson Street, New York, New York 10014, U.S.A. • Penguin Group (Canada), 90 Eglinton Avenue East, Suite 700, Toronto, Ontario, Canada M4P 2Y3 (a division of Pearson Penguin Canada Inc.) • Penguin Books Ltd., 80 Strand, London WC2R 0RL, England • Penguin Ireland, 25 St. Stephen's Green, Dublin 2, Ireland (a division of Penguin Books Ltd.) • Penguin Group (Australia), 250 Camberwell Road, Camberwell, Victoria 3124, Australia (a division of Pearson Australia Group Pty. Ltd.) • Penguin Books India Pvt. Ltd., 11 Community Centre, Panchsheel Park, New Delhi – 110 017, India • Penguin Group (NZ), 67 Apollo Drive, Rosedale, North Shore 0632, New Zealand (a division of Pearson New Zealand Ltd.) • Penguin Books (South Africa) (Pty.) Ltd., 24 Sturdee Avenue, Rosebank, Johannesburg 2196, South Africa

Penguin Books Ltd., Registered Offices: 80 Strand, London WC2R 0RL, England

Published by Plume, a member of Penguin Group (USA) Inc. Previously published in an NAL edition.

First Plume Printing, May 1991
First Plume Printing (second edition), August 2008
10 9 8 7 6 5 4 3 2

 REGISTERED TRADEMARK—MARCA REGISTRADA

LIBRARY OF CONGRESS CATALOGING-IN-PUBLICATION DATA

Roth, Harriet.
  [Cholesterol-control cookbook]
  Harriet Roth's cholesterol control cookbook / by Harriet Roth. — 2nd ed.
    p. cm.
  Includes bibliographical references and index.
  ISBN 978-0-452-28968-0 (trade pbk.)
  1. Low-cholesterol diet—Recipes. I. Title.
  RM237.75.R67 2008
  641.5'638—dc22   200805147

Printed in the United States of America

This revised and updated book is dedicated to the millions of enthusiastic readers whose pursuit of better health through healthful eating is an ongoing proactive process. Your words have fueled my work on this new edition.

Thanks,
HR

Acknowledgments

The past thirty years have been the most challenging and rewarding period of my professional life. The ever-changing face of the food world and the discoveries and advancements made in the fields of food and nutrition are a constant and stimulating challenge. However, it is because of my ongoing support system that my books have become a reality. The cast of characters has changed somewhat, but I have met and worked with people all over the United States and, indeed, the world.

Dr. John Farquhar, Bob Diforio, my agent, and Emily Haynes, my new editor, have been encouraging at all of the right moments. Also at Plume, I thank Matthew Boezi, Jason Johnson, and Abigail Powers. Sharon Berryhill Waldman, my secretarial assistant for the last thirty years, has left a brilliant legacy to my new assistant, Tracy Ung. Tracy, you had big shoes to fill and you did so with great effort and devotion—thank you.

Always just a phone call away were my previous editor, Molly Allen, and Nadia Kashper, the friendly voice at Plume. Once again I discovered what friends were for in the warmth of Irene Baron, Harriett Friedman, Eva Silver, and Dorothy Hartstein, RD. Cappy Fogel supplied not only her freezer but also her encouragement.

My thanks also to Wendy Hess, R.D., C.D.E., who provided the additional nutritional information that supports the database for my new recipes in this edition. She is the consummate professional. My daughter, Sally, and my son, Larry, still offered their suggestions (and questions). I have, at the risk of being repetitious once again, saved the best for last: my husband, my friend, my life partner, Harold. What would I do without his patience, sense of humor, intelligent honesty, and love? He has been my endless source of the positive energy everybody needs, but few people receive. I love you.

—**HR**

Foreword

by John W. Farquhar, M.D.,

author of *The American Way of Life Need Not Be Hazardous to Your Health* and *How to Reduce Your Risk of Heart Disease*

This splendid revised edition of *Harriet Roth's Cholesterol Control Cookbook* deserves careful reading and abundant praise from all who would want to prevent heart attacks, strokes, diabetes, and high blood pressure. It is really five books in one. To begin with there are more than two hundred fifty well-tested recipes, and each is designed to please the palate and protect all of the body's blood vessels, including those of the heart. Secondly, these recipes are blended into more than one hundred very helpful menus for breakfast, lunch, and dinner, with each providing balance in flavor and pleasure.

Harriet Roth has also added a splendid counterattack to our country's obesity epidemic with her two-week diet for weight loss and cholesterol lowering. Imagine the pounds melting away during a time of eating with **pleasure**. This is food portion control and easy weight loss on a silver platter!

We all know the difficulties of navigating hard-to-read food labels and counting calories, sodium, cholesterol, and saturated fat. Harriet makes these easy by using tables that give these components for many commonly available foods. She has added information on trans fat and on dietary fiber—both important in controlling runaway cholesterol levels. The book also provides a very valuable description of the "cholesterol-control story," including, for example, how diet can raise blood levels of the "good" cholesterol (HDL) and lower the harmful cholesterol fraction (LDL).

Two other issues of great importance are well covered: The role of heredity on cholesterol levels, and an extremely valuable section on the benefits versus the potential harm of cholesterol-lowering medications, such as the "statins." All features of this book prove that Harriet Roth has once again presented a system of practical knowledge that meets the needs of any person, responsible to themselves and others, in the pursuit of better health.

—John W. Farquhar, M.D.

Contents

PART I
The Cholesterol-Control Story

PART II
Choosing a Cholesterol-Control Lifestyle

Introduction: Newly Noted

I can hardly believe that thirty years have passed since my husband developed a coronary problem and we made a conscious choice to eliminate damaging overly fatted, high-cholesterol foods from our lives. It was a wise decision although it would have been better if we had reached it years before my husband's problem developed. However, it is important to realize that it is never too late to adopt good food habits and change your lifestyle—whether this decision is used as prevention or cure.

Back in 1978, I was a person who "thought food." I had a deep appreciation of and devotion to fine foods, and I prided myself on being a gourmet cook. I guess I was one of those people who "lived to eat." Although I was a nutrition professional, when I taught others how to cook I used butter, egg yolks, heavy cream, and animal protein with a generous hand. In fact, one of my eminent instructors, a prominent French restaurateur, had told me when I once questioned the use of all these high-cholesterol ingredients: "Harriet, if the ingredients are fresh and natural, you don't have to worry about the cholesterol."

But in my house we *did* have serious cause for worry, for while I was cooking all those fatty, high-cholesterol, high-saturated-fat foods with abandon, I was helping to build up a problem that affected my family directly.

My husband loved my cooking, and, oh, how I enjoyed preparing all his favorite foods. Suddenly and unexpectedly the endless "banquet" came to a halt—he had a serious coronary condition and dangerously high levels of cholesterol. What were we to do?

The doctors all suggested medication and, ultimately, bypass surgery. However, bypass surgery is not a cure, only a temporary aid. Nor are drugs alone a solution, for *without a change in lifestyle, plaque buildup in vein grafts and arteries can continue*. None of the professionals who saw my husband emphasized the importance of a shift to low-fat, low-cholesterol eating. There was no *nutritional* guidance.

In spite of my involvement with gourmet delights, my background in nutrition plus my common sense told me that somehow diet had to be important. I began to read everything I could get my hands on, and I was particularly influenced by the philosophy of Nathan Pritikin with his emphasis on a low-fat, low-cholesterol diet. (I subsequently became director of the Pritikin Longevity Center Cooking School.)

I began to make some changes in our eating habits. I started with the foods I bought at the market and the way I prepared them in the kitchen. I loved my husband dearly and I wanted him to savor the food I prepared—but more important, I wanted to share our lives, and I wanted him to be well enough to enjoy our family life as well as the tennis, the exercise, the professional life, the travel, all the many happy times that made up our life together. I knew there had to be a way to enjoy meals without a cost to health. I was determined to find a way to make low-cholesterol, low-fat dishes taste good so that mealtimes would be a pleasure, not a sentence or punishment.

I stopped teaching classes in classic French and Italian cuisine, and started modifying my recipes and creating exciting new ones. I must admit that in the beginning it wasn't easy to eat in the new style without feeling deprived. It took a while, but everyone in my family adjusted. Today, those traditional recipes, with their cloying sauces, high in fat and cholesterol, seem heavy and not at all appealing to the palate.

From the beginning I had decided I would not cook separate dishes for my husband—we would all eat together as a family and enjoy the same foods and, subsequently, the same good health. For my children and me, it would be prevention; for my husband, it would be an urgently needed cure. We had to forget the bread slathered with butter, margarine, or mayonnaise, the frequent large servings of animal protein, the rich sauces, and the cakes, cookies, and desserts, all filled with saturated fat, trans fat, and cholesterol.

At the time, our two children were teenagers. In the beginning, they would open the refrigerator and complain, "There's nothing to eat, Mom!" What they meant was, "There's no junk food to eat." Our pantry was soon filled with nourishing whole grain cereals and breads, fruits, vegetables, salads, nonfat yogurt and milk, muffins, and other healthful foods and snacks. I reversed the traditional ratio of large servings of protein and limited complex carbohydrates, serving instead small portions of animal protein and large servings of vegetables, salads, and grains.

And it wasn't just family dining that changed. Company meals, too, reflected our new way of life. These days I'm delighted to find that friends look forward to a dinner invitation to our home. They say the food I serve them tastes great, and I'm always told how wonderful they feel afterward—no sensation of being uncomfortably overstuffed and no guilt because their dinner was damaging to their health. I love it when they say, "This is delicious; is it from one of your books?"

Years ago, reliable information was not available about the dangers of cholesterol, trans fat, and saturated fat in food. Today, we have so much documentation and *constantly updated* good information that it would be sheer folly not to listen to what the experts say and follow their advice.

I continue to do just that, and today we are a family who *eats to live*, while still enjoying the pleasures of delicious healthful meals—perhaps enjoying them even more because after thirty years we know now that the foods we eat are helping us to lead healthier and more productive lives.

In the following pages I will explain just what cholesterol is, where it is found, how saturated fat and trans fat dangerously affect your cholesterol levels. How do we avoid these risks and hazards? For those who need to take immediate action, I offer a two-week diet plan that will reduce cholesterol levels and take off pounds. To help with everyday meal planning, I have provided delicious, complete menus with flavorful recipes to tempt your palate—recipes and menus that will *not only lower but also maintain low levels* of cholesterol.

By following my suggestions you will enjoy the rewards of *preventive nutrition* and, in addition, reduce any existing problems of atherosclerosis and heart disease. Research shows that by reducing the harmful ingredients in your diet you not only may be staving off future problems, but actually may be reversing present damage by decreasing the plaque that has already accumulated in your arteries.

Given the current research on nutrition and medicine, *physicians are emphasizing prevention as a means of treatment instead of only treating the disease itself*. While routine exercise, not smoking, and stress management are all important factors in avoiding heart disease, meals low in saturated fat, trans fat, and cholesterol and high in fiber provide the key that opens the door to good health.

Of course, in advanced cases medication may also be indicated, but *in no instance* is a sensible diet not absolutely necessary. Admittedly it does take a little more effort to change your lifestyle than to "pop a pill"—but with a change in lifestyle the only side effects will be a healthier, more vital you.

Cooking and eating healthy meals does not have to be boring. Remember, this is not a fat-free, taste-free style of eating that I am recommending. It's just the bad fats that you avoid. You can include all fresh fruits and vegetables, cereals, whole grains, pastas, poultry (turkey, chicken, Cornish game hen, duck breast—all without the wings and skin), and all fish and shellfish in limited amounts. You can still have 2 to 3 eggs per week (not swimming in butter). Although your food is not salt free, there are endless seasonings and spices (both fresh and dried) to pique and tantalize your taste buds. And yes, there is still the occasional indulgence of a piece of Mom's apple pie or a hot fudge sundae made with frozen yogurt and Orchard Farms' fudge topping with toasted almonds. Try the wonderful chocolate cake on page 344 or the coffee cake on page 340.

What you are doing is limiting portions and eating in moderation. The wide variety of different foods from which you can choose at home or while dining out is ever increasing. Even fast-food restaurants are offering a few healthy alternatives!

As a reward you will have that indescribable feeling of waking up in the morning and just feeling good, knowing that you have taken control of your health.

I started out trying to help someone I love. Then I began to do nutritional counseling to help others. With my books I am reaching out to a larger audience worldwide and enjoying all the positive feedback that I receive.

Like you, I love good food. But more important, I know how what you eat daily can affect your health now and in the future—and in the battle against heart disease, a low-saturated-fat, low-trans-fat, and low-cholesterol diet is a major weapon. Heart disease is the leading cause of death in *both men and women*. Make sure you are not included.

Remember, staying alive is not boring, it is a privilege.

My warmest wishes for your good health and longevity.

—HR

Today is the tomorrow that you planned for yesterday.

PART I

▼

The Cholesterol-Control Story

▼ 1 ▼

Learning About Trans Fat, Saturated Fat, and Cholesterol

Hardly a day has passed without the appearance of new and revolutionary scientific reports on the changing role of saturated fats and trans fats in our diet, and their deadly affect on raising critical cholesterol levels. How do these two types of fat contribute to elevating our cholesterol levels? We have known that genes and lifestyle determine our susceptibility to heart disease; however, we now learn that saturated and trans fat are even more critical in raising cholesterol than the cholesterol that we were consuming. Heart disease is now the number-one cause of death for *both* men and women in the United States. The twenty-first century will emphasize not only the cause, but also the cure, of this deadly disease. We know that there is no such thing as a sudden heart attack—they are usually in the works for years. As a thinking public, can we be more proactive and assume more responsibility for improvements in our health? I believe we *should* and I believe we *can*.

In 1978, when my husband first learned he had a coronary problem, cholesterol was only casually linked to heart trouble, although its role as a culprit was recognized by many cardiologists. Now, however, cholesterol is a household word and we are constantly bombarded in the media with new information about the connection between high cholesterol levels, saturated fat, trans fat, and heart disease.

This concern is also reflected by food manufacturers who proudly proclaim on labels, in newspapers, and on television that their products are low in cholesterol and contain no trans-fatty acids. These companies spend millions of dollars to develop low-cholesterol, no-trans-fat crackers, cookies, cakes, ice creams, mayonnaise and salad dressings, cheeses, and sour cream.

The menus of many restaurants offer low-cholesterol selections, and now fast-food chains feature salads or salad bars, fish, and skinless cuts of chicken, or use of polyunsaturated canola vegetable oil instead of saturated animal fats, hydrogenated oils, partially hydrogenated oils, palm oil, or coconut oil for frying. McDonald's even offers a mushroom burger.

New York City and Philadelphia have gone so far as to require restaurants to eliminate oils that contain trans-fatty acids in their cooking, and to post the trans fat contents of all the foods offered on their menus. KFC has proudly proclaimed that as of July 2007, their chicken is no longer fried in fat that contains partially hydrogenated or hydrogenated oils, which are high in trans-fatty acids. Trans fat content is now a required listing on all food labels. Crystal and Carnival cruise lines have stated that their ships are now trans fat free. These are just a few examples of how the world of nutrition is becoming more concerned about the health of the public. Pediatricians are testing cholesterol levels in children, particularly in families where there is a history of heart disease.

While the findings about cholesterol have changed substantially in the last few years, people's attitudes about addressing this problem have changed even more. There is an increased awareness that what you eat has a definite role in staving off the heart attacks and strokes associated with blocked coronary arteries. In fact, some arterial blockage may even be reversed with a heart-wise lifestyle: no smoking, routine exercise, and, of course, healthful eating.

Yet, even knowing this, for those of us who want to be healthy, creating a healthful style of eating is not easy. This is what I want to help you achieve. This book will provide you with the necessary facts so that you can understand the dangers of high blood cholesterol levels and the important health advantages of low cholesterol levels. You will find menus, recipes, a two-week jump start weight-control diet, and many tips so that you can effectively lower and control your cholesterol. *Each chapter in this book is a link in improving your lifestyle plan. Remember to consult your physician about any treatment that you may pursue.*

What Is Cholesterol and Where Do We Get It?

In combating the problems of too much cholesterol, it helps to know a little about what it is. Cholesterol per se is not bad—in fact, it is essential to life. A fatty, waxlike material, cholesterol forms protective sheaths around the nerves, helps make hormones and vitamin D, and combines with the bile acids that aid in the digestion of fat. Everyone needs cholesterol in correct amounts for good health, but too much cholesterol encourages the development of heart and blood vessel disease.

Our bodies obtain cholesterol in several ways: from our genes; from the liver, which manufactures it; and from the food we eat. The liver synthesizes enough cholesterol for our body's needs—about 75 percent of the cholesterol in the average person's body; any we get from food is extra. The body can dispose of some of the extra cholesterol, but not all. Cholesterol is circulated through the body in the bloodstream. As cholesterol levels in the blood rise, excess cholesterol is deposited as plaque in the lining of the arteries, eventually narrowing them and impeding the blood flow. To avoid this, we need to be careful about the amount of cholesterol we eat. Moreover, there are some people whose bodies tend to produce excessive amounts of cholesterol. This is where your genes kick in. These people in particular must limit the amount of cholesterol—saturated fat and trans fat—they get from food.

The average American consumes about 400 to 500 milligrams or more of cholesterol a day, a range that is in excess of the 100 to 300 milligrams *or less* that is generally advocated. The American Heart Association suggests an allowance of 100 milligrams of cholesterol for every 1,000 calories you consume (not to exceed 300 milligrams). I believe that limiting dietary cholesterol to about 100 milligrams per day, *regardless of the number of calories consumed*, is the safest rule for a low-cholesterol lifestyle.

To many people, a "low-cholesterol diet" suggests simply avoiding egg yolks and organ meats. Although these foods *are* extremely high in cholesterol, it would be a gross oversimplification to assume that you can solve the cholesterol problem merely by eliminating them. Unfortunately, many other foods are laden with cholesterol (*and all are foods from animal sources*). You must also be wary of any foods containing saturated fats and trans fat, because the liver creates additional cholesterol from these fats.

Foods high in saturated fats are not merely those from animal sources, such as meat, poultry (especially the skin), cheeses, whole milk, butter, and ice cream. *Some vegetable oils (particularly coconut and palm oils), cocoa butter (found in chocolate), partially hydrogenated fats, and hydrogenated fats also contain high levels of saturated fat and trans-fatty acids, which can raise cholesterol to a dangerous degree.* Thus, to be effective, a low-cholesterol diet must cut down on or eliminate certain foods, especially limiting saturated fat and practically eliminating trans fat from our diets.

The American Heart Association's Updated Dietary Recommendations Issued in 2006

The AHA now says that trans fats should make up just 1 percent or less of your total daily calories. For example, on 2,000 calories daily, that's about 2 grams of trans fat per day (approximately half of a small bag of the average fast-food French fries).

To summarize, the following are recommendations for a healthy lifestyle:

1. Stop smoking.
2. Increase daily physical activity.
3. Use nonfat or low-fat dairy products, lean cuts of meat, and *eat smaller portions.*
4. Include more vegetables and fruits daily.
5. Eat two fish meals per week. Best choices are oily fish, high in healthful omega-3 fatty acids, such as herring, sardines, salmon, lake trout, mackerel, and albacore tuna.
6. Trim the saturated fat to 7 percent of total calories and limit trans fats to 1 percent of total calories.
7. Avoid foods made with hydrogenated or partially hydrogenated fat.
8. Eat cereal, bread, crackers, and pastas that are whole grain and high fiber, at least six servings per day.

9. Soy foods are recommended to replace high-fat animal products; however, soy will not reduce blood cholesterol or other heart-related risk factors.

To lower your intake of saturated fat, trans fat, and cholesterol, see the following chart to compare similar foods and choose those with lower combined saturated fats, trans fat, and cholesterol.

Total Fat, Saturated Fat, and Trans Fat Content Per Serving

PRODUCT	COMMON SERVING SIZE	TOTAL FAT (GRAMS)	SATURATED FAT (GRAMS)	% DV FOR SAT. FAT	TRANS FAT (GRAMS)	COMBINED SAT. & TRANS FAT	CHOLESTEROL (MG.)
French Fried Potatoes (fast food)	Medium (147 grams)	27	7	35%	8	15	0
Butter	1 tbsp	11	7	35%	0	7	30
Margarine, stick	1 tbsp	11	2	10%	3	5	0
Margarine, tub	1 tbsp	7	1	5%	0.5	1.5	0
Mayonnaise (soybean oil)	1 tbsp	11	1.5	8%	0	1.5	5
Shortening	1 tbsp	13	3.5	18%	4	7.5	0
Potato Chips	small bag (42.5 grams)	11	2	10%	3	5	0
Milk, whole	1 cup	7	4.5	23%	0	4.5	35
Milk, skim	1 cup	0	0	0%	0	0	5
Donut	1	18	4.5	23%	5	9.5	25
Cookies (cream filled)	3 (30 grams)	6	1	5%	2	3	0
Candy Bar	1 (40 grams)	10	4	20%	3	7	less than 5
Cake, pound	1 slice (80 grams)	16	3.5	18%	4.5	8	0

Nutrient values based on FDA's nutrition labeling regulations.

Your Cholesterol Level and What It Means

The first step in cholesterol control is to find out what your own cholesterol picture is by having your cholesterol level tested by your physician. The amount of cholesterol in the body is measured by determining the amount of cholesterol in the blood—referred to as the serum cholesterol level. Both the National Institutes of Health and the American Heart Association recommend that you have your serum cholesterol level checked at least every five years after the age of twenty, or every year if there is a history of heart disease in your family. You should take nothing by mouth except water for at least 12 hours prior to testing. To ensure the accuracy of test results, your physician should seek a laboratory that participates in a suitable standardization program. Because cholesterol levels can fluctuate considerably from day to day depending upon what you have eaten, it is also suggested that more than one cholesterol measurement be obtained and then the averaged values are used as your baseline.

The Total Cholesterol (TC) Count

When you have a routine cholesterol test at the doctor's office, the reading you are given is referred to as your total cholesterol. Optimally, your total cholesterol reading should be well under 200 milligrams per deciliter of blood (200 mg/dl). Dr. Basil M. Rifkind of the National Heart, Lung and Blood Institute has said that "there is no safe level of blood cholesterol above 175 milligrams. . . . It might be necessary to get down to 150 milligrams." Certainly it is clear that the further below 200 it is, the better for you.

If your cholesterol level is under 200, you probably need not be concerned. However, if it is between 200 and 239, you are borderline, or at moderate to high risk. If your cholesterol is above 240, then you are at high risk and should take corrective measures immediately.

The Kinds of Cholesterol: "Good" and "Bad"

If your total cholesterol reading is 200 or over, you need to learn more about the different types of cholesterol. It is important to know what your specific cholesterol makeup is.

Because cholesterol is a sterol and not soluble in water, the body combines it and other fats with protein to form complexes known as lipoproteins so it can be carried in the bloodstream. For our purposes, there are two lipoproteins that are of concern—high-density lipoproteins and low-density lipoproteins. The high-density lipopro-

WHAT IS YOUR RISK FACTOR?

Total Cholesterol Level

Less than 200 mg/dL	Desirable
200–239 mg/dL	Borderline High
240 mg/dL and above	High

LDL Cholesterol Level

Less than 100 mg/dL	Optimal
100–129 mg/dL	Near Optimal
130–159 mg/dL	Borderline High
160 and above	High

HDL Cholesterol Level

Less than 50 mg/dL	Low
60 mg/dL and above	Desirable

teins, or HDLs, are often called "the good cholesterol" because they carry cholesterol away from the body tissues and return it to the liver for recycling. The function of the low-density lipoproteins, or LDLs, is to carry cholesterol to the cells where it is deposited. However, if they transport more than the cells can use, the excess collects, forming plaque which builds up within the arteries, producing a condition known as atherosclerosis, the precursor to heart attacks and strokes. Thus, LDLs are often called "the bad cholesterol."

Since your total cholesterol count does not tell you whether your cholesterol is the "good" or the "bad" kind, you also need to know what your level of HDLs is and the ratio of HDL to total cholesterol, known as the heart-risk ratio. Dr. William Castelli, medical director of the pioneering Framingham Study on Heart Disease, has suggested that to survive in America you should know three numbers: your total cholesterol, your HDL/LDL ratio, and your Social Security number. Unfortunately, most of us know only the third one.

I would add another number to this—your LDL number. We still have a great deal to learn about HDL's role in preventing heart disease; however, there is substantial evidence that lowering total cholesterol and LDL cholesterol levels can reduce the incidence of coronary heart disease.

To determine your HDL and LDL numbers you should have another blood test taken. Ask for a written copy of your blood chemistry, not just a verbal report over the phone.

The High-Density Lipoprotein (HDL) Count

Because higher levels of HDLs may promote healthier arteries, the higher your HDLs, the lower your risk of developing heart disease. Recent studies suggest that HDL cholesterol even has the ability to remove plaque previously deposited on artery walls, thereby reversing atherosclerosis.

The National Heart, Lung and Blood Institute recommends an HDL count above 50. In general, HDLs are found to be higher in thin people, nonsmokers, people who exercise regularly, and those who drink moderate amounts of alcohol (about one drink per day). They are also higher in premenopausal women; for this reason some doctors recommend administering and monitoring *low* levels of estrogen in menopausal and postmenopausal women with high cholesterol counts.

HOW TO RAISE YOUR LEVEL OF HDL—
THE GOOD CHOLESTEROL

1. Stop smoking.
2. Limit your consumption of foods that are high in saturated fat, trans fat, and cholesterol.
3. Engage in regular aerobic exercise.
4. Eat more fish (at least two to three times a week). Select coldwater fatty fish because they have high levels of omega-3 fatty acids (see pages 18–20.)
5. Use canola and/or extra-virgin olive oil (both monounsaturated) in limited amounts as fats of choice (see page 20).
6. Lose weight if you are overweight. Maintaining a healthy body weight is essential to keeping total cholesterol down, thereby raising HDLs and lowering LDLs.

The Low-Density Lipoprotein (LDL) Count

Most of the cholesterol in blood serum is found in the LDLs. Since the low-density lipoproteins deposit cholesterol on the artery walls, the higher the level of LDLs in the blood, the greater your risk of heart disease. The National Heart, Lung and Blood Institute recommends an LDL count under 100. A count over 160 is considered to put you at serious extra risk.

The Heart-Risk Ratio

Ideal cholesterol test results would show:

1.   a total cholesterol count of under 200 milligrams
2.   an LDL count that is as low as possible (under 100)
3.   an HDL count that is as high as possible (50 or over)

In addition, the test results also carry a determination of the heart-risk ratio, the ratio of HDL to total cholesterol, which is obtained by dividing the TC count by the HDL count. The target or ideal number for this ratio is 4.5 or under. For example, if your TC is 180 and your HDL is 40, your heart-risk ratio would be 4.5.

$$180 \div 40 = 4.5$$

Although some experts believe that even if your total cholesterol is higher than 200 a high HDL level may result in an acceptable heart-risk ratio, I believe that you should still try to reduce the total cholesterol count to at least under 200.

YOUR HAPPY HEART FORMULA

lower levels of total cholesterol and lower LDLs

+

higher levels of HDLs

= a lower risk of coronary heart disease

The Triglyceride Count (The Forgotten Lipid)

In addition to the three cholesterol measurements, your blood chemistry tests should also measure the triglyceride count. Triglycerides are blood fats that transport energy to the cells of the body. *There is increasing evidence that connects triglycerides with atherosclerosis.* The optimal average triglyceride levels for men are about 140–150 mg/dl; for women, about 100–120 mg/dl. When these levels are elevated, *they become risk factors, particularly in people with heart disease, diabetes or who are obese.* They are, however, certainly not as critical as elevated total cholesterol or LDL levels.

A study at the National Institutes of Health has indicated that for every 1 percent decrease in blood cholesterol there is a 2 percent decrease in the chance of coronary artery disease.

The Next Step—Cholesterol Control

If your cholesterol readings show that you are at risk, you will need to reduce your cholesterol level and then work to keep it under control by making some changes in your diet and lifestyle. If you are not at risk, you will still need to watch your cholesterol intake so that you can maintain your safety margin. If your lifestyle includes daily exercise (45 minutes five times per week), no smoking, and the healthy food pattern suggested in this book, then you can look forward to many healthy, happy years.

How Dietary Fats, Both Saturated and Trans Fat, Contribute to Cholesterol Levels

That the foods we eat can have a major role in increasing or decreasing cholesterol levels is an established fact. Twenty years ago, however, health professionals only emphasized the importance of avoiding foods high in cholesterol. Today we know that other elements come into play as well, and one of the most important is the amount and kinds of fat we eat. There are different kinds of fat in our food: saturated fat, polyunsaturated fat, monounsaturated fat, and trans fat. Since they all—*particularly saturated fat and trans fat*—can have a direct bearing on high cholesterol levels, it pays to know something about them.

At present, 40 percent of the calories in the diet of the average American comes from fat. Although many experts feel that this figure should be lowered to 30 percent, I believe that ideally it should be a safer 20 percent. Others, like Pritikin followers, insist on no more than 10 percent, but for many people this restriction is too rigid. In my nutrition counseling practice, I have found that an allowance of 20 percent is more realistic for people to be satisfied and stay with a healthful eating program—and after all, that's what cholesterol control is all about. (A guide to reducing your total dietary fat is included in the Appendix.)

But whether it's 10 percent or 20 percent, not more than 10 percent of your total daily fat calories should come from both saturated and trans fats. Saturated fats can cause problems by raising the level of the "bad" low-density lipoproteins.

Trans Fat and Saturated Fat—The Dangerous Culprits

We know that diets high in saturated fat contribute to heart disease by raising cholesterol levels. All saturated fats raise cholesterol. Saturated fats, which are generally solid at room temperature, are found primarily in foods of animal origin such as whole milk dairy products (butter, cream, milk, sour cream, ice cream, and cheeses), and in lard and chicken, beef, and other meat fat. Saturated fats are found also in tropical oils such as coconut oil, palm oil, palm kernel oil, cocoa butter, and *any vegetable oil that has been hydrogenated or partially hydrogenated*, such as solid vegetable shortening and stick margarine. Remember, the softer the margarine, the less saturated fat it contains. However, *when any oil is hydrogenated, it becomes more solid, saturated, and it also forms trans fat*. It is thus more likely to raise your cholesterol level. Tropical oils (e.g., palm or coconut oil), partially hydrogenated, and hydrogenated fats are used commercially because they are inexpensive and the process increases the shelf life and flavor stability of the foods. But this resulting trans fat, like saturated fat, also

---

Remember, eating food high in saturated fat and trans fat raises total blood cholesterol levels more than dietary cholesterol does.

raises the LDL (bad cholesterol) in the blood. Moreover, unlike saturated fat, *trans fat lowers HDL (good cholesterol) in the blood*.

Nothing in our food supply is more dangerous than trans-fatty acids
(trans fat). "By our most conservative estimate, replacement of partially hydrogenated fat in the U.S. diet with natural unhydrogenated
vegetable oils would prevent approximately 30,000 premature coronary deaths per year, and epidemiologic evidence suggests this number is closer to 100,000 premature deaths annually," according to the
Harvard School of Public Health.

Major Food Sources of Trans Fat

The American Heart Association recommends limiting trans fat to
about two grams per day, based on a 2,000-calorie diet.

Trying to count saturated fat, trans fat, and total fat can become a
burden that can be discouraging. Counting total fat is simple! If you
limit your total fat to 20 percent of your calories, you will automatically
be limiting your saturated fat intake. However, remember, saturated fat
and trans fat together should be no more than 10% of total calories.

We consume relatively small amounts of trans fat compared to saturated fat, but *its impact is large*. Small amounts of trans fats occur natu-
rally in foods of ruminant animal origin, but most of the trans fat we
eat comes from partially hydrogenated and hydrogenated vegetable oils
used in processed foods such as vegetable shortening, stick margarine,
store-bought cakes, cookies, and crackers, fried foods from fast-food
chains and restaurants, and supermarket frozen foods. Nondairy creamers, flavored coffees, and whipped toppings also contain trans fat.

In 2003, Denmark became the first country to strictly regulate trans
fat, making it illegal for trans fat to make up more than 2 percent of
the total fat content of a processed food.

Can you believe that a large order of French fries and chicken
nuggets at a McDonald's in New York City has 10.2 grams of
trans fat compared with 0.33 grams in Denmark (according to
the *New England Journal of Medicine*)?

Food manufacturers have changed Nutrition Fact labels to list the
amount of trans fat in their products. This labeling change applies to

all packaged foods that enter interstate commerce in the United States as of January 1, 2006. However, a "zero trans fat" label does not tell the whole story—*food may contain up to 0.5 mg of trans fat per serving and still list it on the label as "0 mg trans fat."* We know that trans fat is not good for us; however, most of us do not understand that replacing it with saturated fats is a *terrible* option and, in some instances, this is just what the food industry is doing.

Beware: If entries in the ingredient list are "partially hydrogenated" or "hydrogenated" oils, a serving could contain up to 0.5 mg of trans fat and still be labeled as "zero grams of trans fat"—adding up quickly if you have several servings!

Think of it this way—if you were driving down the road and saw a stop sign, you wouldn't think twice about stopping. The following list of fats indicates the "stop signs" that you should look for before you give yourself the "green light" to purchase a specific product:

Partially hydrogenated vegetable oils/shortenings
Coconut oil (it has more saturated fat than any other fat)
Palm oil, palm kernel oil, and fractionated palm oils
Butter

Dietary supplement manufacturers must also list trans fat on the Nutrition Facts panel when their product contains trans fat. Examples of supplements containing trans fat are some energy and nutrition bars.

Products Containing Trans Fat

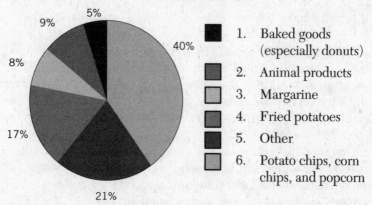

40%

5%

9%

8%

17%

21%

1. Baked goods (especially donuts)
2. Animal products
3. Margarine
4. Fried potatoes
5. Other
6. Potato chips, corn chips, and popcorn

LABEL LOGIC

♦ Read your label for a listing of trans fat and look for partially hydrogenated or hydrogenated oil as one of the ingredients. If present, choose another product.

♦ Use a more healthful spread. The softer a margarine, the better—it means it is lower in trans fat. Look for one that is labeled "trans fat free." Caution: Legally, processed foods may have up to 0.5 mg of trans fat in a serving and still list it on the label as "0 mg" trans fat.

♦ Choose canola oil or olive oil over margarine or butter, and certainly choose canola or olive oils for any frying or sautéing.

♦ We live in a busy time, but try to opt for more healthful home cooking. *Americans get more than 35 percent of their calories dining away from home.*

♦ If you understand the danger of trans fat, cholesterol, and saturated fat, if you read labels carefully and avoid restaurant and bakery baked goods, nondairy creamers, and fried foods—*if you understand that you have options*—you can enjoy a healthier and longer life.

The New Nutrition Facts Label

As of January 2006

In 1994, the Center for Science in the Public Interest, a consumer advocacy organization, filed a petition with the U.S. Food and Drug Administration requesting that the agency take steps to require "trans fat" be listed on nutrition labels and claims. On January 1, 2006, new federal food labeling requirements went into effect to include trans fats.

Accurate food labels are critical for millions of consumers who are overweight; have diabetes, high blood pressure, or food allergies; or are on restricted diets that require careful monitoring of the fats, carbohydrates, sugar, and calories they consume.

Nutrition Facts

Serving Size   1 cup (228g)
Servings Per Container 2

Amount Per Serving

Calories 260   Calories from Fat 120

	% Daily Value*
Total Fat 13g	**20%**
Saturated Fat 5g	**25%**
Trans Fat 2g	
Cholesterol 30mg	**10%**
Sodium 660mg	**28%**
Total Carbohydrate 31g	**10%**
Dietary Fiber 0g	**0%**
Sugars 5g	
Protein 5g	

Vitamin A 4%	*	Vitamin C 2%
Calcium 15%	*	Iron 4%

* Percent Daily Values are based on a 2,000 calorie diet.
Your Daily Values may be higher or lower depending
on your calorie needs:

	Calories	2,000	2,500
Total Fat	Less than	65g	80g
Sat Fat	Less than	20g	25g
Cholesterol	Less than	300mg	300mg
Sodium	Less than	2,400mg	2,400mg
Total Carbohydrate		300g	375g
Dietary Fiber		25g	30g

Calories per gram:
Fat 9   Carbohydrate 4   Protein 4

Ingredients: Enriched (*wheat*) flour, malted barley, sugar, whey (*milk*), eggs, vanilla, lecithin
(*soy*). Contains wheat, milk, and soy.

A word of caution: When fat content in processed foods is reduced, sodium or sugar content is generally increased. Check your food labels.

Polyunsaturated Fats

The good news about polyunsaturated fats is that they lower LDL cholesterol. Since the body does not manufacture these fats, they can *only* be obtained from the food you eat. Good sources are most nuts and seeds (however, they also contain saturated fats), soybeans, corn, and most vegetable oils, such as safflower, soy, corn, sunflower, and sesame oils (see chart on page 23).

Unlike saturated fats, polyunsaturated fats are liquid or soft whether they are kept at room temperature or under refrigeration. The softer the fat, the more polyunsaturates it contains (for example, soft margarine contains more polyunsaturates than does stick margarine and is therefore a better choice *in moderation*).

While polyunsaturated fats can be beneficial, even here don't go overboard. You must limit them as well if you are to stay within the recommended daily amounts for total fat. Too much of any fat has been linked to cancer and definitely produces weight gain.

The Omega-3s in Seafood

Omega-3 fatty acids, which are found in fish and shellfish, are still receiving a good bit of attention. Some research indicates that they may be useful in lowering blood triglycerides and cholesterol levels and may actually help prevent atherosclerosis and clotting, lowering the risk of heart attacks and strokes. Because of the special benefits associated with these particular polyunsaturated fats, it's a good idea to eat fish two to three times a week. Select those that live in deep, cold water, for they are particularly high in omega-3s. Among them are salmon, Atlantic herring, albacore and bluefin tuna, sablefish, sturgeon, Atlantic mackerel, and lake trout. (Don't forget easily available salmon and tuna canned in water.) Wild or line-caught fish is preferable to farm-raised because of fewer pollutants in the water.

A *word of caution:* Because of the current interest in omega-3s, many people have begun to take fish oil capsules. Because the long-term safety of these supplements has not been determined, they are still considered experimental. What we do know is that fish oil supplements add calories and fat. My advice is to skip the capsules and take the safer and healthier route by adding fish to your meals.

The following chart will help you see at a glance the total fat, omega-3 fatty acids, and cholesterol of a selection of fish and shellfish. Interestingly, the fact that saturated fat has been targeted as a culprit has led to some revised thinking about shellfish, most of which were once considered totally off-limits because of their high cholesterol content. Today, however, because they are known to be *very low* in saturated fat, most shellfish are allowed on a low-cholesterol diet *in limited portions*, provided no cream, butter, or cheese is used in their preparation. Shellfish are the vegetarians of the sea.

Fish is not a source of trans fat.

The Total Fat, Omega-3s, and Cholesterol in Commonly Used Seafood

Fish

PORTION: ABOUT 3 OZ. RAW	TOTAL FAT (GRAMS)	OMEGA-3 FATTY ACIDS (GRAMS)	CHOLESTEROL (MILLIGRAMS)
Mackerel, Atlantic	11.81	2.5	60
Herring, Atlantic	7.68	1.6	51
Rainbow trout	2.85	1.6	45
Tuna, bluefin	4.17	1.6	32
Sablefish	13.00	1.5	42
Sturgeon	3.43	1.5	NA
Salmon, sockeye	7.27	1.3	53
Sardines, Atlantic (24 gm, about 2 sardines with bones, oil drained)	5.91	1.2	3.4

Avoid fish that is fried or processed with salt.

Shellfish

PORTION: ABOUT 3 OZ. RAW	TOTAL FAT (GRAMS)	OMEGA-3 FATTY ACIDS (GRAMS)	CHOLESTEROL (MILLIGRAMS)
Mollusks			
Abalone	0.64	0.04	72
Clams	0.83	0.12	29
Mussels, blue	1.90	0.37	24
Oysters, eastern	2.08	0.40	46
Scallops	0.64	0.17	28
Squid	1.18	0.30	198

Shellfish (cont.)

PORTION: ABOUT 3 OZ. RAW	TOTAL FAT (GRAMS)	OMEGA-3 FATTY ACIDS (GRAMS)	CHOLESTEROL (MILLIGRAMS)
Crustaceans			
Crab, Alaska King	0.51	0.40	35
Crab, blue	0.92	0.40	66
Crab, Dungeness	0.83	0.40	50
Crayfish	0.90	0.15	118
Lobster, northern	0.76	0.07	81
Shrimp	1.47	0.40	130

Seafood lovers may rejoice—all shellfish are low in fat! Jacob Exler, Ph.D., the principal author for the USDA's handbook on fish, reports that only 0.05 to 2 percent of all shellfish is fat, and much of that is omega-3 fatty acids. However, some shellfish are high in cholesterol, particularly crayfish, squid, and shrimp. Frequently these shellfish are also fried, adding fat calories as well as saturated fat and trans fat if the oil used for frying contains palm or coconut oil.

A form of omega-3 fatty acids (alpha-linolenic acid) is found in canola oil, soy oil, flax seed, and walnuts. Although this source is less effective, it may be valuable to people who do not eat fish.

Monounsaturated Fats

Because monounsaturated fats may raise the HDL level, they may offer an effective way to decrease your total heart-risk ratio (the ratio of HDLs to total cholesterol). The best source of monounsaturated fat is olive oil, a discovery triggered by the observation that people in the Mediterranean area, who use olive oil in their cooking almost exclusively, have a lower incidence of cardiac disease. Other good sources of this kind of fat are canola oil, olives, almonds, and avocados. Here, too, however, you could overdose if you aren't careful: The amount of monounsaturated fat must also be limited, both to stay within the daily recommended fat allowance and to monitor calories.

How to Choose Fat Wisely

The chart on page 23 compares the fatty acid content of commonly used fats and oils. Notice the difference in the saturated fat content, even in polyunsaturated and monounsaturated vegetable oils. In my recipes, I have recommended using canola oil, cold-pressed safflower oil, and sunflower oil because of their low saturated fat content, and extra-virgin olive oil because of its high monounsaturated fat content and wonderful flavor. *Regardless of your choice, limit the amount of any fat that you use.*

How to Calculate the Percentage of Total Fat in the Recipes in this Book

The diet plan and all the menus and recipes in this book focus on helping you lower your saturated fat, trans fat, and total fat intake as well as your cholesterol intake. Since your goal is to derive no more than 15 to 20 percent of your *daily total calories* from all fat, use the following formula to calculate the *percentage of fat calories* in each serving of any recipe in this book.

Multiply the number of grams of fat listed in each serving by 9 (since there are about 9 calories in each gram of fat). Divide this number by the total number of calories per serving. The resulting figure is the percentage of fat calories per serving.

EXAMPLE: *Mini Turkey Loaves with Piquant Salsa* (page 198)

Grams of *fat* per serving: 4.7×9 calories = $42 \div 210$ (total calories) = 20 percent of total calories from saturated fat

Grams of *saturated fat* per serving: 0.97×9 calories = $8.73 \div 210$ = 4 percent of total calories from saturated fat.[*]

Remember that no more than 7 to 8 percent of your total daily calories should come from saturated fat and no more than 2 grams of trans fat per day.[*] The recipes in this book list the grams of total fat as well as saturated fat and trans fat per serving, when possible.

[*]Refer to **Harriet Roth's Revised Fat Counter,** 2006 edition.

> Trans fats cause an even higher risk of heart disease than satu-
> rated fats. Trans fats not only *raise* the bad cholesterol (LDL),
> but also *lower* the good cholesterol (HDL).

How Dietary Fiber Affects Cholesterol

Foods that contain large amounts of soluble fiber offer another way
to help control cholesterol and your weight. A few years ago, if I had
told you that eating fresh fruit, vegetables, and whole grains would
help lower your risk of heart disease and diabetes, you would probably
have thought I was a health food faddist. Today, however, because of
reliable research by experts like Dr. James W. Anderson, Professor of
Medicine and Clinical Nutrition at the University of Kentucky Medical Center, and others, we know that some of these foods do indeed
help lower cholesterol as well as stabilize blood sugar.

Dietary fiber is that portion of fruits, vegetables, and whole grains
that your body does not break down during digestion. This fiber falls
into two categories: insoluble and soluble. Insoluble fiber (cellulose,
hemicellulose, and lignin), which does not dissolve in water, is found
in the plant walls of all vegetables, fruits, and whole grains. Soluble
fiber (pectins and gums), which is soluble in water, is found in large
amounts in oat bran and oatmeal and the husks of psyllium seeds* and
also in barley, legumes (dried peas, beans, and lentils), okra, apples,
pears, figs, corn, peas, eggplant, and the pulp of citrus fruits.

Insoluble fiber helps principally to expedite the passage of foods
through the gastrointestinal tract. It also helps prevent constipation.
Soluble fiber, with its gel-like pectins and gums, helps to lower serum
cholesterol by as much as 10 percent by trapping the bile acids needed
to make cholesterol and carrying them to the large intestine where
they can no longer be absorbed and are subsequently excreted. Moreover, as a "bonus," when you increase your intake of fiber, which is filling, you generally decrease your intake of other foods, some of which
undoubtedly would contain saturated fat, trans fat, and cholesterol.
A chart showing the dietary fiber content of many common foods is
included in the Appendix (p. 396).

---

*Sold under the brand names Metamucil, Konsyl, Fiber-all, Modane Bulk, etc.

Comparison of Dietary Fats

DIETARY FAT	SATURATED FAT	MONOUNSATURATED FAT	POLYUNSATURATED FAT Alpha-Linolenic Acid (an Omega-3 Fatty Acid)	Linoleic Acid (an Omega-6 Fatty Acid)
Canola oil	7	61	11	21
Safflower oil	8	77	1	14
Flaxseed oil	9	16	57	18
Sunflower oil	12	16	1	71
Corn oil	13	29	1	57
Olive oil	15	75	1	9
Soybean oil	15	23	8	54
Peanut oil	19	48	*	33
Cottonseed oil	27	19	*	54
Lard	43	47	1	9
Palm oil	51	39	*	10
Butterfat	68	28	1	3
Coconut oil	91	7		2

Fatty acid content normalized to 100 percent

*Trace

SOURCE: POS PILOT PLANT CORPORATION

How Much Fiber Do We Need?

We should try to consume 30 to 35 grams of dietary fiber (both soluble and insoluble) daily. Ironically, the American diet of 100 years ago was in some ways more healthful than it is today because high-fiber unprocessed foods were a more integral part of the diet. Unfortunately, it is estimated that the average American today consumes only 10 to 15 grams of total fiber a day. Our "Western diet," which relies heavily on processed and highly refined foods and is lacking in fiber, has been linked to atherosclerosis and to a variety of other health problems as well, among them diabetes, colon cancer, and diverticulitis.

Good sources of dietary fiber (both soluble and insoluble) include:

Fiber is the dieter's best ally because it is not calorically dense. High-fiber foods are low in saturated and trans fat and contain no cholesterol. They are also high in vitamins, minerals, and complex carbohydrates. They slow down digestion and take up room, making you feel fuller. High-fiber foods also require more chewing, so that your body has more time to get the message from the brain (if you listen!) that you've had enough to eat.

♦ Whole grain bread (not white bread)
♦ Whole fruits, including *pulp* and skin when possible (not just the juice)°
♦ Sweet potatoes, okra, eggplant, and other vegetables with edible skins or stems
♦ Whole grain, high-fiber cereals, and whole grain, spelt, or soba pastas
♦ Brown rice, barley, bulgur wheat, quinoa, and buckwheat
♦ Corn tortillas, whole wheat pita, and whole grain crackers
♦ Fresh vegetable salads (not just lettuce)
♦ Dried fruits (more fiber, but also more calories)
♦ Dried peas, beans, and lentils
♦ Air-popped popcorn

Because soluble fiber is so important in combating cholesterol, a large portion of the fiber you consume each day should be soluble.

If you haven't already been eating a high-fiber diet, it may take a few weeks for your body to adjust. Initially some people have complained of gas, but this problem usually levels off quickly. You generally need not worry about getting too much fiber—the very bulk of the food will keep you from overeating. Nor should you be concerned about an abnormal loss of vitamins and minerals on a high-fiber diet resulting when food moves quickly through the digestive tract, because the increased intake of vitamins and minerals in whole grains, fruits, and vegetables means additional nutrients that will more than take care of any losses.

°Wash fruit before eating, not before storing.

GOOD SOURCES OF SOLUBLE FIBER

To maintain a diet that is *high enough in soluble fiber to lower cholesterol*, you should eat daily:

♦ One serving of oat bran (⅓ cup uncooked) and two Oat Bran Muffins (page 108) or two servings of Cheerios daily, or Quickie Breakfast Beverage (p. 111)
♦ At least two to three servings of whole fruits (unwaxed apples, pears with skin, oranges or tangerines with pulp)
♦ At least one serving of legumes: dried or canned peas, beans, or lentils (include these in soups, salads, or casseroles)
♦ 1 heaping teaspoon of psyllium in 8 ounces of liquid

WHAT COUNTS AS A SERVING?

Amount per serving, by food group:

Bread, Cereal, Rice, and Pasta
1 slice of bread
1 oz. ready-to-eat cereal
½ cup cooked cereal, rice, or pasta

Vegetables
1 cup raw leafy vegetables
½ cup other vegetables (cooked or raw, chopped)
¾ cup vegetable juice

Milk, Yogurt, and Cheese
1 cup milk or yogurt
1½ oz. natural cheese
2 oz. processed cheese

Meat, Poultry, Fish, Dry Beans, Egg, and Nuts
2–3 oz. cooked lean meat, poultry, fish, or seafood
½ cup cooked dry beans, 1 egg, or 2 teaspoons peanut butter
1 oz. lean meat

Fruit
1 medium apple, banana, or orange
½ cup chopped, cooked, or canned fruit
¾ cup chopped fresh fruit

▼ 2 ▼

Preventing the Hazards of High Cholesterol

Today we know that the primary cause of coronary artery disease is atherosclerosis—the accumulation of plaque along the inner walls of an artery that transports blood from the heart to the organs and tissues of the body. This plaque is composed of cholesterol, fat, fibrous tissue, and in the late stages, some calcium. When it accumulates, the artery thickens and becomes narrowed, blocking the normal flow of blood to the heart. This restriction may cause damage to the heart, and, ultimately, a heart attack or stroke. So it's clear that having a high cholesterol level puts you at serious risk of coronary problems, circulatory disorders, strokes, and intermittent claudication (a severe blockage of the blood vessels in the legs that produces pain on walking). However, while high cholesterol levels are the major factor in causing atherosclerosis, there are other causes as well, as the list that follows shows.

Risk factors that contribute to atherosclerosis and heart disease include:

1. Smoking
2. High blood pressure (over 120/80)
3. Elevated blood cholesterol (over 200 mg/dl)
4. Diabetes (A1C more than 6%)
5. Obesity (being more than 30 percent overweight)
6. Inactivity or sedentary lifestyle
7. Stress
8. High LDL levels: 100 or above
9. Low HDL levels: 50 or under
10. Elevated blood triglycerides (over 120 for women and over 150 for men)

11.   Having a parent or sibling who suffered a heart attack or died suddenly of heart disease before the age of 65
12.   Waist circumference: over 35" women; over 40" men.

If your total cholesterol is under 200 milligrams as an adult, you are at relatively low risk from cholesterol-related heart disease. If it is above 240 milligrams, you are at high risk. Indeed, your risk is almost double the risk of someone with a count of 200 or under.

Today, *more than half of all American adults have cholesterol levels over 200, and one out of every four Americans has a cholesterol level that puts him at serious risk* (see page 9). In plain numbers, that means that there are 60 million people in the United States who are at risk because their counts exceed 200; these are people who should actively be taking steps to lower their cholesterol levels.

Under the most recent guidelines issued in 2004 by the National Cholesterol Education Program, it is recommended that all Americans follow a prudent diet plan (no more than 300 mg of cholesterol and 7 percent of calories from saturated fat daily). It is further suggested that doctors treat all those patients with serum cholesterol counts in excess of 200, first by using a special diet for six months and then, if diet therapy alone is not sufficient, ultimately with drugs and diet. *It is now recognized that making nutritional changes is the first and most important weapon in combating elevated serum cholesterol levels.*

Indeed, among health experts, the focus has shifted from emphasizing nutritional deficiencies to the role nutrition can play *in preventing disease*. That we are now entering *the age of prevention* is reflected in the U.S. government's 1990 Health Goals, which have been partially achieved.

1.   Lowering serum cholesterol in the adult population to below 200 mg/dl.
2.   Identifying recommended foods that are low in fat and sodium and high in fiber, as well as warning people about foods that are high in calories and sugar.
3.   Labeling all packaged foods with calorie counts and nutrition information, including saturated and trans fat content, so that consumers can make more intelligent choices.

In the United States today the typical diet is about two-thirds foods of animal origin and one-third plant foods. Years ago, Frances Moore

Lappe, in her book *Diet for a Small Planet*, encouraged us to eat lower on the food chain (i.e., more plant foods)—and she was right. By reversing the ratio and returning to a diet in which two-thirds of calories are derived from plant foods (that is, complex carbohydrates like whole grains, cereals, vegetables, and fruits) and the remainder a balance between protein and fat (I recommend a maximum of 15 to 20 percent fat), we could help erase heart disease as the nation's number-one killer.

Changing our eating habits in order to reduce serum cholesterol and the risk of heart attacks "is no longer hypothesis or theory but very sound science," according to Scott M. Grundy, M.D., PhD., chairman of the panel that drafted the National Cholesterol Education Program's new cholesterol guidelines.

Heredity and What You Can Do to Help Your Children

Heredity plays an important role in determining which of us will develop atherosclerosis. The diet I am suggesting to avoid heart disease (low fat, high fiber) may also help prevent obesity and, very likely, certain major adult-onset cancers such as breast and colorectal cancer. As I mentioned earlier, your genes also have something to do with how you handle cholesterol. Some people seem to be "cholesterol sensitive"; that is, their cholesterol level is raised much more readily by eating foods high in cholesterol, saturated fats, and trans fat. Obviously, we cannot change our genes, at least not at this point in medical history. However, we now know that what we eat, how much we eat, and how we live are of enormous importance in determining our cholesterol levels.

Studies have shown that children with high cholesterol will probably grow up to be adults with cholesterol problems and therefore have a greater chance of developing heart disease unless we change their food and exercise patterns. About 30 percent of American children already have cholesterol levels that many experts consider abnormally high. *In the last three decades, obesity in American children between the ages of five and eleven has increased by 54 percent*, according to federal nutrition surveys. This is attributed to an increase in sedentary activities like TV watching, surfing the Internet, and obsession with computer games, a reduction in exercise programs in schools, and a higher consumption of convenience foods and high-fat fast foods.

A low-saturated-fat, low-trans-fat, low-cholesterol diet will:

♦ Prevent new lesions and plaque from forming in the arteries
♦ Stabilize old lesions
♦ Eventually contribute to the reversal of existing lesions or plaque

---

As parents, we are constantly concerned about our children's education, morality, and general development. What about their food habits and long-term health? Are the consequences of frequent fast-food restaurant meals, frozen dinners high in cholesterol and fat, and snacks of hot dogs, hamburgers, French fries, cheese-laden pizzas, ice cream, donuts, cookies, and candy worth the time saved in the kitchen? Is that convenience worth the ultimate increased risk of heart disease?

As early as 1984, the National Institutes of Health Consensus Conference on Cholesterol recommended a prudent diet lower in fat and higher in complex carbohydrates for *all Americans over the age of two.* This is a true public health approach. You can start to control your children's nutritional environment by limiting and moderating their cholesterol and fat intake, by setting a good example buying and stocking healthful food, and by preparing healthful meals.

Today's children are overfed and underexercised, resulting in childhood obesity that has reached epidemic proportions. Unless we reverse this trend, our children may have *shorter* rather than longer life expectancies that we now enjoy as adults.

In order to aid this cause, Kellogg and Kraft have recently unveiled tougher advertising guidelines for advertising to children under the age of twelve.* In order to be advertised to kids, products must meet specific nutrition guidelines. The new standards are: One serving of food must

---

*Michael F. Jacobson, executive director of Science in the Public Interest, and Susan Lynn, the cofounder of Campaign for a Commercial Free Childhood, head the two advocacy groups that spearheaded the campaign to abolish mindless advertising to children under the age of twelve.

have no more than 200 calories, no trans fat, no more than 2 grams of saturated fat, no more than 230 milligrams of sodium, and no more than 12 grams of sugar. Kellogg will introduce "nutrition at a glance" labeling that will appear in the upper right corner of all cereal products. Already introduced in Europe and Australia, the new labels will highlight the important parts of the nutrition label on the front of the box. These voluntary changes will be made throughout 2007 and 2008, and apply to about half of the products that Kellogg markets to children worldwide, including products such as Apple Jacks, Fruit Loops, and Pop Tarts.

My strong beliefs in the fundamentals of a healthful diet are unchanged. Eat fewer foods that contain saturated fat or trans fat, limit added sugar, cholesterol, and salt. Include fruits, vegetables, and whole grains—foods that you know contain the nutrients you need to keep healthy. Limit your consumption of animal protein. Finally, *watch what you eat and especially how much you eat.*

Are You Sabotaging Your Health?

If it seems frightening that there can be a genetic predisposition to heart attacks or that they can even be predicted, the good news is that they can also be prevented. According to *Preventive Medicine* (12:868, 1983), fibrous plaques first appear in the coronary arteries between the ages of fifteen and twenty. There is no such thing as a "sudden heart attack"; it has been in the works for years. Unfortunately, too many people have just not made the effort to head it off.

Make sure you aren't in that group by answering these questions honestly.

♦ Are you someone who eats everything you feel like eating, someone who "lives to eat" and does not control portions?

♦ Do you refer to yourself as a meat-and-potatoes person? Do you include animal protein at every meal and avoid whole grains, salads, fresh vegetables, and fruits as much as possible?

♦ Do you think of bread'n'butter as one word?

♦ Do you never miss a chance to have a rich dessert?

♦ Are your pantry shelves filled with processed and refined foods?

♦ Do you seldom read the labels on foods to check what they contain?

♦ When you eat fast foods, are they fat-laden hamburgers, hot dogs, French fries, malts, tacos, donuts, and cheesy pizzas?

♦ Do you feel that a low-cholesterol diet just means avoiding egg yolks and red meat?

♦ Are you a couch potato? If you get the urge to exercise, do you just relax until the feeling passes over?

♦ Do you count on the fact that if you ever develop a coronary problem there will be a drug or some other medical miracle to rescue you?

♦ Do you think the fuss about trans fat is transitory?

♦ Are you "eating" or "cheating" more than you think?

If you answer *yes* to all or most of these questions, it is probably time to make some changes.

Calories Count!

In 2007, the American Heart Association distributed this handy chart to help you estimate how many calories you burn each day.*

		ACTIVITY LEVEL AND ESTIMATED CALORIES BURNED		
GENDER	AGE (YEARS)	SEDENTARY[1]	MODERATELY ACTIVE[2]	ACTIVE[3]
FEMALE	19–30	2,000	2,000–2,200	2,400
	31–50	1,800	2,000	2,200
	51+	1,600	1,800	2,000–2,200
MALE	19–30	2,000	2,000–2,200	2,400
	31–50	1,800	2,000	2,200
	51+	1,600	1,800	2,000–2,200

1. Sedentary means you have a lifestyle that includes only the light physical activity associated with typical day-to-day life.
2. Moderately active means you have a lifestyle that includes physical activity equivalent to walking about 1.5 to 3 miles per day at 3 to 4 miles per hour, in addition to the light physical activity associated with typical day-to-day life.
3. Active means you have a lifestyle that includes physical activity equivalent to walking more than 3 miles per day at 3 to 4 miles per hour, in addition to the light physical activity associated with typical day-to-day life.

*Reprinted with permission © 2007 American Heart Association.

What You Can Do to Help Yourself

Step One: Have at least two blood tests taken. Average the results to determine your average total cholesterol. (The results may vary due to lab error or biological variation; cholesterol is like blood pressure—it changes from day to day.) If the final average is 200 or over, have a fasting blood test taken (i.e., nothing other than water for at least 12 hours prior to testing) in order to determine what your HDL, LDL, and triglyceride levels are.

Step Two: If your cholesterol is at a safe level and you want to maintain it, follow the guidelines for a low-cholesterol lifestyle in Chapter 5. If you find you have a cholesterol problem:

1. Switch to a diet higher in fiber and low in saturated fat, trans fat, and cholesterol and high in soluble fiber. Follow my two-week diet plan described in Chapter 4.
2. Try to reach and maintain your optimum weight—the diet plan is designed to help you lose weight as well as lower your cholesterol.
3. Engage in regular aerobic exercise—30 minutes a day four times a week or build to walking 3 miles in 45 minutes.

Step Three: If after six months of your new lifestyle, you still have a problem and your physician recommends it, drug therapy may be necessary.

Statins: Friend or Foe?

In view of the statistics that name heart disease the number-one cause of death for both men and women in the United States, continuing research by pharmaceutical companies has shown that statins can markedly reduce heart attacks and strokes.

The most effective drugs commonly used to lower cholesterol are the following (in no particular order):

PRESCRIPTION STATINS	GENERIC STATIN EQUIVALENTS
Lipitor	Atorvastatin
Zocor	Simvastatin
Mevacor	Lovastatin
Crestor	Rosuvastatin
Lescol	Fluvastatin
Pravachol	Pravastatin

Statins are the first choice among cholesterol-lowering drugs to be used by people who have *high LDL* cholesterol, especially if those individuals are also diabetic. Statins reduce the liver's production of cholesterol and increase the ability of the liver to remove LDL cholesterol from the blood. Statins significantly reduce the level of LDL cholesterol as well as *moderately* decreasing triglyceride levels and increasing HDL cholesterol levels.

New studies in statins have shown that they have benefits that far outweigh their risks, generally speaking. The risks included with statins pertain to a possible negative interaction with several other drugs and can cause neuropathy and other side effects. In fact, long-term use of statins can cause poly-neuropathy. *Certain antibiotics* and *grapefruit juice can adversely interfere with statins* and increase the risk of muscle damage. For example, Lipitor and Zocor may increase the effects of Coumadin, a blood-thinning medicine.

Remember, if taking statins, do so under a physician's direction and guidance. Obviously, there are situations in which some drug therapy is absolutely necessary; however, if you can avoid resorting to drugs by changing your lifestyle in conjunction with your physician's guidance, that is a more satisfactory route to take. It is far more economical, too; the cost of some of the drugs may run as high as $1,000 a year, although many of the statins are currently available in a generic, less expensive form. Check with your pharmacist and physician to see if there is a safe, alternative, generic drug for you. It is important for you to realize that when you stop taking any cholesterol-lowering drug, your cholesterol levels will rise again!

If ongoing research confirms that statins do indeed build bone, increase health, and maintain mental abilities, further research will be needed to learn the differences among the different statins and determine which statins work best. In conclusion, *statins alone are not a cure-all in the battle against heart disease*—you must not forget the importance of healthful eating, food choices, and daily exercise!

What About Niacin (Nicotinic Acid)?

This drug works in the liver by affecting the production of blood fats—it's used to lower LDL cholesterol and increase HDL cholesterol. It comes in prescription form and as a dietary supplement. Dietary supplement niacin is not regulated by the Food and Drug Administration the way that prescription niacin is. Therefore the amount of niacin may vary from pill to pill in a single brand of dietary supplement.

Dietary supplement niacin *must not* be used as a substitute for prescription niacin. It should not be used for lowering cholesterol because of potential, yet very serious, side effects. Note: *If you are taking any of the medications discussed here, it is important that you do not stop or start taking any of them without consulting a doctor.*

Can This Book Help You?

I know that it is possible to prepare easy, appealing healthful meals that are neither Spartan nor "dietetic" because I've done it for my family and I have shown others how to do it both in my consulting practice throughout the world and in my previous books, *Deliciously Low*, *Deliciously Simple*, *Deliciously Healthy Jewish Cooking*, and *Harriet Roth's Fat Counter*.

This book will help you lower and control your cholesterol—*and teach you to help yourself*—by changing the way you eat. It has more than 350 low-cholesterol dishes and more than 100 menus to keep you on course. The recipes employ many of the culinary tricks I have discovered that cut the amounts of cholesterol, saturated fat, and now trans fat while not lowering taste.

It provides a guide to selecting low-cholesterol, low-fat products for your pantry and alerts you to the cholesterol, saturated fat, and trans fat content of many foods. (Remember to read your labels!)

And it presents a special two-week diet that is designed to substantially *lower your cholesterol* if you need to take immediate action and at the same time *lower your weight*.

Remember, it is not the occasional indulgence that raises cholesterol levels. *It is the foods you buy, keep on hand, cook, and have available* for your family on a daily basis that determine the state of your health. The best way to live longer is to start eating and exercising right—right now.

Regardless of your cholesterol level or your age, by following the suggestions in this book, you can begin today to lower your cholesterol and keep it under control. It is never too late to start to reduce your risk of heart disease and lead a healthier lifestyle. The sooner you begin, the better.

Cholesterol control is up to you.

A RECIPE FOR GOOD HEALTH

Changes in your lifestyle will lower your risk of heart disease and stroke.* Physical activity, weight control, and healthful eating have many positive effects on your health. In addition to lowering your LDL "bad" cholesterol, they can help raise your HDL "good" cholesterol, lower your triglycerides, lower your blood pressure, and reduce your chance of developing diabetes.

In conclusion, the average life expectancy for women is 80 years; for men, it's 74.8—unless you live in Okinawa, where it's 81.2 years, and with the highest percentage of people living more than 100 years.

So, if you knew you were going to live so long, would you have taken better care of yourself?

Although the following paragraphs have nothing to do with lowering your cholesterol and losing weight—directly—they do greatly concern all of us.

Each year 76 million Americans can get sick from food; more than 300,000 end up in the hospital and 5,000 die, according to the Centers for Disease Control and Prevention. The consumer's confidence in the safety of supermarket food has reached an eighteen-year low, according to the Food Market Institute. The Food and Drug Administration is responsible for monitoring 80 percent of our food supply—everything

---

*Buy a pedometer! Try to reach 10,000 steps per day.

but meat, which the U.S. Department of Agriculture supposedly oversees. The food inspection program has been sorely underfunded for years and has little enforcement capability beyond asking for voluntary recalls. *It is able to inspect less than 1 percent of the $60 billion worth of food we import each year.*

What is a hungry consumer to do? "If you want 100 percent safety, you would have to stop eating," said Marian Nestle, a professor of nutrition at NYU and author of *What to Eat.* Food-safety experts advocate providing enough funding to do more inspections and grant the FDA the authority to require food recalls.

Until these actions are in the works, the best defense against food-borne illness starts in your kitchen.

1.   Wash your hands and wash all foods. All produce, whether organic or not, home grown, or imported, *should be washed under running cold water just before it is eaten.* Drying with a clean towel or paper towel may also remove lingering contaminants.
2.   A refrigerator thermometer is essential. It should be kept at 40°F.
3.   Produce should be stored separately from uncooked meat, poultry, fish, and eggs.
4.   Cutting boards need to be washed in hot, soapy water or in the dishwasher.
5.   Cooking is the best way to kill bacteria—160°F for hamburgers (well past pink).
6.   Frozen foods are cooked in processing, making them a safer bet than fresh berries and spinach.
7.   More people have turned to buying certified organic fruits and vegetables. They do carry less pesticide and herbicide residue than conventionally grown products. Under federal law, organic milk, meat, and produce cannot contain added growth hormones, antibiotics, or genetically modified organisms.
8.   When possible, buy locally grown food in season or at farmers' markets. This would also be environmentally friendly—burning fewer fossil fuels. It is believed that domestically grown foods are inherently safer (15 percent of the food eaten in the United States comes from other countries; the top five countries that export food into the United States are: *Canada, Mexico, China,*

Thailand, and *Chile* [U.S. Census Bureau, 2006]). There are now 4,000 farmers' markets throughout the United States.

9. The bottom line, meanwhile, is that everybody should be shouting about the lack of oversight of our food supply. Talk to your government representatives. Continue pushing for more information and required country-of-origin labeling for all foods. According to the *Washington Post*, the average American eats about 260 pounds of imported foods a year.

Centuries ago, people feasted principally on nuts, seeds, and grains. As time passed we became more of a "meat 'n' potatoes" society—which was more indicative of one's economic and social status. Today, our future predicts more of a vegan-based society and increasing population. Two-thirds of the world's population still exists on rice. The pressure to "go green" becomes more acceptable worldwide.

It's no secret—*Americans love to eat.* In fact, last year the average person consumed:

- ♦ 27 pounds of hamburger
- ♦ 73 pounds of chicken
- ♦ 15 pounds of fish
- ♦ 10 pounds of cheddar cheese
- ♦ 12 pounds of chocolate

PART II

▼

Choosing a Cholesterol-Control Lifestyle

▼ 3 ▼

Stocking the Low-Cholesterol Kitchen

In this new edition of the *Cholesterol Control Cookbook* we will reap the rewards of the continuous addition of new foods available to us in the marketplace that are lower in saturated fat, trans fat, and cholesterol, in addition to having lowered sodium and sugar content. This greatly improves our healthy food choices in the stores as well as the finished products in our kitchens.

Choosing a low-cholesterol lifestyle doesn't mean that you have to forgo all your favorite foods forever, but it does mean that you have to both exercise physically as well as show good judgment in your daily food selections.

It's important to always have the most healthful foods close at hand. If you don't—and you make do with unhealthy foods just because they're there on the shelf—all your best intentions of eating properly to lower your cholesterol will come to naught.

To help you make low-cholesterol cooking a reality in your home, I have listed the healthful foods you should have on hand or choose in your menu planning and the unhealthful high-cholesterol, high-saturated-fat, trans-fat foods you should avoid. If you are diabetic, hypertensive, or concerned about weight control, you will also want to avoid foods with added sweeteners or high sodium content. To make your shopping easier, I have included a section on deciphering labels.

Staples for a Low-Cholesterol Lifestyle

In the Refrigerator

Nonfat, skim, or 1% milk—use with whole grain cereals, in cooking and baking, or just to drink. (Light Silk Soymilk may be substituted.)

Nonfat plain or fruit yogurt—use in salad dressings, cooking, or as a food itself. (Fage Greek Yogurt)

Tofu—use in limited amounts in stir-fries, salad dressing, soups, or as a food.

Part-skim or nonfat ricotta cheese—use sparingly as a spread on bread or in limited amounts in cooking.

1%-fat cottage cheese—use in limited amounts.

Galaxy Veggie slices—tofu cheese in six flavors

Part-skim mozzarella cheese—use in limited amounts or substitute with soy cheese.

Low-calorie Italian or vinaigrettes—the calorie count should be *no more than 10 calories per tablespoon.* Check the sodium content, because often in lowering calories, excess salt is added for flavor.

Weight Watchers, Spectrum, Hellman's, Best Foods, and Smart Balance—all make reduced-fat or no cholesterol mayonnaise.

Extra-virgin olive oil—it is expensive, but a little goes a long way. Olive oil is believed to raise your HDLs.

Cold-pressed canola oil, sunflower oil, or safflower oil—cold-pressed means that no chemicals have been used to extract the oil. Canola oil* has the lowest amount of saturated fat of any oil and the best fatty-acid ratio.

Extra-large or jumbo eggs—since generally you will be using only the white, they're a better buy.

Eggland eggs—25 percent lower in saturated fat and contain omega-3 fatty acids

Egg substitute (low-fat, trans-fat free, and cholesterol free)—
Eggbeaters, Publix Eggstirs, Eggmates, Better'n'Eggs, Ener-G
Liquid Egg Whites—all whites

---

*The FDA has currently ruled that 1½ tablespoons of Canola oil per day MAY reduce the risk of coronary heart disease when used *in place of* saturated fat.

Chopped or crushed garlic—a readily available seasoning for many foods, also available in some frozen food sections

Sugar-free preserves (and apple butter)—a good substitute spread for butter or margarine

Corn or whole wheat tortillas—flour tortillas, only if they are low-fat and lard free

Whole wheat pita bread—great for pocket sandwiches, chips, wraps, and pizzas

Fruits—*use seasonal fresh fruit*, preferably, particularly apples, pears, oranges, and tangerines because they are higher in the soluble fiber that lowers cholesterol. If fresh is not available, use frozen unsweetened fruit and fruit juice concentrate, canned fruit without sugar added, or dried fruit. Have lemons or limes on hand as a seasoning or for salads. Organically certified fresh fruits are also lower in insecticides and pesticides.

Vegetables—whenever possible use fresh, seasonal, certified organic vegetables. Their flavor and safety is preferable due to the lack of pesticide and insecticide residue. However, for convenience, frozen (without sauces) are certainly acceptable. Salad greens, asparagus, celery, green, yellow, orange, and red peppers, okra, red cabbage, carrots, tomatoes, jicama, radishes, eggplant, broccoli, cauliflower, and cucumbers are particularly good because they are high in insoluble fiber, which aids digestion. Prepare by steaming or microwaving. Try using local farmers' markets for both fruits and vegetables. Wash before using!

In the Pantry

Choose whole grain, unrefined carbohydrates such as whole grain breads, cereals, and pastas, as well as legumes, potatoes, and corn. They are all low in fat but high in vitamins, minerals, and fiber.

Canned goods that have added fat, meat, or high sodium levels should be avoided. Use only those that contain no preservatives, MSG, or sugar. Sugar appears on labels under many different names: syrup, sucrose, dextrose, maltose, lactose, invert sugar, honey, high fructose corn syrup, fructose, fruit juice concentrate, corn syrup, corn sweetener, sugar alcohol, and others.

Salt is the most frequently used additive in foods. Select salt-reduced products if salt free is not available. Rinse salted canned products to remove added salt.

Nonstick cooking spray *(without fluorocarbons)*—use in cooking pan instead of butter or oil.

Dried split peas, beans, and lentils—high in soluble fiber

Brown rice, wild rice, barley, bulgur, pilaf mix, polenta, and other whole grains—high in insoluble fiber (If brown rice is kept a long time, store it in the refrigerator to keep it from becoming rancid.)

Pasta—whole grain, spelt, soba, or those made with semolina and no egg yolks (Asian style noodles)

Oat bran—a great source of soluble fiber; use as a hot cereal or in baking and cooking whenever possible

Oatmeal, steel-cut oats, oat bran cereal (such as those made by: Erewhon, Arrowhead Mills, Roman Meal, Quaker, Lundberg, McCann's, Nabisco, Nature's Path, Mother's, and Kashi)

Cold cereals: Cheerios, Kashi

Shredded wheat and bran—a salt-free, sugar-free whole grain cereal high in insoluble fiber

Sweet potatoes, shallots, onions, green garlic, and garlic

Canned Goods

Albacore tuna in water—contains omega-3 fatty acid that lowers cholesterol (preferably wild or line caught)

Crabmeat

Salmon (pink or red)—high in omega-3 fatty acid that lowers cholesterol (preferably wild or line caught)

Sardines in olive oil

Unsweetened fruit in natural juice

Artichokes, quartered or bottoms, canned in water

Hearts of palm in water

Whole-kernel corn (preferably sodium-reduced)—high in soluble fiber

Kidney, cannelini, pinto, garbanzo, and black beans—high in soluble fiber

Sauerkraut (such as Cascadian Farms, which is low in sodium)

Black-eyed peas—high in soluble fiber

Sodium-reduced Swanson's chicken broth defatted, Wolfgang Puck's vegetable broth

Sodium-reduced or salt-free tomato paste, tomato sauce, diced to-
matoes, Italian plum tomatoes, and any San Marzano tomatoes
Sodium-reduced marinara sauce (no meat added)—Newman's
Own, Muir Glen
Vegetarian Anderson's split-pea soup or lentil soup—high in soluble
fiber
Amy's, Healthy Choice, Campbell's Healthy Request, and other
low-fat, low-sodium soups
Sodium-reduced vegetable juice (V-8)

Seasonings

Balsamic, red or white wine, and brown rice vinegars
Japanese rice vinegar
Sodium-reduced soy sauce
Wishbone salad spritzers—no fat
Dijon mustard
Worcestershire sauce (use in limited amounts)
Salt-free vegetable seasonings
Fresh garlic, fresh ginger
Garlic and onion powders (not salts)
Italian herb blend
Herbes de Provence
Crushed red pepper flakes
Fresh or dried thyme, dill, bay leaves, and any other of your favorite
herbs and spices
Black or assorted peppercorns (in mill for fresh grinding)
Dehydrated onion, garlic, shallot, and vegetable flakes
Hungarian paprika (once opened, it should be stored in the
refrigerator—sweet or spicy)
Nutmeg (preferably whole, to be used with a grater or grinder)
Ground cinnamon and ground ginger
Pure vanilla extract

Dairy Products

Nonfat or 1% lowfat evaporated milk—also called evaporated skim
milk; use for cooking or baking
Nonfat powdered milk—also called dried skim milk; use as a lightener in coffee instead of most nondairy creamers that may be
high in tropical oils and/or saturated fat or trans fat

Snacks

Brown rice crackers, Finn-Crisp, TLC crackers, low-fat Triscuits, Trader Joe's Pita Chips, whole wheat matzo wafers, Melba toast, matzo, bagel chips, Stacy's Pita Chips, Wasa bread, Unseasoned Rye-Krisp, Kavli, or other crackers that are whole grain with no fat added are good for snacking.

Popcorn—low calorie, high in insoluble fiber; make in an air popper or microwave; make sure it has no added oil, butter, or salt

Snack bars—Nature Valley Oats-n-Honey, Quaker Oats Chocolate Chip Chewy, Quaker Muffin

In the Freezer

The freezer offers an "emergency shelf" of items that can help you put together healthful meals without having to make a trip to the store. While fresh fruits and vegetables in season have wonderful flavor and are certainly preferable to frozen, foods properly frozen and stored still have good flavor, food value, and convenience.

Frozen vegetables—particularly corn, peas, okra, and mixed beans, which are high in soluble fiber and can be added to salads as well as served as vegetables; spinach, broccoli, and cauliflower and other cruciferous vegetables can also be used; avoid any vegetables frozen in butter or other sauces

Frozen pasta and vegetable mix—use as salad, hot pasta (add sauce), or stir-fry.

Veggie burgers—Gardenburger, sausage patties; Morning Star Farms, Lightlife Smart Bacon and Smart Links; Yves veggie bacon and Yves veggie sausage links (in limited amounts)

Natural fruit juice bars (no sugar added)—an acceptable, non-nutritive, no-cholesterol snack

Frozen unsweetened fruit juice concentrates—apple, pear, grape, pineapple, or orange (to be used in cooking, not as juice)

Unsweetened frozen fruit

Freshly grated Reggiano Parmesan cheese—use sparingly as a seasoning (or there is a vegan Parmesan cheese).

Soups, Tabashnik—frozen split pea or black bean soup

Nonfat frozen yogurt—an acceptable occasional dessert, also Soy Delicious soy products and Skinny Cow

Almonds or walnuts—limited use in baking or sometimes as a garnish; they do contain fat, although the fat is principally polyunsaturated

Whole wheat flour—because the germ has not been removed, it will become rancid if stored a long time at room temperature.

Whole grain breads, preferably those without added fat and sugar, such as rye, pumpernickel, spelt, Thomas' whole grain English muffins, Orowheat whole grain no sugar bread, Milton's whole grain bread and Ezekiel Bread; I suggest freezer storage since no preservatives are added

Oat Bran Muffins (recipe, page 108) and waffles (recipe, page 117)— prepare a double recipe and store in freezer for future use.

Skinned chicken breast fillets or turkey breast slices (4 or 5 ounces raw*)—a ready convenience for quick cooking

Turkey breast—Trader Joe's fresh, but stored in the freezer

Ground turkey breast (skin and fat removed)

Skinned chicken and turkey legs

Skinned 2-pound broiler, quartered, with excess skin and fat removed

Large or colossal tail-on cooked or raw shrimp or scallops

Salmon fillets (cut into 4 to 5 ounce serving portions) or whole fillets, microwave ready, from Trader Joe's

---

The Great Cholesterol Challenge: Foods to Enjoy, Foods to Limit

EAT THIS	LIMIT

Meats

If you eat meat occasionally after you have lowered your cholesterol to a safe level, try to limit it to twice a month. Limit all servings to no more than 4 or 5 ounces raw (3 or 4 ounces cooked), with all visible fat removed. Try to use the leanest cuts; buy Grade "Good" or "Select"—both have less fat.

EAT THIS	LIMIT
Beef—round, sirloin, tenderloin, or flank steak	Most beef, pork, veal, lamb, and other meats such as cold cuts, sausage, bacon, spare ribs, frankfurters, and canned meats
Lamb—leg	
Ostrich	
Pork—tenderloin	All organ meats (heart, liver, kidney, brains, sweetbreads, and tongue)
Veal—round, cutlet, or loin chop	
Venison	
Beefalo	

*4 ounces raw if on the two-week diet.

The Great Cholesterol Challenge (cont.)

EAT THIS	LIMIT

Poultry

Limit all servings to no more than 4 or 5 ounces raw° (3 or 4 ounces cooked) and remove all skin and visible fat.

EAT THIS	LIMIT
Chicken or turkey, breast or leg	Duck, goose, squab, quail
Cornish hen	All giblets and poultry skin
Duck breast, no skin, wild	Turkey bacon and turkey sausage
	Chicken sausage

Fish

Limit all servings to no more than 4 or 5 ounces raw° (3 or 4 ounces cooked).

EAT THIS	LIMIT
All fresh or frozen fish	Crayfish and squid
Fresh oysters, mussels, crab, clams, scallops, and shrimp	Sardines in olive oil
Canned fish in water, mustard, or tomato sauce (no oil)— particularly good are crab, salmon, albacore tuna, herring, and mackerel	

Eggs and Dairy Products

EAT THIS	LIMIT
Eggwhites, low-fat, cholesterol-free egg substitutes (Eggbeaters)	Egg yolks (one per week)
Liquid egg whites	Eggland Eggs
Nonfat (skim) or 1% fat milk, nonfat evaporated milk, nonfat dried milk	All whole milk and whole-milk dairy products (yogurt, evaporated milk, half-and-half, heavy cream, sour cream)
Nonfat or lowfat sour cream	All powdered and liquid nondairy creamers, especially those containing coconut, palm, palm kernel oil, or hydrogenated fat
Nonfat plain or fruit yogurt (no sugar added)	
Part-skim mozzarella cheese and grated Parmesan cheese, in limited amounts	
Galaxy tofu cheeses	

°4 ounces raw if on the two-week diet.

The Great Cholesterol Challenge (cont.)

EAT THIS	LIMIT
Cream cheese, lowfat, nonfat, or soy Part-skim or nonfat ricotta cheese Low fat cottage cheese Nondairy substitutes, low-fat Silk Soy milk and rice milk	Whole-milk cheeses or cheeses that have more than 5 grams of fat per ounce

Fruits

All fresh fruits Unsweetened applesauce Any unsweetened frozen fruit Any unsweetened canned fruit in natural juice Frozen unsweetened fruit juice concentrate Avocado, olives (enjoy but limit)	Dried fruit (high in sugar)

Vegetables

Any fresh vegetables Frozen vegetables	Prepared vegetables that have butter, cream, or cheese sauces added or are fried (especially in saturated fats) Vegetables frozen in butter or sauces

Grains and Grain Products

Whole wheat or whole grain flour Brown rice, wild rice, pilaf mix, or any other whole grain rice Bulgur wheat, barley, quinoa, spelt Oat bran Whole grain cereals without sugar added, such as Shredded Wheat and Bran, oatmeal, oat bran flakes, Ralston, Roman Meal, Uncle Sam's, Cheerios	White flour White rice Refined cereals with sugar, coconut or palm oil added Granola or muesli cereals with coconut, coconut oil, palm oil, or *any* hydrogenated or partially hydrogenated oil added Cereals with more than 6 grams of sugar per serving, muesli

The Great Cholesterol Challenge (cont.)

EAT THIS	LIMIT
Whole grain breads without sugar added, such as whole wheat, rye, pumpernickel; whole wheat pita; corn tortillas; water bagels; whole grain English muffins	Breads made from refined flours
	Breads made with egg yolk or whole eggs, butter, partially hydrogenated or hydrogenated fat, palm or coconut oil: egg bread, egg bagel, pastries, croissants, donuts, biscuits; commercial muffins, waffles, and pancakes, flour tortilla with added fat
Homemade muffins, pancakes, waffles, and cornbread°	
Air-popped popcorn	
Rye or whole wheat melba toast, Finn Crisp, flatbread, matzo crackers, whole wheat bread sticks, brown rice or Flax crackers	Buttered popcorn or popcorn with palm or coconut oil added
Kashi—TLC crackers	High-fat crackers like cheese or butter crackers; any crackers made with any tropical oil (coconut oil, palm oil), partially hydrogenated, or hydrogenated fat

Pasta

Whole wheat, soba, spelt, or any pasta made from whole grain or semolina flour	Fettuccine, or any pasta made with whole eggs
Asian noodles	Prepared pastas with cream or cheese sauces
Suggested sauces: marinara (no meat added), fresh tomato and basil, primavera, red clam°	

Beans and Legumes

All dried and canned beans, (red or green) lentils, and split peas

°Recipes to follow in this book.

The Great Cholesterol Challenge (cont.)

EAT THIS	LIMIT

Nuts and Seeds

Chestnuts
(Almonds, walnuts, pistachios, and hazelnuts in limited amounts)

Cashews, macadamia nuts, pine nuts, and Brazil nuts
Pumpkin, sunflower, and sesame seeds (used only in very limited amounts)

Fats and Oils

Vegetable oils like canola, cold-pressed safflower oil, sunflower oil, walnut oil, and extra-virgin olive oil, all in limited amounts
Soft margarines without trans fat (Benecol, Take Control, Promise, and Smart Best)

Tropical oils such as coconut oil, palm oil, palm kernel oil, cocoa butter (watch for especially in bakery products, commercially fried foods, processed foods, and candy)
Partially hydrogenated and hydrogenated vegetable oils and shortening, butter, lard, stick margarine, peanut oils, cottonseed oil, meat drippings, and chicken fat

Salad Dressings

Low-calorie (about 10 calories per tablespoon or less), preferably oil-free, or those made with reduced oil, nonfat yogurt, or buttermilk
Wishbone salad spritzers—fat free
"No oil" dry salad dressing mixes that require only the addition of vinegar and water
Walden Farms Soy Dressing
Weight Watchers Spectrum, Best Foods, Smart Balance, Hellman's reduced-calorie, low- or no-cholesterol mayonnaise

Any salad dressing made from whole eggs (Caesar), cheese, cream, or mayonnaise combinations
Mayonnaise

The Great Cholesterol Challenge (cont.)

EAT THIS	LIMIT

Soups and Broths

Homemade or canned vegetarian split-pea or lentil, minestrone, bean, barley, or vegetable soups, or red (tomato-based) fish chowders, or organic chicken or vegetable broths (*reduced sodium* and *fat removed*)

Frozen; Amy's or Tapatchnik vegetarian; Progresso low-sodium; Campbell's Healthy Request

LIMIT:

Cream soups and meat-based soups

Desserts and Snacks

Nonfat frozen yogurt, frozen natural fruit juice bars (no coconut), fruit sorbets or ices

Fresh fruit

Canned fruit in juice

Unsweetened frozen fruit

Homemade cakes or cookies, custards or puddings made with skim milk, egg whites, and safflower, sunflower, or canola oil

Klondike Slim-a-Bear (no sugar added)

Tropicana real fruit, no sugar added, bars

Baked salt-free corn or potato chips, pita chips

Nonfat popcorn

Kellogg's All-Bran Bars

LIMIT:

Ice cream (especially chocolate with cocoa butter or eggs added)

Skinny Cow

Tofutti Cuties

Tofu Soy Delicious ice cream in limited amounts

Whipped cream

Commercial cakes, cookies, ice cream mixes, pies, custards, puddings, or Jell-O with sugar

Homemade cakes or cookies with butter and/or eggs

Any fried chips or snacks

Most granola bars

The Great Cholesterol Challenge (cont.)

EAT THIS	LIMIT

Beverages

Mineral water

Water-processed decaffeinated coffee, green tea, or herb tea

Hot cereal beverages (Postum)

Fruit juices without added sugar (in limited amounts—has calories and provides no fiber)

Pomegranate juice

Sodium-reduced vegetable juice (V-8)

Nonalcoholic beer

Water—6 to 8 8-ounce glasses of water per day

Coffee, tea, whole milk, cream, or creamers

Limit alcoholic beverages to 1 serving per day (1 serving = 1 ounce liquor, 8 ounces beer, or 6 ounces wine)

Alcoholic beverages with coconut, cream liqueurs, heavy cream (piña colada), syrups, and salt

Kaiser Permanente Center for Health and Research found that participants who kept a food diary were the single best predictors of successful weight loss.* (List everthing that passes your ruby-red lips.)

*Refer to *Harriet Roth's Fat Counter*

▼ 4 ▼

Lose Pounds While You Lower Your Cholesterol: A Two-for-One Diet for Immediate Action

Nothing catches the popular fancy more than an easy solution to a tough problem—and generally nothing is farther from reality. People who need to lose weight are happy to find a diet that promises they can become sylphlike simply by eliminating a few foods. And many people who have to lower their cholesterol like to think they will be home free if they just cut out eggs, whipped cream, steaks, and butter. Alas, it isn't so.

Where cholesterol is concerned, the truth of the matter is that you have to make major changes in the foods you eat and the way you exercise, and those changes have to be permanent—it's really a lifestyle change, with the emphasis on *life*.

For those of you who want to lower your cholesterol level, I have put together a special diet plan. The diet is based on years of experience with clients who have been referred to me by their physicians in order to correct cholesterol levels and obesity without resorting to drugs. In many instances, excess weight has contributed to their problems, so a low-calorie diet has been in order initially as well as one that is low in cholesterol, saturated fat, and trans fat, and high in complex carbohydrates and fiber. Thus, this diet will give you two benefits for the price of one: It will help you lose up to three pounds a week and lose them safely—and it will lower your cholesterol levels.

The diet has the added advantage that it does not demand that you be preoccupied with food or how to prepare it. It does not call for exotic or expensive foods. The meals are nutritious and simple and can be prepared without difficulty. Many of them can also be easily ordered in restaurants—for let's face it, most of us have some meals out, if not for pleasure, simply out of necessity.

Obviously, when I consult privately with clients I can take into consideration different individual requirements and food preferences. However, the more generalized basic diet in this book should give you good results quickly and safely. It allows no more than 100 milligrams of cholesterol a day and about 1,000 calories daily for women and 1,200 calories for men. (The suggested calories for women are lower because women tend to lose weight less readily than do men, and also because women can generally operate on fewer calories due to their size.)

The diet may seem restrictive, but remember that it produces results because it imposes limits. I have found that clients prefer a diet plan that is simple, with meals that do not require too much effort to prepare. And I have had constant positive feedback: The people who have gone on my diet regimen say they are never hungry and have never felt better or more energetic. Once your cholesterol has been brought down to a safe level, you can progress to a much more varied maintenance diet *while still limiting your cholesterol to no more than 100 milligrams per day and trans fat to no more than 2 grams per day.* °

The people who have come to me for consultation generally stay on their individualized diets for a minimum of six weeks, or until their desired goals of lowered cholesterol and/or weight are reached. Once they have reached their goals, they are given low-cholesterol lifestyle menus like the ones in Chapter 5. Of course, my clients have been referred to me because their cholesterol levels are dangerously high. You may simply want to bring your cholesterol (and weight) down a bit to fall within the safe range. The diet in this book is less drastic, designed to be practiced for only two weeks at a time, followed by a week on your choice of the menus in Chapter 5. If you find after that that you still have a way to go, return to the diet for another two weeks. Repeat this rotation until you have reached a cholesterol level that is under 200 and are at your optimal weight.

Once you have your cholesterol and weight under control, you can maintain both by following the ongoing cholesterol lifestyle plan in

---

° Refer to *Harriet Roth's Fat Counter*, 2006 edition, for current information.

Chapter 5. You will be consuming more calories than on the diet, but you won't be overdosing on foods that will raise your cholesterol.

Remember, the two-week diet is designed to be a quick way to lower cholesterol and lose weight, and is meant to be followed for only two weeks at a time. The menus and recipes in the lifestyle plan are suggested for a way of eating that will keep your cholesterol low and excess pounds off for the rest of your life.

Caution: Although this diet is nutritionally sound and conforms to the recommended dietary allowances, I do not suggest *unsupervised* weight loss if you are taking medication for diabetes, hypertension, or cardiac problems or if you are pregnant. Before you try any restricted diet, you must *first consult your physician.* If he or she approves, then you are ready to start to take control of your health.

WHAT THIS TWO-WEEK DIET OFFERS YOU

1. Reduced amounts of cholesterol, saturated fat, and trans fat
2. Increased amounts of complex carbohydrates and fiber, *particularly cholesterol-reducing soluble fiber*
3. No empty calories—portion control!
4. A nutritionally sound plan that you can *live* with—no mindless eating!

Directions for
Following the Two-Week Jump Start Diet

1. The diet prescribes complete menus and recipes for two weeks. Follow the diet plan exactly as directed and *never skip meals* or *snacks.* When you miss a meal, you place unnecessary strain on your body and also run *the risk of eating larger portions at the next meal.*
2. Exercise portion control—don't exceed the amounts listed.
3. Eat *all* the foods listed.
4. Make sure you always get adequate oat bran daily—1⅓ cups oat bran cereal (⅓ cup uncooked) plus two oat bran muffins.
5. Take a heaping teaspoon of psyllium in an 8-ounce glass of water each day before breakfast.

6. Drink six to eight 8-ounce glasses of water a day (particularly since you are taking psyllium), including one full glass before each meal and snack.

7. Take a multivitamin, multimineral supplement every day *after* breakfast.

8. Include at least 30 to 45 minutes of walking, swimming, or bicycling for a minimum of five days a week. (If walking, try to build up to three miles in 45 minutes.) *Physical activity is a very important factor in both weight and cholesterol reduction, control, and longevity.* Exercise throws your metabolism into high gear while it *dampens* your appetite.

9. Do not drink alcoholic beverages. Alcohol is off-limits because it produces dehydration and adds calories that have no nutritive value. (When you go to the everyday "lifestyle" menus, try to limit your intake for the same reasons.)

Crucial Components That Make the Diet Work

Limited Protein: The maximum amount of animal protein allowed daily is about 4 to 5 ounces of raw (which translates into 3 to 4 ounces cooked). Three days a week are basically vegetarian days—one strictly vegetarian and one allowing minuscule amounts (1 to 1½ ounces) of animal protein.

Oat Bran: Because oat bran, a soluble fiber, has been found to be especially effective in lowering cholesterol, it is included in the diet every day. For optimal results, you need to eat about ⅔ cup (or 2 ounces) of oat bran daily in some form. The basic diet calls for cooked oatmeal or oat bran cereal for breakfast with two oat bran muffins daily as snacks. If you do not like cooked cereal or don't want to take the time to make it, the note on breakfasts, page 61, will give you some alternative suggestions.

Psyllium:° For an additional quick and easy source of lots of soluble fiber to lower cholesterol, I prescribe as part of the diet a heaping

---

° See footnote, page 22, for brand names.

teaspoon of unsweetened psyllium in an 8-ounce glass of water each day, preferably before breakfast or with it, followed by several additional glasses of water throughout the day. The active ingredient in psyllium is the plant fiber which is derived from the husks of psyllium seeds. According to a study by Dr. James W. Anderson at the University of Kentucky College of Medicine, it may lower cholesterol by increasing the excretion of bile acids, digestive substances that are made from cholesterol. Normally, bile acids are reabsorbed from the intestines, but if they are excreted instead, the body then takes cholesterol from the blood to make a new supply, thus lowering cholesterol levels. Unlike potent cholesterol-reducing drugs, psyllium generally has no undesirable side effects if taken as prescribed above with lots of water. And, as an added bonus, psyllium is a bulking agent so it helps in weight reduction and aids regularity.

Adequate Water: On the diet drink one glass of water *before* each meal and snack, with *a total of six to eight 8-ounce glasses of water every day*, particularly when you are using psyllium. Drinking a glass of water before each meal helps you feel a bit full before you start to eat. (Coffee, tea, or soft drinks don't count.) The more water you drink, the less fluid your body retains. Adequate water prevents fluid retention, gives a feeling of satiety, and aids regularity.

Whole Fresh Fruit: The diet calls for lots of unpeeled pears and apples and whole oranges with the pulp because of the fiber they supply. Never select juice if the whole fruit is available. In addition to valuable fiber the fruit gives you fewer calories. For example, one small apple contains only 60 calories plus fiber, while 8 ounces of apple juice contain 118 calories and no fiber.

Vitamins: While on the diet, since the calories are limited, you must take a multivitamin, multimineral supplement once a day *after* breakfast to ensure that your individual vitamin and mineral requirements are met. Make certain that these supplements contain no sugar, sodium, or added preservatives (such as Centrum).

What You Will Need
for the Two-Week Jump Start Diet

To help make it easy for you to follow the diet plan, I have prepared a shopping list for each of the two weeks so that with only one shopping trip a week you can be sure you will have everything on hand that you will need. But to ensure that you "stay on the straight and become narrow," it might help to rid your pantry of any high-fat, high-cholesterol, high-saturated-fat and trans-fat foods (see the list of foods to avoid in Chapter 3).

Before shopping, you should read the entire diet to get a feeling for what you will be doing. In some cases there are choices to be made. When you shop, follow the guidelines for stocking a healthy kitchen in Chapter 3.

In general, in my menus and recipes, I prefer to use fresh fruits and vegetables. However, I know that convenience is part of staying on a diet even for just two weeks, and for that reason, I have also suggested frozen fruits and vegetables and sodium-reduced canned soups and beans. If time permits, you can prepare your own beans and soup and freeze the leftovers for future use. If you use canned beans, rinse them with cold water first to remove as much added salt as possible.

Further Advice About How to Proceed

When You Eat Matters, Too

As in other areas of life, timing is everything when you are dieting. It is important to have meals at regular times: ideally, breakfast between 7 and 9, lunch between 12 and 2, and dinner early, between 6 and 7.

Of course, this isn't always possible. Dinner time is the most common problem. If you find it is necessary to eat your evening meal later than 7:00, then switch lunch and dinner menus on the diet and eat the larger meal at noon, so that you can work it off. For people who are working, this is often more convenient—the business lunch, which can undermine a diet plan, can then become the day's dinner, leaving the evening meal a light one.

Try not to eat after dinner. Although the diet contains optional evening snacks, it is best if you can avoid eating anything after dinner. Try drinking salt-free bottled water or seltzer with a wedge of lime, lemon, or orange instead. If a snack is absolutely necessary, limit yourself to the air-popped popcorn (without fat or salt), a natural sugar-free fruit juice bar, or ½ cup Cheerios cereal the diet provides. Although a snack at night is more a psychological need than a nutritional necessity, if you feel the urge it is better to indulge it wisely than to give in to a midnight raid on the refrigerator.

Switching Meals

Just as you will sometimes want to switch lunch and dinner menus, feel free to exchange the midmorning and midafternoon snacks.

But whatever you do, *do not skip any meals or snacks*; it is important to eat all the foods listed each day for optimal results.

A Word About Breakfast

The diet plan breakfast is simple and unvaried. It calls for fresh fruit rather than fruit juice because of the fiber content, and includes oat bran or oatmeal every day. Since oat bran is such a good source of the soluble fiber that helps lower cholesterol, you should try to consume the equivalent of ⅔ cup uncooked oat bran daily. You can meet this goal by eating two Oat Bran Muffins (page 108) a day plus 1⅓ cups of hot cooked oat bran cereal or old-fashioned oatmeal (no instant oatmeal).

Some Alternative Breakfasts

If you find cooked oat bran cereal not to your liking, try:

Plain Oatmeal: Substitute oatmeal made by combining ⅓ cup of uncooked rolled oats with 2 tablespoons of oat bran prepared according to package directions. (Although oatmeal contains oat bran, the bran isn't concentrated enough to give you your quota by itself.)

Oat Bran Muffins: Substitute two additional oat bran muffins for the hot cooked oat bran cereal, but remember, if you do this you will add about 100 calories to your diet.

A Quick Breakfast Beverage: If you simply don't have time to prepare cooked cereal, try the Oat Bran Quickie Breakfast Beverage or Quick Breakfast in a Bowl (page 111).

Coffee and Tea

Go slow on coffee. If you drink coffee or tea for breakfast, choose a water-processed decaffeinated coffee, green or herbal tea, or roasted cereal beverage (such as Postum). If you use a lightener in your coffee, tea, or beverage, use powdered or liquid nonfat milk. *Avoid nondairy creamers*—unless they are nonfat.

Eating Out

If you are eating out, order fruit and cooked oatmeal. Eat the oatmeal with nonfat or 1% milk.

Before You Begin . . .

You will notice that I suggest that you start your diet on Saturday. This is deliberate since weekends are often conducive to "falling off the wagon"—a time when you consume too many high-calorie foods or simply eat too much. By starting on Saturday, you head this problem off at the pass.

I have deliberately put salads first on many of the menus because, like a glass of water taken before you eat, they help fill you up so that you do not feel deprived of food. One cup broth or vegetable soup may also be used.

One final word of advice: Don't "weigh yourself down" by getting on the scale every day. Instead, weigh yourself when you start the diet and not again until the end of the first week. For a more accurate reading, always weigh yourself at the same time of day, with the same mode of dress or undress. And keep a journal of what, how, and when you eat!°

Remember, *a serving* is the standard amount of food listed on a label; a *portion* is the larger amount you choose to put on your plate and eat.

°Refer to an online journal such as myfooddiary.com for additional help.

Eat Smarter

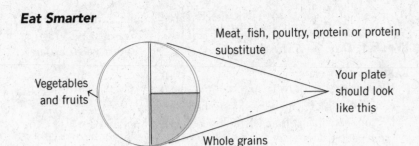

Move More and Eat Less

A FACT OF LIFE

We tend to gain only an average of one pound a year after the age of twenty-five; after fifty our metabolism slows down even more, so we need fewer calories. For this reason, the nutritional quality of each bite is more important than ever. *We cannot afford wasted calories or huge portions.*

The Two-Week Jump Start Diet for Cholesterol and Weight Reduction

Recipes for dishes in the daily menus begin on page 84.

When a salad is called for, be sure to eat it first—not with or after the meal. Salads help fill you up so that you are satisfied with the more reduced portions on the diet.

Note: I have added six simply delicious soup recipes, starting on page 272. *As an option*, you may serve three-quarters cup before any lunch or dinner in the diet plan.

Remember to include psyllium every day as a part of your two-week diet: 1 heaping teaspoon of unsweetened psyllium dissolved in an 8-ounce glass of water. You *must* drink four more glasses of water daily.

WEEK ONE DIET

Week 1, Day 1—Saturday

ABOUT 1,000 CALORIES

BASIC BREAKFAST

1 glass water

1 small orange, ½ cup berries, or ½ banana

1⅓ cups cooked oat bran (⅓ cup uncooked oat bran) or oatmeal,° with cinnamon

½ cup nonfat or 1% fat milk, or Light Silk Soymilk

MIDMORNING SMART SNACK

½ small apple, unpeeled, or 1 ounce Galaxy Veggie slice cheese†

1 Oat Bran Muffin (page 108)

LUNCH

1 glass water

3 cups mixed vegetable salad: 1 tablespoon Marinated Kidney Beans (page 84) or plain kidney beans *and* a combination of your choice of the following: artichoke hearts, broccoli, red cabbage, zucchini, cauliflower, mushrooms, radishes, cucumber, green or red pepper, pea pods, baby spinach, romaine and/or other leafy lettuces, cherry tomatoes, watercress, and a few onions if you like, mixed with 2 tablespoons low-calorie oil-free Italian dressing, lemon juice, balsamic vinegar, or salsa, and 1 slice Galaxy Veggie cheese

2 Finn Crisp crackers or 1 unseasoned Rye-Krisp

MIDAFTERNOON SMART SNACK

6 ounces plain nonfat yogurt (mixed with 1 teaspoon sugar-free jam or 2 tablespoons fresh or frozen berries, 1 teaspoon vanilla extract, if desired) or 1 cup nonfat milk

1 Oat Bran Muffin (page 108)

DINNER

1 glass water

2 cups mixed green salad topped with 1 shredded carrot and 2 cherry tomatoes, mixed with 1 tablespoon low-calorie oil-free Italian dressing, or lemon juice, or balsamic vinegar, or salad spritzer

---

°For alternative suggestions, see page 61.

†This principally soy cheese is also lactose free.

3 ounces broiled or poached salmon (4 ounces raw) brushed with 1 teaspoon mustard and ¼ teaspoon chopped garlic (or 3 ounces canned
drained salmon)

1½ cups combined fresh or frozen broccoli, cauliflower, and zucchini

1 clementine

P.M. SNACK (OPTIONAL)

1 cup air-popped popcorn (no salt or fat added) or ½ cup Cheerios with
⅓ cup nonfat milk or 1 package Blue Diamond almonds

OPTIONAL EXPANSION TO 1,200 CALORIES FOR MEN:

♦ *Breakfast:* Add 1 slice whole wheat,° rye, or pumpernickel toast (*or*
½ whole grain English muffin) with 1 teaspoon sugar-free jam or
apple butter

♦ *Midmorning snack:* Eat 1 whole *small* apple or pear instead of ½

♦ *Dinner:* Increase salmon to 5 ounces raw

Note: Be sure you have eaten two Oat Bran Muffins, and also keep a
food journal.

Week 1, Day 2—Sunday

BREAKFAST

See Day 1, you may substitute a treat of Oat Bran Waffle (page 117) with 1
tablespoon of sugar-free syrup instead of cooked oat bran or oatmeal.

MIDMORNING SNACK

See Day 1

LUNCH

1 glass water

3 ounces drained and flaked, canned albacore tuna or salmon in water
mixed with 2 cups mixed vegetable salad (see Day 1 lunch for vegetable suggestions), mixed with 2 tablespoons low-calorie oil-free Italian
dressing, lemon juice, or balsamic vinegar

½ 6-inch whole wheat pita bread

Note: You can make this into a sandwich if you wish.

°Mitton's 100% whole wheat bread or Ezekiel bread

MIDAFTERNOON SNACK
See Day 1

DINNER
1 glass water
1 cooked fresh artichoke, or 8 slim asparagus spears, with a lemon wedge and 1 tablespoon low-calorie oil-free Italian dressing
1½ cups cooked whole wheat soba or spelt penne with Light Tomato-Mushroom Sauce (page 85)
1 cup sliced zucchini or broccoli, steamed
¼ small cantaloupe

P.M. SNACK (OPTIONAL)
See Day 1

EXPANSION TO 1,200 CALORIES FOR MEN
♦ *Breakfast:* Add 1 slice whole wheat, rye, or pumpernickel toast (or ½ whole grain English muffin) with 1 teaspoon sugar-free jam or apple butter
Optional: 2 slices grilled Canadian bacon *instead* of 1 slice bread
♦ *Midmorning snack:* Eat 1 whole *small* apple instead of ½
♦ *Dinner:* Increase veggies to 2 cups

Week 1, Day 3—Monday   ABOUT 1,000 CALORIES

BREAKFAST
See Day 1

Note: Store-bought oat bran muffin may not be subsituted.

MIDMORNING SNACK
See Day 1

LUNCH
1 glass water
Antipasto Salad (page 86)
2 Finn Crisp crackers or 1 unseasoned Rye-Krisp
1 6-ounce can chilled sodium-reduced V-8 juice with lemon
1 clementine

MIDAFTERNOON SNACK
See Day 1

DINNER
1 glass water
½ cup Vegetarian Lentil Soup (page 87) or canned vegetarian lentil soup
2 cups mixed radicchio, watercress, and hearts of palm mushroom salad with 2 tablespoons oil-free Italian dressing
½ baked yam topped with 1 tablespoon plain nonfat yogurt and chopped green onion
1 cup fresh or frozen French-cut green beans, with water chestnuts if desired
1 Baked Stuffed Tomato (page 86)
¾ cup sliced banana and berries (optional)

P.M. SNACK (OPTIONAL)
See Day 1

EXPANSION TO 1,200 CALORIES FOR MEN:
♦ *Breakfast:* Add 1 slice whole wheat, pumpernickel, or rye toast (or ½ whole grain English muffin) with 1 teaspoon sugar-free jam or apple butter
♦ *Lunch:* Eat 1 whole *small* apple instead of ½
♦ *Dinner:* Increase to 1 whole baked yam or 1 cup lentil soup

Week 1, Day 4—Tuesday   ABOUT 1,000 CALORIES

BREAKFAST
See Day 1

MIDMORNING SNACK
See Day 1

LUNCH
1 glass water
3 cups mixed vegetable salad with 1 tablespoon Marinated Kidney Beans (page 84, see Day 1 lunch for vegetable suggestions), mixed with 2 tablespoons oil-free Italian dressing
2 Finn Crisp crackers or 1 unseasoned Rye-Krisp
1 clementine

MIDAFTERNOON SNACK
See Day 1

DINNER
1 glass water
2 cups watercress and romaine, topped with 2 orange slices
1 tablespoon yogurt combined with 1 tablespoon orange juice for salad dressing
3 ounces broiled (4 ounces raw) fillet of sole (or any lean whitefish), brushed with 1 teaspoon mustard and 1 tablespoon lemon juice
1 cup steamed broccoli, cauliflower, and/or carrots
½ ear corn (save the other half for lunch salad Wednesday)
½ cup fresh fruit salad (optional)

P.M. SNACK (OPTIONAL)
See Day 1

EXPANSION TO 1,200 CALORIES FOR MEN:
♦ *Breakfast:* Add 1 slice whole wheat, rye, or pumpernickel toast (or ½ whole grain English muffin) with 1 teaspoon sugar-free jam or apple butter
♦ *Lunch:* Add 1 cup homemade or canned Vegetarian Lentil Soup (page 87)
♦ *Dinner:* Increase fillet of sole to 5 ounces raw

Week 1, Day 5—Wednesday   ABOUT 1,000 CALORIES

BREAKFAST
See Day 1

MIDMORNING SNACK
See Day 1

LUNCH
1 glass water
2 cups Marinated Broccoli, Corn, Artichoke Heart, and Red Pepper (page 88) or 3 cups mixed vegetable salad (see Day 1 lunch for vegetable suggestions), 1 ounce cheese or turkey breast
2 Finn Crisp crackers or 1 unseasoned Rye-Krisp
1 6-ounce can sodium-reduced V-8 juice
¼ cantaloupe

MIDAFTERNOON SNACK
See Day 1

DINNER
1 glass water
1 cup Spicy Cold Tomato Soup (page 88)
Seafood Salad Vinaigrette (page 89)
½ 6-inch toasted whole wheat pita bread
1 sliced kiwi with 2 tablespoons berries

P.M. SNACK (OPTIONAL)
See Day 1

EXPANSION TO 1,200 CALORIES FOR MEN:
 ♦ *Breakfast:* Add 1 slice whole wheat, rye, or pumpernickel toast (or ½ whole grain English muffin) with 1 teaspoon sugar-free jam or apple butter
 ♦ *Lunch:* Add 1 cup homemade or canned Anderson's Vegetarian Lentil Soup (page 87)
 ♦ *Dinner:* Increase seafood in salad by 2 large shrimp or 2 scallops

Week 1, Day 6—Thursday
(Vegetarian Day)   ABOUT 1,000 CALORIES

BREAKFAST
See Day 1

MIDMORNING SNACK
See Day 1

LUNCH
1 glass water
½ cup homemade or canned Vegetarian Lentil Soup (page 87)
3 cups mixed vegetable salad (see Day 1 lunch for vegetable suggestions), mixed with 2 tablespoons low-calorie oil-free Italian dressing
2 Finn Crisp crackers or 1 unseasoned Rye-Krisp
½ cup blueberries

MIDAFTERNOON SNACK
See Day 1

DINNER
1 glass water
Caesar Salad (page 91) with 3 grilled shrimp (optional)
2 cups Quick Vegetable Lo Mein (page 90)
3 cantaloupe slices

P.M. SNACK (OPTIONAL)
See Day 1

EXPANSION TO 1,200 CALORIES FOR MEN:
♦ *Breakfast:* Add 1 slice whole wheat, rye, or pumpernickel toast (or ½ whole wheat English muffin) with 1 teaspoon sugar-free jam or apple butter
♦ *Lunch:* Eat 1 whole *small* apple instead of ½
♦ *Dinner:* Add ¼ cup lowfat cottage cheese to fruit and 1 cup Campbell's Healthy Request tomato soup

Week 1, Day 7—Friday   ABOUT 1,000 CALORIES

BREAKFAST
See Day 1

MIDMORNING SNACK
See Day 1

LUNCH
1 glass water
½ Tuna-Apple Salad Sandwich on whole grain bread (page 91)
Crudités: 2 carrot sticks, 2 red pepper sticks, 2 broccoli or cauliflower florets, 3 cucumber sticks, 3 radishes
1 6-ounce can sodium-reduced V-8 juice

MIDAFTERNOON SNACK
See Day 1

DINNER
1 glass water·
1½ cups Artichoke, Mushroom, and Pepper Salad with Yogurt Dressing (page 92)

2 ounces sliced roast turkey breast or 2 ounces grilled turkey breast with salsa

1 cup steamed spinach with lemon juice

1 cup steamed yellow crookneck squash

½ cup mixed fresh fruit (use any fruits left over from week)

P.M. SNACK (OPTIONAL)
See Day 1

EXPANSION TO 1,200 CALORIES FOR MEN:
 ♦ *Breakfast:* Add 1 slice whole wheat, rye, or pumpernickel toast (or ½ whole wheat English muffin) with 1 teaspoon sugar-free jam, or 1 Oat Bran Muffin (page 108)
 ♦ *Lunch:* Add another slice of whole grain bread to the sandwich
 ♦ *Dinner:* Increase to 4 ounces roast turkey breast with salsa

WEEK TWO DIET

One week down and another to go. If you've cheated just a bit, don't give yourself a hard time. Remember, the occasional urge to indulge won't wreck your long-term efforts for a low-cholesterol lifestyle and weight control. Treat it as a temporary diversion and don't feel you are doomed to overeat forever.

Week 2, Day 1—Saturday   ABOUT 1,000 CALORIES

BREAKFAST
 1 glass water
 1 small orange, ½ cup berries, or ½ banana
 1⅓ cups cooked oat bran (⅓ cup uncooked oat bran) or oatmeal,° with cinnamon
 ½ cup nonfat or 1% fat milk, or Light Silk Soymilk

MIDMORNING SNACK
 1 small apple, unpeeled
 1 Oat Bran Muffin (page 108)

° For alternative suggestions, see page 61.

LUNCH

   1 glass water

   ½ water, pumpernickel, or whole wheat bagel (no egg) scooped out and
      filled with 2 tablespoons each chopped tomato and green onion and
      1 Galaxy Veggie slice, lightly broiled

   12 *assorted* crudités (3 each): broccoli florets, green pepper sticks, cu-
      cumber sticks, radishes, or raw vegetables of your choice

   1 6-ounce can chilled sodium-reduced V-8 juice with lemon

MIDAFTERNOON SNACK

   1 6-ounce nonfat yogurt or 8-ounce nonfat milk

   1 Oat Bran Muffin (page 108)

DINNER

   1 glass water

   ½ cup Vegetarian Split Pea Soup (page 93) or canned vegetarian split
      pea soup

   2 cups mixed greens with red onion rings and pepper strips, with 2
      tablespoons low-calorie oil-free Italian dressing

   Pronto Pasta Primavera (page 94)

   10 seedless grapes

P.M. SNACK (OPTIONAL)

   1 cup air-popped popcorn (no salt or fat added) or ¼ cup cereal with ¼
      cup nonfat milk

EXPANSION TO 1,200 CALORIES FOR MEN:

   ♦ *Breakfast:* Add 1 slice whole wheat, rye, or pumpernickel toast (or
      ½ whole wheat English muffin) with 1 teaspoon sugar-free jam or
      apple butter

   ♦ *Lunch:* Add additional ½ scooped, filled bagel

   ♦ *Dinner:* Increase to 1 cup split pea soup

Note: Be sure you have eaten two Oat Bran Muffins.

Eating lunch in a restaurant? Try to choose one with a salad bar
and refer to the salad suggestions in the menu for Week 1, Day 1,
so that you will know what to select.

Week 2, Day 2—Sunday   ABOUT 1,000 CALORIES

BREAKFAST
See Day 1. You may substitute Spinach Frittata (page 160) for cooked oat bran.

MIDMORNING SNACK
See Day 1

LUNCH
1 glass water
1 cup Tomato Bouillon (page 95)
Choose 1 Quesadilla (page 95) *or* Pronto Pasta Primavera salad (page 94)
12 *assorted* crudités (3 each): snow peas, red pepper strips, broccoli florets, cucumber sticks
¼ cantaloupe

MIDAFTERNOON SNACK
6 ounces plain nonfat yogurt (mixed with 1 teaspoon sugar-free jam or 2 tablespoons fresh or frozen berries, if desired) or 1 cup light plain soy milk
1 Oat Bran Muffin (page 108)

DINNER
1 glass water
2 cups mixed greens with shredded red cabbage, mixed with 2 tablespoons low-calorie oil-free Italian dressing
4 ounces broiled tuna or salmon brushed with balsamic vinegar (or 3½ ounces canned albacore tuna in water or salmon, drained)
1 cup cooked spinach
2 small steamed new potatoes
½ cup berries

Note: Broil 8 ounces of fish at dinner and save 2 ounces (¼) for lunch salad on Monday.

P.M. SNACK (OPTIONAL)
1 natural fruit juice bar, 1 cup air-popped popcorn (no salt or fat added), or ½ cup Cheerios and ¼ cup nonfat milk

EXPANSION TO 1,200 CALORIES FOR MEN:

- *Breakfast:* Add 1 slice whole wheat, rye, or pumpernickel toast (or ½ whole wheat English muffin) with 1 teaspoon sugar-free jam or apple butter
  Optional: 2 slices Canadian bacon
- *Lunch:* Use 2 corn tortillas instead of 1 in the Quesadilla (see page 95)
- *Dinner:* Increase berries to 1 cup

Week 2, Day 3—Monday   ABOUT 1,000 CALORIES

BREAKFAST
See Day 1

MIDMORNING SNACK
See Day 1

LUNCH
1 glass water
1 6-ounce can chilled sodium-reduced V-8 juice with lemon
Tuna or Salmon Niçoise Salad (page 96)
1 unseasoned Rye-Krisp cracker
1 clementine

MIDAFTERNOON SNACK
See Day 1

DINNER
1 glass water
½ cup Vegetarian Split Pea Soup (page 93) or canned vegetarian split pea soup
3 ounces baked sweet potato
1 cup steamed broccoli
Vegetable Kebab: 3 chunks each squashes, cherry tomatoes, and mushrooms brushed with low-calorie oil-free Italian dressing and broiled
½ cup fresh fruit salad with 1 tablespoon plain nonfat yogurt, sprinkled with cinnamon.

P.M. SNACK (OPTIONAL)
See Day 1

EXPANSION TO 1,200 CALORIES FOR MEN:
 ♦ *Breakfast:* Add 1 slice whole wheat, rye, or pumpernickel toast (or
   ½ whole grain English muffin) with 1 teaspoon sugar-free jam or
   apple butter
 ♦ *Dinner:* Increase to 1 cup split pea soup and 1 cup fresh fruit salad
   with 6 ounces of plain nonfat yogurt

Week 2, Day 4—Tuesday   ABOUT 1,000 CALORIES

BREAKFAST
  See Day 1

MIDMORNING SNACK
  ½ *small* apple, unpeeled
  1 Oat Bran Muffin (page 108)

LUNCH
  1 glass water
  3 cups mixed vegetable salad with 1 tablespoon Marinated Kidney Beans
    (page 84, *and* a combination of your choice of the following: broccoli,
    red cabbage, zucchini, cauliflower, celery, carrot, mushrooms, radishes,
    cucumber, green or red pepper, spinach, romaine and/or other leafy veg-
    etables, and a few onion slices if you like, mixed with 2 tablespoons low-
    calorie oil-free Italian dressing, salsa, lemon juice, *or* balsamic vinegar)
  2 Finn Crisp crackers or 1 unseasoned Rye-Krisp
  1 clementine

MIDAFTERNOON SNACK
  See Day 2

DINNER
  1 glass water
  Parsley and Tomato Salad with Basil Vinaigrette (page 96)
  9–10 ounces boneless chicken breast broiled and glazed with ½ tea-
    spoon Dijon mustard and 1 teaspoon frozen apple juice concentrate
    (defrost breast in refrigerator the night before)
  1 cup fresh or frozen French-cut green beans
  1 cup crookneck squash
  1 sliced kiwi with 1 tablespoon berry puree

  Note: Save one-third of chicken breast for Thursday lunch.

P.M. SNACK (OPTIONAL)
See Day 2

EXPANSION TO 1,200 CALORIES FOR MEN:
♦ *Breakfast:* Add 1 slice whole wheat, rye, or pumpernickel toast (or ½ whole wheat English muffin) with 1 teaspoon sugar-free jam or 1 cheese veggie slice
♦ *Lunch:* Add ½ cup Vegetarian Split Pea Soup (page 93) and 1 hard-cooked egg
♦ *Dinner:* Add 1 slice whole wheat bread and ½ cup berries

Week 2, Day 5—Wednesday   ABOUT 1,000 CALORIES

BREAKFAST
See Day 1

MIDMORNING SNACK
See Day 1

LUNCH
1 glass water
Vegetarian Chop Suey Salad Sandwich in pita bread (page 98)
6 ounces sodium-reduced V-8 juice
1 clementine

MIDAFTERNOON SNACK
See Day 1

DINNER
1 glass water
½ cup Vegetarian Split Pea Soup (page 93)
Seviche Salad (page 97)
½ 6-inch pita bread, toasted
½ papaya with lime

P.M. SNACK (OPTIONAL)
See Day 1

EXPANSION TO 1,200 CALORIES FOR MEN:
♦ *Breakfast:* Add 1 slice whole wheat, rye, or pumpernickel toast (or ½ whole grain English muffin) with 1 teaspoon sugar-free jam or apple butter

♦ *Lunch:* Add ¾ cup soup from Simply Delicious Soup Recipes (page 272)
♦ *Midafternoon snack:* Increase apple to 1 whole *small* apple
♦ *Dinner:* Increase scallops in seviche to 6 ounces

Avoid fast foods. They are generally high in cholesterol-producing saturated fat, trans fat, cholesterol, and fluid-retaining sodium.

Week 2, Day 6—Thursday   ABOUT 1,000 CALORIES

BREAKFAST
See Day 1

MIDMORNING SNACK
See Day 1

LUNCH
1 glass water
½ papaya with Curried Chicken Salad (page 98)
2 unseasoned Rye-Krisp crackers
12 assorted crudités (3 each): snow peas, red pepper strips, broccoli florets, radishes

MIDAFTERNOON SNACK
See Day 2

DINNER
1 glass water
2 cups mixed greens with 1 tablespoon Marinated Kidney Beans (page 84) and 4 quarters artichoke hearts
1½ cups spaghetti squash or 1 cup cooked pasta, mixed with ⅔ cup salt-free marinara sauce or Light Tomato Mushroom Sauce from Week 1 (page 85)
½ cup each steamed broccoli, eggplant, and carrot
½ cup fresh fruit salad with 1 teaspoon balsamic vinegar and ⅛ teaspoon vanilla

P.M. SNACK (OPTIONAL)
See Day 2

EXPANSION TO 1,200 CALORIES FOR MEN:
- ♦ *Breakfast:* Add 1 slice whole wheat, rye, or pumpernickel toast (or ½ whole grain English muffin) with 1 teaspoon sugar-free jam or 1 veggie cheese slice
- ♦ *Dinner:* Increase to 2½ cups spaghetti squash or 1½ cups pasta with 1 cup sauce; increase to 1 cup fresh fruit salad

Week 2, Day 7—Friday ABOUT 1,000 CALORIES

BREAKFAST
See Day 1

MIDMORNING SNACK
6 ounces nonfat plain yogurt or nonfat milk
1 Oat Bran Muffin (page 108)

LUNCH
1 glass water
1 6-ounce can reduced-sodium V-8 juice
1 cup defrosted Pasta Salad Orientale from Week 1 (or cold cooked spaghetti squash or pasta from night before) mixed with ½ cup each: julienne carrots, zucchini, and red pepper, mixed with 2 tablespoons low-calorie oil-free Italian dressing
1 clementine

MIDAFTERNOON SNACK
See Day 1

DINNER
1 glass water
Broiled eggplant and bell pepper strips on lettuce with basil vinaigrette (dressing from Tuesday dinner, page 75)
4 ounces broiled (5 ounces raw) salmon drizzled with low-sodium soy sauce topped with sautéed, sliced mushrooms
2 small steamed summer squash with grated carrot
½ cup fresh fruit salad

P.M. SNACK (OPTIONAL) TREAT!

2 squares Guylian Dark Chocolate, no sugar added

EXPANSION TO 1,200 CALORIES FOR MEN:

♦ *Breakfast:* Add 1 slice whole wheat, rye, or pumpernickel toast (or ½ whole grain English muffin) with 1 teaspoon sugar-free jam or apple butter

♦ *Lunch:* Increase pasta to 1½ cups

♦ *Dinner:* Add 1 cup soup

Shopping Lists for the Two-Week Diet

Week 1

Before shopping, read the entire diet. Don't be put off by the length of the shopping list for Week 1. You will only have to go to the market once a week, and many of the foods are to be used both in Week 1 and Week 2. Some may be ingredients that you already have in your pantry.

You will notice that these lists specify if perishables like seafood should be frozen. If you prefer not to use frozen items or do not wish to wait for them to thaw, you can simply buy the items on the day you plan to cook them. Remember to wash fruits and vegetables before eating, not before storing.

1 jar multivitamin, multimineral supplement (100 tablets) (Centrum)

21-ounce jar unflavored psyllium (see page 22 for brand names) or Metamucil crackers

1 quart nonfat milk or ½ gallon low-fat soy milk

8 6-ounce containers nonfat plain (Greek Fage) yogurt, or (if you do not eat yogurt) 1 additional quart nonfat milk

1 dozen eggs (for Weeks 1 and 2) or 1 dozen Eggland eggs*

2 ounces freshly grated Parmesan cheese (for Weeks 1 and 2)

2 packages Galaxy Veggie slices—any flavor

2 pounds oat bran (for Weeks 1 and 2)

1 package oatmeal and/or Cheerios (for Weeks 1 and 2)

1 package Finn Crisp crackers or unseasoned Rye-Krisp (for Weeks 1 and 2)

*Contains 25% less saturated fat and 100 mg omega-3 fatty acid

1 package Milton's whole wheat bread (for Weeks 1 and 2) or 1 package Oroweat 100% whole wheat, no sugar, bread

1 package 6-inch whole wheat pita bread (for Weeks 1 and 2)

2 boxes Blue Diamond almonds (7 snack packs)

1 jar Tap-N-Apple apple butter

10 small oranges or clementines

8 small apples

1 small cantaloupe

4 bananas

2 pints blue or seasonal berries, or 1 16-ounce package frozen unsweetened berries

2 lemons and 2 limes

2 cans nonfat evaporated milk

1 package Splenda brown sugar blend

Pure vanilla extract

1 can hearts of palm

8 ounces salmon fillet, or 3 3½-ounce cans salmon (wild or line caught)

5 ounces fillet of sole or any lean whitefish (freeze for Tuesday)

3 ounces canned or fresh bay shrimp, crab, or lobster (if fresh, freeze for Wednesday)

4 ounces cooked sliced turkey breast, or 2 2-ounce slices of raw turkey fillet (freeze for Friday)

3 3½-ounce cans albacore tuna in water

4 slices Canadian bacon (for Weeks 1 and 2)

1 fresh artichoke, or 8 slim asparagus spears

2 bunches (about 3 pounds) broccoli florets or 3 packages frozen broccoli florets

1 head (about 1 pound) cauliflower

1 bunch carrots

1 bunch celery (for Weeks 1 and 2)

1 head each: romaine, red lettuce, endive, and butter lettuce or any other variety

1 small head radicchio

1 bunch watercress

½ small head red cabbage or 1 package shredded red cabbage (for Weeks 1 and 2)

5 small zucchini

3 crookneck squash

2 ears fresh or frozen corn (or 1 can or package frozen corn)

1 pound fresh green beans, or 1 16-ounce package frozen French-cut green beans with water chestnuts

2 small red peppers and 1 small green pepper

1 cucumber, European

8 ounces sliced fresh mushrooms

1 12-ounce package frozen spinach

1 medium tomato

10 fresh Italian plum tomatoes, 2 8-ounce cans salt-free tomato sauce, or 1 16-ounce jar salt-free tomato sauce

1 small red onion

2 small yellow onions and 3 shallots

2 6-ounce sweet potatoes (yams)

1 bunch green onions

Garlic or 1 package frozen garlic (for Weeks 1 and 2), Dorat brand Herbes de Provence or Italian herb blend

1 jar ground cumin

1 16-ounce package frozen edamame beans

1 16-ounce package frozen broccoli, cauliflower, and carrots (for Monday)

1 16-ounce package frozen broccoli, corn, and red peppers (for Wednesday lunch, if not using fresh)

1 16-ounce package frozen Pasta Salad Orientale, or 2 ounces egg-free linguine (if using fresh vegetables for Thursday dinner's Vegetable Lo Mein)

1 pint reduced-fat mayonnaise

1 jar sugar-free jam (optional) and 1 jar cinnamon and 1 jar apple butter (Tap'N'Apple)

1 bottle sodium-reduced soy sauce (for Weeks 1 and 2)

12 6-ounce cans *sodium-reduced* vegetable (V-8) juice

1 can sodium-reduced chicken broth (Swanson's For Goodness Sake)

1 jar Newman's Own salsa (as spicy as you like), or 1 carton fresh salsa (for Weeks 1 and 2)

1 15-ounce can quartered artichoke hearts in water

1 14-ounce can sodium-reduced kidney beans

1 bottle low-calorie Italian, balsamic, or herb salad dressing (for Weeks 1 and 2) or 1 bottle oil-free Italian dressing*

1 bottle balsamic or Japanese rice vinegar and 1 small bottle canola oil.

1 16-ounce jar popcorn for optional snacks (for Weeks 1 and 2)

2 cans vegetarian lentil soup, or for homemade soup, add 1 16-ounce package lentils, 1 onion, and 1 28-ounce can crushed San Marzano tomatoes in puree

*Any Walden Farms *oil-free* salad dressing may be used.

Week 2

Before shopping, *check the list for any leftover ingredients from Week 1* so that you do not purchase unnecessary items.

1 quart nonfat milk
8 6-ounce containers nonfat plain yogurt, or 1 additional quart nonfat milk
4 ounces Galaxy Veggie slices
1 package 6-inch corn tortillas
1 water, rye, or whole wheat bagel (no egg)
1 8-ounce package pasta (penne) (whole grain or spelt)
10 small oranges or clementines
4 small apples
4 bananas
1 pint seasonal berries, or 1 16-ounce package frozen unsweetened berries
2 lemons
2 limes
2 kiwis
1 cantaloupe, wash before cutting!
1 papaya
1 bunch red seedless grapes (16)
8 ounces tuna or salmon fillet, or 2 3½-ounce cans light tuna in water or salmon (line caught)
9–10 ounces skinned, boned chicken breast
5 ounces salmon (freeze until Friday)
4 ounces bay scallops (divide and freeze for Wednesday)
2 bunches broccoli florets or frozen (about 3 pounds)
1 head each: romaine, red lettuce, butter lettuce, radicchio, watercress, or any variety you want or need
1 large bunch fresh Italian parsley
1 bunch fresh basil
1 small spaghetti squash
2 bunches radishes
2 bunches carrots
1 jicama
1 red pepper
1 pint cherry tomatoes or grape tomatoes
1 Italian plum tomato
1 small red onion

2 Japanese eggplant or ½ pound eggplant

1 cucumber

1 12-ounce package frozen spinach

½ pound green beans, or 1 10-ounce package frozen French-cut green beans

4 crookneck squash

3 zucchini

2 summer squash

1 4-ounce sweet potato (yam)

2 small new potatoes

12 snow peas or sugar snap peas

1 16-ounce package frozen broccoli, corn, and red peppers (if not using fresh)

1 16-ounce package frozen broccoli, zucchini, and red peppers (if not using fresh)

1 15-ounce can quartered artichoke hearts in water

2 cans sodium-reduced chicken broth

1 can vegetarian split pea soup, or for homemade, add 1 onion and 16 ounces green or yellow split peas or red lentils

Optional Special Treat

1–3 bars Guylian Dark Chocolate, no sugar added

Remember, no eating between meals unless listed as a Smart Snack!

Recipes for the Jump Start Diet

All recipes are for 1 serving unless otherwise indicated.

Week 1, Saturday

Marinated Kidney Beans Ⓠ

Yield: 1½ cups (1 tablespoon = 1 serving)

1½ cups cooked kidney beans *or* 1
    15½-ounce can kidney beans, or
    1 package frozen edamame (soy
    beans), rinsed and drained
¼ cup low-calorie Italian dressing
½ teaspoon dried Italian herb
    blend, basil, or oregano crushed

1 tablespoon red wine, balsamic,
    or tarragon vinegar (optional)
1 tablespoon chopped red onion
    (optional)

1. Combine the beans with the dressing, herbs, and vinegar and onions
(if desired) and mix well.
2. Place in a covered dish and allow to marinate in the refrigerator.
These beans will keep for up to 2 weeks in the refrigerator, so that they
may be used in both Week 1 and Week 2.

Per serving: 0 mg cholesterol, 0.01 gm saturated fat, 0.3 gm total fat, 0.3 gm fiber,
17 mg sodium, 12 calories, 0 gm trans fat

RECIPE SYMBOLS

Ⓠ indicates recipe may be prepared in 30 minutes or less.

Ⓜ indicates recipe may be prepared in a microwave oven.

Week 1, Sunday

Light Tomato-Mushroom Sauce ⓠ

Yield: 3 cups sauce (1 serving = about 1 cup)

Use 1 cup sauce over 1½ cups cooked pasta and sprinkle with 1 teaspoon grated Parmesan cheese. Freeze the rest to use in Week 2 if desired.

Before freezing, remove ¼ cup sauce (without mushrooms) and refrigerate to use in Week 1 Wednesday's soup.

1 shallot or ¼ small onion, minced
1 clove garlic, minced
3 tablespoons dry white wine or
   defatted chicken broth
1 cup thinly sliced fresh
   mushrooms
8 fresh Italian plum tomatoes,
   diced, or 1 16-ounce can San
   Marzano tomatoes

¼ teaspoon Italian herb blend
Few grains crushed red pepper
   flakes
4 leaves fresh basil, chopped, or 1
   teaspoon dried basil, chopped

1. In a small nonstick saucepan, sauté the shallot or onion, garlic, and wine or broth for 2 minutes. Add the mushrooms and sauté 2 minutes.

2. Add the tomatoes, herb blend, pepper flakes, and basil, combine well, and cook 5 minutes.

NOTE: If you don't want to make your own sauce, substitute about 2 cups of salt-free canned marinara sauce, and add sautéed mushrooms and herbs as directed above.

Per serving: 0 mg cholesterol, 0.09 gm saturated fat, 0.8 gm total fat, 2.8 gm fiber, 26 mg sodium, 75 calories, 0 gm trans fat

Week 1, Monday

Antipasto Salad Ⓠ

6 ounces canned light tuna in oil
   or water, drained and flaked
   (save the other half can for
   Friday lunch)
1 cup mixed fresh broccoli,
   cauliflower, and carrots,
   steamed, or 1 cup frozen mixed
   broccoli, cauliflower, and
   carrots, thawed, drained on
   paper towels

1 tablespoon Marinated Kidney
   Beans (page 84)
2 tablespoons low-calorie oil-free
   Italian dressing
1 cup shredded romaine

1. Mix the tuna, vegetables, and beans with the dressing until combined. Chill at least 30 minutes.

2. Add the romaine and toss, and serve in pita bread.

Per serving: 21 mg cholesterol, 0.39 gm saturated fat, 1.7 gm total fat, 3.2 gm fiber, 409 mg sodium, 142 calories, 0 gm trans fat

Baked Stuffed Tomato Ⓠ

1 medium tomato
¼ cup chopped broccoli, steamed
   or microwaved until crisp
2 tablespoons soft breadcrumbs

½ teaspoon Italian herb blend
½ teaspoon grated Parmesan
   cheese

1. Cut tomato in half; scoop out pulp.

2. Combine pulp, broccoli, breadcrumbs, and herbs.

3. Fill each tomato half with the broccoli mixture and sprinkle with Parmesan cheese.

4. Bake in a preheated 400° oven for 5 minutes.

Per serving: 1 mg cholesterol, 0.29 gm saturated fat, 1 gm total fat, 1.6 gm fiber, 79 mg sodium, 65 calories, 0 gm trans fat

Vegetarian Lentil Soup

Yield: about 6 cups (½ cup = 1 serving)

This quick and easy soup may be prepared ahead and frozen in ½- or 1-cup portions.

1 onion, finely chopped
2 stalks celery with leaves, finely chopped
3 carrots, finely chopped
2 garlic cloves, minced
2 teaspoons extra-virgin olive oil
1 teaspoon dried thyme, crushed
1 teaspoon Italian herb blend, crushed
½ teaspoon crushed red pepper flakes

1 bay leaf
8 ounces lentils, washed and drained
5 cups hot water
1 cup crushed San Marzano plum tomatoes in puree
1 cup fresh sliced mushrooms
⅓ cup barley (optional)

1. Add the onion, celery, carrots, and garlic to the oil in a 6-quart saucepan. Sauté about 5 minutes.
2. Add the thyme, herb blend, pepper, bay leaf, and lentils and stir to combine.
3. Add the hot water, tomatoes, mushrooms and barley if desired, bring to a boil, reduce to simmer, and cook for 1 hour.
4. Taste and adjust seasonings.
5. Remove bay leaf before serving.

NOTE: If you find your time is limited, a good cannned vegetarian lentil soup may be substituted—but don't forget to check the sodium content; high sodium contributes to fluid retention while you are trying to lose pounds.

Per serving: 0 mg cholesterol, 0.12 gm saturated fat, 0.8 gm total fat, 2.2 gm fiber, 35 mg sodium, 66 calories, 0 gm trans fat

A healthy diet rich in fruit and vegetables, plus regular exercise, helps ward off heart disease.

Marinated Broccoli, Corn, Artichoke Heart, and Red Pepper Ⓠ

2 cups fresh chopped broccoli and
   corn, steamed until crisp, or 2
   cups frozen broccoli, corn, and
   red peppers, thawed, drained
   on paper towels
4 thin slices red pepper (unless
   frozen combination is used)

4 quarters canned artichoke
   hearts, rinsed and drained
2 tablespoons low-calorie oil-free
   Italian dressing
¼ teaspoon Dijon mustard

1. Combine the steamed vegetables with red peppers and artichoke hearts.
2. Add salad dressing and mustard and toss to combine.
3. Chill 15 minutes before serving.

Per serving: 0 mg cholesterol, 0.07 gm saturated fat, 0.5 gm total fat, 6.5 gm fiber, 330 mg sodium, 84 calories, 0 gm trans fat

Spicy Cold Tomato Soup Ⓠ

Yield: Serves 1 (¾ cup = 1 serving)

¼ cup nonfat plain yogurt
1 teaspoon lime juice
½ teaspoon curry powder
¼ teaspoon ground cumin
¼ teaspoon spicy salt-free
   vegetable seasoning
Freshly ground pepper
2 drops Tabasco

¼ cup crushed tomatoes in juice
   or puree, or reserved Light
   Tomato-Mushroom Sauce (do
   not add mushrooms) from
   Sunday (page 85)
¼ cup canned sodium-reduced V-8
   juice
Nonfat yogurt for garnish (optional)

1. Whisk the yogurt in a mixing bowl until smooth.
2. Add the remaining ingredients, blend thoroughly, and chill in freezer for 20 minutes.
3. Taste and adjust seasonings before serving.

To Serve: Spoon into a chilled cup or bowl and garnish with a dollop of nonfat yogurt if desired.

Per serving: 0 mg cholesterol, 0.03 gm saturated fat, 0.1 gm total fat, 0.2 gm fiber, 37 mg sodium, 16 calories, 0 gm trans fat

Seafood Salad Vinaigrette Ⓠ

This salad may be prepared without the dressing hours in advance and chilled until serving time.

2 cups mixed torn greens (romaine, red lettuce, spinach, or butter lettuce)
3 ounces precooked or canned bay shrimp, lobster, and/or crab, or 3½ ounces canned albacore tuna in water
½ cup sliced fresh mushrooms
4 quarters canned artichoke hearts, rinsed, drained, and sliced

¼ red pepper, sliced
1 carrot, sliced
½ cup diced cucumber
1 Italian plum tomato
1 slice red onion (optional)
2 tablespoons low-calorie oil-free Italian dressing, lemon juice, or balsamic vinegar

1. Place all ingredients except the dressing in a salad bowl and toss lightly.
2. Add dressing and toss lightly again before serving.

Variation: 4 tablespoons salsa may be substituted for the Italian dressing.

Per serving: 91 mg cholesterol, 0.29 gm saturated fat, 1.9 gm total fat, 5 gm fiber, 935 mg sodium, 200 calories, 0 gm trans fat

---

One tablespoon of sugar has the same number of calories as a three-ounce baked potato.

Week 1, Thursday

Quick Vegetable Lo Mein ⓠ

Serves: 1

As my life gets busier, I'm always looking for easier answers to my cooking that are still healthy. Frozen vegetables are often more nutritious than old or out-of-season produce from the market, and, of course, they are timesavers, so I use them in this recipe. However, if you prefer to use fresh produce, combine 2 ounces linguine or cappellini, cooked and drained, with 2 cups of a mixture of raw sliced asparagus, green beans, broccoli, carrots, water chestnuts, bean sprouts, green pepper, and/or bok choy that have been stir-fried and substitute the combination for the frozen pasta-vegetable mixture. Either way, this recipe fulfills all the nutritional requirements and is delicious—in fact, so delicious that you must watch your portions and stick to the recipe.

½ 16-ounce package frozen Pasta Salad Orientale (pasta, broccoli, Chinese pea pods, water chestnuts, and red bell peppers—save ½ in freezer for Week 2 Friday lunch)
1 cup frozen French-cut green beans and water chestnuts or fresh green beans cut into julienne strips

1 teaspoon cold-pressed canola oil
1 large clove garlic, minced, or ½ teaspoon chopped garlic
1 tablespoon sodium-reduced soy sauce
1 green onion, sliced

1. Place the frozen pasta salad and beans in a colander and defrost under cold running water for 1 to 2 minutes. Drain thoroughly.
2. Heat the oil in a nonstick skillet. Add the garlic and stir-fry for ½ minute.
3. Add the pasta and vegetable mixture and stir-fry for 2 minutes.
4. Add the soy sauce and stir-fry one minute.
5. Sprinkle with green onion and serve immediately.

Per serving: 0 mg cholesterol, 0.53 gm saturated fat, 5.2 gm total fat, 5.9 gm fiber, 512 mg sodium, 214 calories, 0 gm trans fat

Caesar Salad Ⓠ

1 egg white
2 tablespoons low-calorie oil-free
  Italian dressing
⅛ teaspoon minced garlic
½ teaspoon Worcestershire sauce
2 teaspoons fresh lemon juice

2 teaspoons grated Parmesan
  cheese
2 cups chilled romaine leaves
1 cup radicchio or shredded red
  cabbage

1. Place the egg white in a 1-cup glass measure and cook in microwave on high for 25 seconds (or cook whole egg in shell in boiling water for 2 minutes and use only white).

2. Add dressing, garlic, Worcestershire sauce, lemon juice, and 1 teaspoon cheese. Beat with a fork to blend.

3. Put the romaine and radicchio in a bowl, drizzle with dressing, and toss lightly to coat the greens. Sprinkle with 1 teaspoon cheese. Serve immediately.

Per serving: 1 mg cholesterol, 0.45 gm saturated fat, 0.8 gm total fat, 0.8 gm fiber, 378 mg sodium, 65 calories, 0 gm trans fat

Week 1, Friday

Tuna-Apple Salad Sandwich Ⓠ

3 ounces canned light tuna in
  water, drained and flaked
1 tablespoon nonfat plain yogurt
½ small unpeeled apple, washed
  and diced

1 slice whole wheat, rye, or pita
  bread
½ cup shredded romaine
2 chopped walnuts, optional

1. Combine the tuna, yogurt, apple, and walnuts, if using.

2. Spread on the bread, top with the shredded romaine, cut in half, and close sandwich.

Per serving: 19 mg cholesterol, 0.45 gm saturated fat, 2 gm total fat, 3.9 gm fiber, 301 mg sodium, 156 calories, 0 gm trans fat

Artichoke, Mushroom, and Pepper Salad with Yogurt Dressing Ⓠ

4 quarters canned artichoke
  hearts, halved
4 fresh mushrooms, sliced
2 tablespoons diced green pepper
2 tablespoons diced red pepper
2 tablespoons nonfat plain yogurt
1 tablespoon low-calorie oil-free
  Italian dressing
1 teaspoon Worcestershire sauce

⅛ teaspoon dried tarragon or ½
  teaspoon fresh tarragon
Drop of Tabasco
¼ teaspoon Dijon mustard
  Red leaf lettuce

1 red onion, slice, separated in
  rings, for garnish

1. Combine the artichoke hearts, mushrooms, and peppers in a bowl.

2. *To make the yogurt dressing*, mix the yogurt, Italian dressing, Worcestershire, tarragon, Tabasco, and mustard.

3. Add dressing to vegetables, mix well, and serve on lettuce garnished with red onion rings.

Per serving: 1 mg cholesterol, 0.11 gm saturated fat, 0.6 gm total fat, 1.2 gm fiber, 233 mg sodium, 66 calories, 0 gm trans fat

---

If you eat tortillas, try corn or whole wheat—flour tortillas have between 150 and 225 calories from fat, depending upon the brand.

Week 2, Saturday

Vegetarian Split Pea Soup

Yield: 14 to 15 cups (½ cup = 1 serving)

Make your own and freeze in 1-cup portions, or buy canned vegetarian split pea soup. (*Check the sodium content.*)

1 large onion, finely chopped
2 garlic cloves, minced
3 stalks celery with leaves, finely chopped
6 carrots, finely chopped
2 teaspoons extra-virgin olive oil or canola oil
1½ teaspoons dried thyme, crushed
2 teaspoons salt-free vegetable seasoning

½ teaspoon crushed red pepper flakes
2 bay leaves
16 ounces green and/or yellow split peas, washed and drained
2 quarts hot water
Freshly grated nutmeg (optional)
Freshly ground pepper (optional)

1. In a 4-quart saucepan, sauté the onion, garlic, celery, and carrots in oil for 5 minutes, stirring constantly.

2. Add the thyme, seasoning, and pepper flakes and sauté 5 minutes.

3. Add the bay leaves, split peas, and hot water, bring to a boil, reduce to simmer, and cook 2 hours.

4. Remove the bay leaves. (If you desire, the soup may be pureed at this point.)

5. Add freshly grated nutmeg and/or freshly ground pepper to taste if you like.

Per serving: 0 mg cholesterol, 0.08 gm saturated fat, 0.6 gm total fat, 1.3 gm fiber, 11 mg sodium, 65 calories, 0 gm trans fat

---

To kill germs in your kitchen sponges: wet and then microwave them at full power for two minutes.

Pronto Pasta Primavera Ⓠ

Serves: 2 (as an accompaniment or first course)

Today you have a hot, delicious, vegetarian pasta entrée—tomorrow it's a delicious, cold pasta salad!

3 ounces spaghettini or soba pasta
1 cup broccoli florets
1 5-ounce package fresh mixed chopped vegetables, available in the produce department
or 1 16-ounce package frozen mixed cauliflower, broccoli, and carrots

1 cup frozen edamame beans
3 tablespoons low-calorie oil-free Italian dressing, at room temperature
2 teaspoons extra-virgin olive oil, optional
2 teaspoons grated Reggiano Parmesan cheese, optional

1. Add pasta to boiling water. Bring to a second boil, and cook for 4 minutes.

2. Add all vegetables; bring to a boil, and cook for 3 minutes, or until pasta is al dente (firm to the bite).

3. Drain pasta and vegetables thoroughly, and return to pot.

4. Add salad dressing, and olive oil if desired. Toss lightly to blend.

To Serve: Mound hot pasta on a heated platter or in a bowl, and sprinkle with the Parmesan cheese, if desired. Serve immediately.

Variation: Save one-half of recipe to be served as Pasta Primavera salad the next day.

Per serving: 0.37 mg cholesterol, 0.06 gm saturated fat, 1.5 gm total fat, 2.49 gm fiber, 4.87 gm sugar, 260 calories, 49.92 gm carbohydrate, 0 gm trans fat

---

Remember, good nutrition depends on your total diet,
not a single food.

Week 2, Sunday

Tomato Bouillon Ⓠ

⅓ cup sodium-reduced vegetable
juice (V-8)
⅔ cup sodium-reduced chicken
broth (spoon off fat)

1–2 teaspoons lemon juice
¼ teaspoon Worcestershire sauce

1. Combine juice and broth; bring to a boil.
2. Season with lemon juice and Worcestershire sauce and serve.

Per serving: 0 mg cholesterol, 0.28 gm saturated fat, 1 gm total fat, 0.3 gm fiber,
183 mg sodium, 41 calories, 0 gm trans fat

Quesadilla Ⓠ

1 6-inch corn tortilla
3 tablespoons chopped tomato
1 green onion, sliced

1–2 tablespoons salsa
1 slice Galaxy Veggie slices

1. Heat the tortilla briefly in a nonstick skillet.
2. Sprinkle with the tomato, onion, and salsa and top with the veggie
slices. Heat in the nonstick skillet until the cheese is melted.
3. Fold in half and serve.

NOTE: *For men on the diet*: After adding cheese, top with another
tortilla and heat quesadilla on both sides. Cut in half before serving.

Per serving: 12 mg cholesterol, 2.28 gm saturated fat, 4.6 gm total fat, 1 gm fiber,
155 mg sodium, 133 calories, 0 gm trans fat

Week 2, Monday

Tuna or Salmon Niçoise Salad Ⓠ

3 cups torn salad greens
1 3½-ounce can tuna or salmon
   (or flaked fish left over from
   Sunday dinner)
1 tablespoon Marinated Kidney
   Beans (from Week 1, page 84)
½ cup raw broccoli and red
   peppers
2 cherry tomatoes, halved

1 tablespoon capers, rinsed
   (optional)
3 snow peas
Balsamic or red wine vinegar,
   lemon juice, or low-calorie oil-
   free Italian dressing

1 slice red onion for garnish
   (optional)

1. Place the greens in a bowl. Add the fish, beans, broccoli and peppers, tomatoes, capers, and snow peas.
2. Sprinkle with vinegar, toss lightly, and serve, garnished with the red onion slice if you like.

Per serving: 18 mg cholesterol, 0.38 gm saturated fat, 1.7 gm total fat, 4.3 gm fiber, 442 mg sodium, 123 calories, 0 gm trans fat

Week 2, Tuesday

Parsley and Tomato Salad with Basil Vinaigrette Ⓠ

This oftentimes overlooked salad green is not just a garnish—it is high in Vitamin A and flavor and low in calories. It is also a natural diuretic. If you substitute sun-dried tomatoes for cherry tomatoes, let them stand in salad dressing for at least 30 minutes before serving.

2 cups parsley sprigs (stems
   removed)
4 red or yellow cherry or
   grape tomatoes, halved, or 1
   tablespoon sun-dried tomatoes,
   sliced
¼ cup low-calorie Italian dressing

1–2 tablespoons lemon juice
8–10 fresh basil leaves
1 large clove garlic, minced
1 tablespoon grated Parmesan
   cheese
Freshly ground pepper

1. Wash and thoroughly dry the parsley. Toss with the tomatoes.

2. *To make the basil vinaigrette,* combine the Italian dressing, lemon juice, basil, garlic, cheese, and pepper in a blender or food processor mini-mixer and process until pureed.

3. Pour half of dressing° over parsley; toss to blend.

Per serving: 1 mg cholesterol, 0.17 gm saturated fat, 0.8 gm total fat, 1.9 gm fiber, 335 mg sodium, 84 calories, 0 gm trans fat

°Save half dressing to serve Friday on the eggplant and bell pepper salad.

Week 2, Wednesday

Seviche Salad ⓠ

4 ounces *defrosted* bay scallops (or sea scallops, quartered) or firm-fleshed fish (sea bass, halibut, or tuna) cut into 1-inch cubes
2 cups boiling water
Juice of ½ lemon or lime
Juice of ½ orange
2 tablespoons diced red onion
1 teaspoon olive oil
½ clove garlic, minced

1 tablespoon raspberry wine vinegar
4 strips red pepper
4 strips green pepper
4 quarters canned artichoke hearts
1 dash Tabasco
3 cherry tomatoes, quartered
3 tablespoons salsa

Butter lettuce and radicchio leaves

1. Place the scallops or fish in a strainer and pour the boiling water over them. Let stand 2 minutes.

2. In a bowl, sprinkle the juices over the fish. Combine with the remaining ingredients and toss lightly to blend.

3. Marinate 20 minutes at room temperature, stir, and chill, covered, in the refrigerator for at least 20 minutes.

To Serve: Line a soup bowl with butter lettuce and radicchio and spoon the seviche onto the greens.

Per serving: 37 mg cholesterol, 0.13 gm saturated fat, 1.1 gm total fat, 1 gm fiber, 201 mg sodium, 153 calories, 0 gm trans fat

Vegetarian Chop Suey
Salad Sandwich ⓠ

A total of 1½ cups of any raw vegetable mixture that you favor may be substituted for those listed here.

¼ cup chopped fresh broccoli
¼ cup chopped cucumber
¼ cup chopped carrots
¼ cup sliced radishes
¼ cup sliced red or green pepper
1 sliced green onion
¼ cup diced red pepper

3 cherry tomatoes, quartered
¼ cup nonfat plain yogurt or light
  sour cream
1 teaspoon dried dill or 1
  tablespoon chopped fresh dill
½ 6-inch whole wheat pita bread

1. Mix the vegetables with the yogurt and dill until well combined.
2. Stuff into the pita pocket and serve.

Per serving: 1 mg cholesterol, 0.19 gm saturated fat, 1.2 gm total fat, 4.4 gm fiber, 75 mg sodium, 132 calories, 0 gm trans fat

Week 2, Thursday

Curried Chicken Salad ⓠ

1 tablespoon nonfat plain yogurt
1 teaspoon frozen unsweetened
  apple juice concentrate or sweet
  pickle relish
¼ teaspoon curry powder
3 ounces diced chicken (from
  Tuesday dinner)

2 tablespoons chopped celery
2 tablespoons chopped red pepper
½ papaya, seeded and seasoned
  with ¼ lime, juiced

1. Combine the yogurt, apple juice concentrate or relish, and curry powder.
2. Add the chicken, celery, and red pepper; stir with a fork to blend.
3. Spoon into the papaya half and chill until serving time.

Per serving: 48 mg cholesterol, 0.67 gm saturated fat, 2.4 gm total fat, 1.6 gm fiber, 72 mg sodium, 166 calories, 0 gm trans fat

Maintaining a Healthful
Low-Cholesterol Lifestyle

Now that you have been on the diet plan for two weeks, the time has come to take a break and move on to the greater variety of the low-cholesterol lifestyle plan presented in the next chapters. (Of course, you may want to go back to the diet if your cholesterol and/or weight haven't reached the levels you want; stay on the menu maintenance plan for a week, then return to the diet. Remember, you should not be on the diet for more than two weeks at a time.)

The menus and recipes in the lifestyle plan will help you stay on track; by following them you can be sure of keeping your cholesterol consumption around 100 milligrams a day. You should still eat oat bran or oatmeal with 2 tablespoons of oat bran and cinnamon for breakfast five days a week and take psyllium daily. Be sure to include two oat bran muffins or a variation (pages 108–110) in your daily diet so that you will still get enough soluble fiber to maintain the right cholesterol levels.

The twentieth century was focused on improving the treatment of diseases. Now in the twenty-first century, physicians and patients are more focused on prevention—the prevention as well as the cure.

▼ 5 ▼

Menus and Recipes for Low-Cholesterol Meals: An Ongoing Lifestyle Plan

If your total cholesterol reading is under 200, you can't just sit back and rest on your laurels. As we have seen, to be assured of keeping a healthy cholesterol level, you must adopt a whole new approach to eating in which you limit your cholesterol, saturated fat, and trans fat in a conscientious and consistent way—"preventive nutrition," if you will.

The easy-to-prepare, flavor-filled meals that follow are meant to serve as a model for this new way of eating. They are high in complex carbohydrates and fiber and low in cholesterol and fat, and are based on the following recommended total daily calorie distribution:

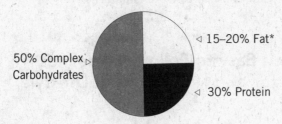

50% Complex ▷
Carbohydrates

◁ 15–20% Fat*

◁ 30% Protein

They allow you to eat varied and appealing meals and still limit your cholesterol to no more than 100 milligrams a day.

This new approach to eating will mean a change not only in your eating habits but also in your shopping and cooking habits—a whole new lifestyle. But it will be worth the effort. When you adopt this lifestyle plan, not only will you reduce your risk of heart disease, stroke, and

*No more than 7 percent of total calories from saturated fat.

even certain kinds of cancer (breast, colon, prostate, and pancreas), but you will find that after following it only a few weeks you'll feel terrific and have more energy.

How the Menus Work

The menus are organized by category: breakfast, lunch or supper (light meals), and dinner (main meals). You simply combine your choice of breakfast, lunch, and dinner menus to make up your daily meals, following the requirements in the guidelines. In the beginning you may find it easier to use the two-week diet plan as a base, substituting recipes from Chapters 5 to 7 as you choose.

No recipes are included for some of the dishes in the menus because they are basic recipes easily found in many cookbooks. It is important that these generic dishes be prepared with low-cholesterol and low-saturated-fat ingredients. On the other hand, many recipes are included in the book that are not called for in the menus. These are meant to be substituted in the menus as you choose. In addition, any of the recipes in my three previous books, *Deliciously Low*, *Deliciously Simple*, and *Deliciously Healthy Jewish Cooking*, can also be used. After you have followed the menus and recipes for a while, you will find it easy to create your own low-cholesterol menus and recipes.

Easy-to-Follow Guidelines
for a Low-Cholesterol Lifestyle

Daily Dos

1. *Limit all animal protein.* Do not eat more than a total of 4 ounces of cooked (5 ounces of raw) meat or fish a day (that's about the size of a deck of cards). This can be eaten at either lunch or dinner, but not both. Select lean meat; although it has as much cholesterol as fatty meat, it is a bit lower in saturated fat.

   TIP: One way to cut down on animal protein is to use it as an accent or seasoning in stir-fried dishes, casseroles, or salads of vegetables and/or grains. Often just a small amount (1 to 1½ ounces) is enough to make an otherwise vegetarian dish acceptable to the most ardent meat lover.

2. Keep in mind that only 15 to 20 percent of your total daily calories should come from fat and *no more* than 7 percent of your total daily calories should come from saturated fat, and 2 percent from trans fat.

3. Include some source of *soluble fiber*—plain oat bran cereal (⅓ cup dry cereal, cooked), 2 oat bran muffins, and three servings from any of the following: barley, dried peas, lentils, or beans, corn, peas, apples, pears, oranges, okra, or eggplant.

4. Include as sources of *insoluble fiber* at least two servings each of whole fresh fruits, vegetables, salads, and whole grains such as bulgur wheat, kamut, brown rice, whole grain breads (wheat, rye, pumpernickel), corn or whole wheat tortillas, or whole grain cereals.

5. *Before breakfast*, take 1 heaping teaspoon of psyllium in 8 ounces of water, and drink six additional glasses of water throughout the day. Current research indicates that this natural soluble fiber helps to lower total cholesterol as much as 10 percent.

Weekly Dos

1. *Serve fish 2 to 3 times a week.* Include some cold-water fatty fishes like salmon, herring, tuna, mackerel, or trout because these fish contain high levels of desirable omega-3 fatty acids.

2. *At least two to three days a week have all vegetarian or mostly vegetarian meals.*

TIP: This doesn't mean just rice and bean sprouts—how about a pasta dinner with a tomato or primavera sauce, a vegetable salad, whole grain bread, and fresh fruit for dessert?

3. Be alert when shopping; *read all labels carefully* and check the guidelines for healthful ingredients in Chapter 3.

4. Try to *include garlic and onions* in your recipes; they contain allicin, a chemical that may inhibit blood clotting. Like olive

oil, these are commonly used ingredients in Greek and Italian dishes, and may account for the lower incidence of cardiovascular disease among Mediterranean people.

Avoid

1. *Egg yolks* (one egg yolk contains 213 milligrams of cholesterol). Use egg whites instead.*

2. *All whole-milk dairy products.* Use nonfat (skim) or at most 1 percent fat products. Select cheeses that are made at least partially from nonfat milk, such as part-skim ricotta or part-skim mozzarella, or veggie soy cheese, and use them only very sparingly.

3. *Butter, stick margarine, lard, and chicken fat.* When choosing fats, select vegetable oils like canola, cold-pressed safflower oil, or sunflower, olive, corn, or walnut oil.

4. *Coconut and palm oils, hydrogenated or partially hydrogenated fats, or any foods that contain them or are fried in them.*

5. *Fried food.* Broil, bake, poach, steam, or grill instead, and use a nonstick frying pan or nonstick spray when cooking instead of butter or oil.

A Note on Sodium and Sugar

The average American is addicted to sodium. It is an acquired taste, and with all the emphasis on lowering the sodium in our diets, many people are gradually weaning themselves away from unnecessary sodium by not adding salt in cooking, not using salt shakers on cooked foods, and by judiciously reading product labels to determine the sodium content.

In my recipes I recommend using many sodium-reduced or low-sodium products and generally add no salt in cooking.

If you are hypertensive, have cardiac or kidney problems, or are just prone to fluid retention, keep your sodium consumption to a moderate amount (about 1600 milligrams per day).†

---

*The AHA currently allows three eggs per week! Try Eggland's Best.
†Do not use a salt substitute without your physician's approval!

Remember, too, that although we all know sugar has only "empty calories," excessive amounts may also raise triglyceride levels, which can contribute to cardiac disease. Here, again, I use limited amounts of sugar in all my recipes, if I use it at all.

RECIPE SYMBOLS

Ⓠ indicates recipe may be prepared in 30 minutes or less.

Ⓜ indicates recipe may be prepared in a microwave oven.

Breakfast and Brunch

You owe it to yourself to take a few minutes to enjoy a heart-healthy breakfast—one that's high in cholesterol-lowering soluble fiber. The two Basic Breakfasts in this section include high-fiber fruit (berries or orange) and oat bran cereal or muffins to give you the advantage you need to keep your cholesterol low. The other breakfast menus will give you some variety as well as the proper nutrition.

Because brunches can be deadly, I have suggested some ways you can be good to yourself without being denying. The average brunch as found in restaurants (and those served in homes, too) are often terribly high in fat, cholesterol, and calories. Consider eggs Benedict (599 milligrams of cholesterol, 10.7 grams of saturated fat, and about 1040 calories), cheese omelettes with fried potatoes (924 milligrams of cholesterol, 20.1 grams of saturated fat, and about 850 calories), corned beef hash with poached eggs (706 milligrams of cholesterol, 11.8 grams of saturated fat, and about 600 calories). Request some bacon, sausage, or ham on the side and you add on 200-plus calories and loads of sodium, to say nothing of more artery-clogging fat and cholesterol. This doesn't include the fat-laden muffins, croissants, pastries, or rolls with butter—never mind the dessert! It really adds up. To help avoid these problems, I have created some taste-tempting brunch menus and recipes for you, your family, and your friends.

Try to avoid breakfast buffets—they encourage overeating!

Recipes

Breakfasts (beginning on page 107)

Hot Oat Bran Cereal
Basic Oat Bran Muffins with 13 Variations
Oat Bran Quickie Breakfast Beverage
High-Fiber Granola
Triple Oat Porridge with Raisins
Buckwheat Blueberry Pancakes
Oatmeal Pancakes with Orange Slices
Whole Grain French Toast
Oat Bran Waffles

Brunches (beginning on page 118)

Scrambled Eggs with Zucchini, Red Onion, and Red Pepper
Vegetarian Frittata
No-Yolk Spinach and Mushroom Omelette
Assorted Vegetable Platter with Dill Sauce
Salmon Hash
Pasta and Vegetable Casserole
Cheese Bread Soufflé
Frittata Loaf
Breakfast Burritos

BASIC BREAKFAST I

Orange slices (with all the fiber)
♦ Hot Oat Bran Cereal or Oatmeal ♦
Nonfat Milk or Low-fat Soy Milk

Hot Oat Bran Cereal Ⓠ Ⓜ

Serves: 1

Oat bran cereal or oatmeal is the best low-cholesterol breakfast you can have. Because oat bran is high in soluble fiber it not only lowers your cholesterol level, but also helps you maintain the desired level once you have reached it.

1 cup cold water or nonfat milk or low-fat soy milk
⅓ cup oat bran
Nonfat milk or low-fat soy milk, served w/ cereal

½ teaspoon cinnamon *or* 1 teaspoon sugar-free apple butter (optional)

1. Place the cold water or milk and oat bran in a heavy saucepan; mix well.
2. Bring to a boil over high heat, stirring occasionally.
3. Reduce heat to low and cook 1 to 2 minutes or until desired consistency is reached.

To Serve: Serve with nonfat milk or low-fat soy milk. Sweeten with Splenda or sugar-free apple butter if you like and sprinkle with cinnamon.

To Microwave: Combine the cold water and cereal in a microwave-proof cereal bowl. Cook on high for 2 to 2½ minutes. Stir and serve.

Per serving: 0 mg cholesterol, 0 gm saturated fat, 2.8 gm total fat, 7.3 gm fiber, 3 mg sodium, 111 calories, 0 gm trans fat

BASIC BREAKFAST II

Orange Wedges
♦ Basic Oat Bran Muffins ♦
Nonfat Milk or Low-fat Soy Milk

Basic Oat Bran Muffins Ⓠ

with 13 variations

Yield: 12 muffins (1 muffin = 1 serving)

Because oat bran is high in soluble fiber that lowers cholesterol, you should eat two Oat Bran Muffins (or any of the variations) *each day* in addition to other foods high in soluble fiber. If you are really on the run, two Basic Oat Bran muffins may also be substituted for hot oat bran cereal at breakfast, giving you a total of four Oat Bran Muffins that day.

2½ cups oat bran*
½ cup whole grain pastry flour
1½-2 teaspoons ground cinnamon
1 tablespoon baking powder
3 tablespoons Splenda Brown Sugar Blend
2 extra-large egg whites and 1 Eggland's Best egg, slightly beaten
1¼ cups 1% fat milk, nonfat evaporated milk, or soy milk

⅔ cup sugar-free applesauce
1 tablespoon canola or cold-pressed safflower oil
2 teaspoons pure vanilla extract
½ cup dark raisins, chopped dates, chopped figs, dried tart red cherries, or chopped walnuts (optional)

1. Preheat the oven to 425° and coat muffin tins with nonstick cooking spray or line with paper baking cups.

2. Combine the dry ingredients in a mixing bowl and blend with a fork.

3. Beat the remaining liquid ingredients except fruit in a separate bowl with a fork.

4. Add the liquid ingredients to the dry and stir with a slotted spoon until flour disappears. (Optional dried fruit and/or nuts may be added now.)

5. Fill the muffin tins, place in the preheated oven and lower the temperature to 400°.

6. Bake 17 to 20 minutes or until lightly browned. Cool slightly before removing from tins.

Suggestion: Since I recommend that you eat two muffins a day, make a double recipe and freeze some for future use. These muffins will also keep fresh in the refrigerator for three to four days. I feel they taste a little better if they are heated briefly in a toaster oven or microwave before serving.

Per serving: 1 mg cholesterol, 0.15 gm saturated fat, 2.9 gm total fat, 4.7 gm fiber, 107 mg sodium, 126 calories, 0 gm trans fat

*Substitute 1 cup Old-Fashioned Oats for 1 cup oat bran and soak in milk for 10 minutes before proceeding with recipe.

VARIATIONS

For Banana Bran Muffins: Substitute two very ripe bananas (⅔ cup mashed) for the sugar-free applesauce and add 1 teaspoon banana extract.

For Spicy Apple Bran Muffins: Add 1 cored chopped organic apple with skin to the liquid ingredients, and 1½ teaspoons cinnamon, ½ teaspoon ground nutmeg, and 2 tablespoons chopped almonds or walnuts to the dry ingredients.

For Blueberry Bran Muffins: Add 1 cup frozen (not defrosted) or fresh blueberries after liquid and dry ingredients are combined.

For Banana-Blueberry Bran Muffins: Add 1 cup frozen or fresh blueberries to the Banana Bran Muffin mixture.

For Pear Bran Muffins: Substitute 1 small ripe pear, peeled and mashed, for the sugar-free applesauce in the recipe and add 1 cored chopped pear.

For Cranberry Bran Muffins: Add 1 cup chopped raw cranberries mixed with 1 tablespoon Splenda Sugar Blend to liquid ingredients.

For Boysenberry or Raspberry Bran Muffins: Add 1 cup berries after the liquid and dry ingredients are combined.

For Jelly Bran Muffins: Fill each muffin cup ⅓ full with batter, add 1 teaspoon sugar-free jam on top of the batter, and top with the remaining batter.

For Honey Double-Bran Muffins: Add 1 cup All-Bran to the dry ingredients and substitute ¼ cup honey or 3 tablespoons Splenda Brown Sugar Blend for 3 tablespoons sugar.

For Streusel-Topped Oatmeal Bran Muffins: Substitute 1 cup rolled oats for 1 cup oat bran and soak in the 1¼ cups milk called for in the recipe for 10 minutes. Combine with the other liquid ingredients before adding to dry ingredients. To make streusel topping: Chop ¼ cup rolled oats, ¼ cup walnuts, 2 tablespoons oat bran, and 2 tablespoons Splenda Brown Sugar Blend in the food processor and sprinkle on top of the muffins before baking.

For Pineapple Bran Muffins: Add 1 5½-ounce can crushed pineapple sweetened with its juice.

For Upside-Down Prune Bran Muffins: In the bottom of each muffin well, place 1 stewed, drained, and pitted prune. Cover with batter and bake as directed.

For Wild Rice Bran Muffins: Substitute 1 cup cold cooked wild rice for 1 cup of the oat bran and omit the sugar, cinnamon, and vanilla. Because these are not sweet, they are delicious served as a dinner roll.

One of my clients who chooses not to make and eat two Oat Bran Muffins each day compensates for this by doubling his serving of hot oat bran cereal in the morning. To some this may seem an enormous amount, but it works for him.

Oat Bran Quickie
Breakfast Beverage Ⓠ

Serves: 1

Perhaps you are one of those people who doesn't start your day by sitting down to breakfast, enjoying your food, and relaxing. Some hurried (or harried) people who don't have the time or inclination to bake muffins, cook hot cereal, or even serve cold cereals may be interested in preparing this breakfast beverage, which contains as much soluble fiber as a serving of Hot Oat Bran Cereal (page 107) or two Basic Oat Bran Muffins (page 108). It also makes a great afternoon pick-me-up.

1 cup *cold* nonfat milk, 1% milk,
   or low-fat soy milk
⅓ cup oat bran
½ large *ripe* banana, sliced
½ orange, peeled and cubed
¼ cup blackberries or blueberries,
   fresh or frozen

1 teaspoon pure vanilla or almond
   extract
Dash of ground cinnamon or
   freshly ground nutmeg
½ cup nonfat yogurt

1. Blend all the ingredients except the cinnamon or nutmeg together in a blender for 6 seconds or until foamy. (A stick blender may be used.)
2. Pour into a glass and sprinkle with cinnamon or nutmeg and serve immediately.

Variation: 1 small ripe sliced peach, nectarine, or pear, ½ orange, peeled and cubed, ½ cup fresh or frozen strawberries, or ¼ ripe sliced papaya or mango may be substituted for the banana. You may also add ½ cup nonfat yogurt to the basic recipe.

For Quick Breakfast in a Bowl: Serve 1½ cups cold Oat Bran Crunch (Kellogg's Heartwise), Quaker Oat Squares, or General Mills Cheerios or Kashi, high protein, sprinkled with 2 tablespoons of oat bran, ½ banana, sliced, ¼ cup blueberries, and 1 cup nonfat milk.

Per serving: 5 mg cholesterol, 0.45 gm saturated fat, 3.6 gm total fat, 10.4 gm fiber, 131 mg sodium, 294 calories, 0 gm trans fat

BASIC BREAKFAST III

Papaya with Fresh Lime
♦ High-Fiber Granola ♦
with Sliced Banana and Nonfat Milk

High-Fiber Granola

Yield: 4 cups (½ cup = 1 serving, 1 tablespoon = 1-snack)

Here's another quick breakfast that requires no cooking. Unlike most commercial granolas, which have coconut and/or coconut and palm oil added (high in *saturated fat*), this granola recipe is high in fiber, particularly soluble fiber, with *no added fat*.

2 cups rolled oats	**½ cup almonds, chopped**
1 cup 7-grain cereal	**2 tablespoons ground cinnamon**
½–⅔ cup pomegranate juice or	**1 teaspoon freshly ground nutmeg**
papaya juice, no sugar added	**½ cup dark seeded Manuka raisins**
1 red apple with skin, cored and	**or dried cranberries**
grated	**1 split vanilla bean**
2 cups Cheerios and 1 cup Kashi	

1. Place the oats and 7-grain cereal in a bowl; mix. Add pomegranate juice and apple; mix with a fork.
2. Add the dry cereal, cinnamon, and nutmeg. Mix thoroughly with a fork.
3. Place on a nonstick baking sheet (15½" × 10") and bake in a pre-heated 350° oven for 30 minutes or until lightly browned. Mix halfway through baking time.
4. Add the raisins; cool and store in a tightly sealed jar to which you have added a split vanilla bean for flavor.

To Serve: Serve as a cold cereal topped with nonfat milk or Light Silk Soymilk and sliced bananas. In winter you may decide to use warm milk instead of cold.

Variation: Use blueberries or sliced fresh peaches, strawberries, mango, or other fruit instead of banana.

NOTE: Any of the cold oat bran cereals recommended in Chapter 3, page 44, may be substituted for High-Fiber Granola.

Per serving: 1 mg cholesterol, 0.55 gm saturated fat, 2.2 gm total fat, 4.2 gm fiber, 112 mg sodium, 208 calories, 0 gm trans fat

Sliced Bananas and Blueberries
with Nonfat Yogurt
♦ Triple Oat Porridge with Raisins ♦

Triple Oat Porridge with Raisins Ⓠ

Servies: 4 (1 cup = 1 serving)

By starting to cook your cereal in cold water and milk you get a creamier consistency.

2½ cups cold water
½ cup nonfat milk or low-fat soy
  milk
1 cup rolled oats

½ cup oat bran
¼ cup steel-cut oats
¼ cup dark raisins

1. Put the cold water and milk into a saucepan. Add all the cereals and mix thoroughly.
2. Place over medium heat, stirring occasionally, until the mixture starts to boil. Reduce to a simmer, cover, and cook for 12 to 15 minutes, add raisins and cook 2 minutes.

To Serve: Serve hot with cold nonfat milk.

Per serving: 1 mg cholesterol, 0.34 gm saturated fat, 2.7 gm total fat, 4.8 gm fiber, 19 mg sodium, 177 calories, 0 gm trans fat

---

Because of the danger of salmonella, eggs should not be eaten when runny or undercooked.

Orange Wedges
♦ Buckwheat Blueberry Pancakes ♦
with
Veggie Sausage

Buckwheat Blueberry Pancakes Ⓠ

Yield: 12 3-inch pancakes (3 pancakes = 1 serving)

These light and luscious whole grain pancakes are well worth the time and effort it takes to beat the egg whites.

½ cup buckwheat flour
¼ cup unbleached white flour or
    whole wheat flour
¾ cup oat bran
2 teaspoons baking powder
2 tablespoons Splenda
1 extra-large egg, slightly beaten
1 cup nonfat plain yogurt
¼ cup soy milk

2 extra-large egg whites, beaten
    until stiff
1 cup fresh or frozen blueberries

¼ cup nonfat plain yogurt
    mixed with ½ teaspoon pure
    vanilla extract and 1 cup fresh
    blueberries, for garnish

1. Mix the flours, oat bran, baking powder, and Splenda in a bowl.
2. Blend 1 slightly beaten egg, yogurt, and milk.
3. Add the yogurt mixture to the flour mixture and blend with a fork.
4. Fold the stiffly beaten egg whites and the blueberries into the mixture.
5. Immediately cook on a hot nonstick griddle or skillet coated with nonstick spray, using ¼ cup batter for each pancake.

To Serve: Place the hot pancakes on warm plates and garnish with a dollop of yogurt and fresh blueberries.

NOTE: Leftover batter does not give fluffy pancakes because of beaten egg whites that are used.

Per serving: 18 mg cholesterol, 0.14 gm saturated fat, 2.1 gm total fat, 5.5 gm fiber, 261 mg sodium, 185 calories, 0 gm trans fat

Baked Apple with Nonfat Milk
♦ Oatmeal Pancakes with Orange Slices ♦
Sugar-free Boysenberry Syrup or Preserves

Oatmeal Pancakes with Orange Slices ⓠ

Yield: 15 3-inch pancakes (3 pancakes = 1 serving)

These pancakes are a low-cholesterol quadruple header—the 1%-fat buttermilk and egg whites (no yolks) keep cholesterol intake down, and the rolled oats and oat bran help to reduce serum cholesterol levels. Best of all, they taste delicious.

1 cup rolled oats
1¾ cups buttermilk, strained, or
   nonfat evaporated milk
1 tablespoon Splenda
¾ cup whole wheat flour
2 tablespoons oat bran
1 teaspoon baking powder

½ teaspoon baking soda
½ teaspoon cinnamon
2 extra-large egg whites, slightly
   beaten

1 orange, sliced, for garnish

1. Combine the rolled oats, buttermilk, and Splenda and let stand for 5 minutes.
2. Mix together the flour, oat bran, baking powder, baking soda, and cinnamon and stir into the oat mixture.
3. Add the egg whites, mix with a spoon, and let rest 10 minutes. If batter is too thick, thin with a little more buttermilk.
4. Cook on a hot nonstick griddle or skillet coated with butter-flavored nonstick spray, using ¼ cup batter for each pancake.

To Serve: Place the hot pancakes on warm plates, garnish each plate with an orange slice, and serve with boysenberry syrup or preserves.

NOTE: Leftover batter may be refrigerated and used the next day.

Per serving: 3 mg cholesterol, 0.7 gm saturated fat, 2.2 gm total fat, 1.9 gm fiber, 258 mg sodium, 188 calories, 0 gm trans fat

Cantaloupe Wedges
♦ Whole Grain Raisin French Toast ♦
with
Sugar-free Applesauce
Morning Star Farms veggie sausage patty, optional

Whole Grain French Toast ⓠ

Yield: 16 half pieces (4 halves = 1 serving)

In a restaurant, French toast usually means *egg bread*, dipped in an *egg batter* and *deep-fried in oil* (that usually contains palm or coconut oil that is highly saturated) or *fried in butter*. At home, instead of the usual bread, I use whole wheat bread (sometimes raisin bread), and the batter has no whole eggs, oil, or sugar added. I then grill the French toast in a nonstick pan sprayed with butter-flavored nonstick spray—with tasty results!

4 extra-large egg whites, or 1 carton Eggbeaters
1 cup low-fat soy milk, or fresh orange juice

2 teaspoons Splenda
2 teaspoons pure vanilla extract
8 slices whole grain raisin bread, sugar free

1. In a shallow pan, beat all ingredients except the bread with a fork.
2. Soak both sides of the bread in the mixture.
3. Heat a nonstick skillet coated with nonstick spray over medium-high heat; add four slices of the bread. Reduce to medium heat and brown both sides. Repeat this process.
4. Remove the toast to a heated serving dish and serve with applesauce.

Variation: Instead of applesauce, serve with fresh berries.

To Freeze for Future Use: Place single browned slice of toast in an airtight plastic bag and freeze.

Per serving: 4 mg cholesterol, 0.34 gm saturated fat, 1.6 gm total fat, 4.2 gm fiber, 344 mg sodium, 182 calories, 0 gm trans fat

Sliced Fresh Fruit with Yogurt
♦ Oat Bran Waffles ♦
with
Sugar-free Boysenberry Syrup
2 Slices Turkey Bacon, optional

Oat Bran Waffles Ⓠ

Yield: 8 waffles (½ waffle = 1 serving)

This is a delicious way to incorporate more oat bran (soluble fiber) into your daily diet as a breakfast or brunch dish or a snack. The oat bran gives the waffles a crispy texture. It is one of my family's favorites.

1¼ cups oat bran
¾ cup whole grain or Kamut flour
1½ teaspoons baking powder
½ teaspoon baking soda
3 extra-large egg whites, slightly beaten, or 2 extra-large egg whites plus ¼ cup egg substitute

2 cups nonfat evaporated milk
1½ tablespoons canola oil
2 tablespoons Splenda Brown Sugar Blend
1 teaspoon vanilla extract

1. Coat a waffle iron with butter-flavored nonstick spray and preheat.
2. Combine the oat bran, flour, baking powder, baking soda, and Splenda in a mixing bowl.
3. Combine the egg whites, milk, oil, vanilla and add to the dry ingredients. Blend thoroughly.
4. Pour about 1 cup waffle mixture into the preheated waffle iron, close lid, and bake according to manufacturer's directions, or until steaming stops. Repeat until all batter is used.

To Serve: Place on a warm plate and serve with sugar-free boysenberry syrup.

Variation: Instead of boysenberry syrup, serve with sugar-free pancake syrup and/or fresh fruit with yogurt.

To Freeze for Future Use: Place single browned, cooled waffle squares in an airtight plastic bag and freeze. To use, remove from plastic bag and heat in toaster oven or toaster.

Per serving: 3 mg cholesterol, 0.24 gm saturated fat, 4.1 gm total fat, 4.7 gm fiber, 212 mg sodium, 174 calories, 0 gm trans fat

Brunches

Prunes and Apricots, Stewed in Green Tea with Lime Wedges
♦ Scrambled Eggs with Zucchini, Red Onion, and Red Pepper ♦
Sliced Tomatoes, Green Onions, and Carrot Sticks
Toasted Whole Wheat or Rye Bagels with
Nonfat Whipped Cream Cheese with Chives

Scrambled Eggs with Zucchini, Red Onion, and Red Pepper Ⓠ

Serves: 8

If you are going to eat an egg occasionally, this dish is relatively low in cholesterol. One serving has less cholesterol than a 4-ounce serving of chicken! Of course, you can eliminate the yolks and cholesterol entirely by using only egg whites.

½ tablespoon extra-virgin olive oil
1 medium red onion, thinly sliced and separated
2 large garlic cloves, minced
2 small zucchini, thinly sliced
½ red pepper, seeded and cut into ¼-inch strips
2 whole eggs (Eggland)

8 extra-large egg whites, plus 1 tablespoon water
Freshly ground black pepper
2 teaspoons salt-free vegetable seasoning
1 tablespoon grated Parmesan cheese

1. Place the oil in a nonstick skillet; add the onion and garlic and stir-fry 5 minutes.
2. Add the zucchini and red pepper and sauté for 3 minutes.
3. Place the eggs and egg whites in a large bowl, add the pepper and vegetable seasoning, and beat thoroughly with a whisk until foamy. Add the sautéed vegetable mixture and cheese and blend well.
4. Heat a nonstick skillet and pour in the egg mixture. Cook over medium heat, lifting the cooked portion as it sets.
5. Serve immediately, while hot.

Per serving: 50 mg cholesterol, 0.77 gm saturated fat, 2.9 gm total fat, 0.4 gm fiber, 75 mg sodium, 63 calories, 0 gm trans fat

Assorted Melon Slices
♦ Vegetarian Frittata ♦
Broccoli Crown Vinaigrette (page 305)
Toasted High-Fiber Whole Grain Onion Bread (page 332)
Blueberry Bran Muffins (page 109) with Sugar-free Jam

Vegetarian Frittata Ⓠ

Serves: 6 (1 slice = 1 serving)

This frittata contains no egg yolks, yet its taste does not suffer. One serving of a traditional eight-egg frittata contains about 360 milligrams of cholesterol. One serving of *this* frittata has *no* cholesterol.

1 medium onion, peeled, halved, and diced
1 large clove garlic, chopped
2 teaspoons extra-virgin olive oil
4 mushrooms, cleaned and sliced
1 small zucchini, thinly sliced
½ cup red bell pepper, diced
6 slim asparagus spears, cut into 1-inch pieces (set tips aside for garnish)

1 8-ounce carton egg substitute
2 extra-large egg whites
1 Italian plum tomato, diced
¼ teaspoon white pepper
4 teaspoons thinly shredded Parmesan cheese

Cherry tomatoes and asparagus tips, for garnish

1. Sauté the onions and garlic with oil in a nonstick skillet for about 5 minutes or until wilted and *lightly* browned.
2. Add the mushrooms, zucchini, red pepper, and asparagus and sauté 3 minutes.
3. Beat the egg substitute and egg whites with a whisk or fork until well blended. Add the tomato, white pepper, 2 teaspoons of the cheese, and the sautéed vegetables. Blend well.
4. Pour the egg mixture into a hot nonstick skillet that has been coated with nonstick spray and arrange the asparagus tips in spokelike fashion on top.
5. Cook over medium heat until bottom is lightly browned.
6. Sprinkle with the remaining 2 teaspoons cheese and place under a preheated broiler until the top is golden brown and the mixture is set.
7. Loosen the bottom and slide onto a warm serving plate.

To Serve: Cut into six pie-shaped pieces and surround with cherry tomatoes.

Per serving: 0 mg cholesterol, 0.52 gm saturated fat, 3.1 gm total fat, 0.8 gm fiber, 142 mg sodium, 96 calories, 0 gm trans fat

Assorted Melon Chunks with Grapes
♦ No-Yolk Spinach and Mushroom Omelette ♦
Wild Rice Bran Muffins (page 110)

No-Yolk Spinach and Mushroom Omelette Ⓠ

Serves: 1

In this omelette, I combine egg substitute with egg whites. The egg whites give it a much better flavor than egg substitute alone.

3 mushrooms, cleaned and sliced
1 clove garlic, minced
1 teaspoon extra-virgin olive oil
2 cups fresh spinach leaves, washed and drained, stems removed
1 teaspoon lemon juice

½ cup egg substitute, or 3 extra-large egg whites
2 extra-large egg whites
⅛ teaspoon white pepper
⅛ teaspoon salt, optional

1 green onion, sliced, for garnish

1. Sauté the mushrooms and garlic in olive oil in an 8-inch nonstick skillet for 2 to 3 minutes. Add the spinach and lemon juice and sauté until the spinach is wilted. Remove mixture from pan and keep warm.
2. Beat the egg substitute, egg whites, and pepper with a fork until foamy.
3. Add egg mixture to a heated nonstick skillet that has been coated with butter-flavored nonstick spray.
4. When the egg mixture becomes firm around the edges, lift and push the solid portion toward the center of the pan, allowing the uncooked portion to flow to the edge of the pan and set.
5. When slightly brown on the bottom, turn the egg over to just dry.

6. Flip the egg onto a warm plate, place the drained spinach and mushroom mixture on one half, and fold over the other half.

To Serve: Sprinkle with green onion and serve immediately.

Per serving: 1 mg cholesterol, 1.53 gm saturated fat, 9.1 gm total fat, 4.9 gm fiber, 429 mg sodium, 226 calories, 0 gm trans fat

Mixed Fresh Berries with Banana Slices
Poached Salmon with Lemon Wedge
♦ Assorted Vegetable Platter with Dill Sauce ♦
Whole Wheat or Rye Bagels with Nonfat Whipped Cream Cheese
Assorted Oat Bran Muffins (page 108) with Sugar-free Jam

Assorted Vegetable Platter with Dill Sauce ⓠ

Serves: 4

For a change, it's nice to have your serving of fish for brunch. Of course, this means your food choices for the remaining meals that day should exclude any animal protein: Select from soups, salads, vegetables, whole grains, or pastas in the Mix and Match section or a vegetarian dish from this section.

12 fresh or frozen asparagus
  spears, steamed or roasted
8 radishes
1 10-ounce package frozen baby
  corn, steamed, or 1 16-ounce
  can baby corn, drained
4 green onions
12 grape tomatoes
1 red onion, very thinly sliced
1 bunch Belgian endive

Dill Sauce:

1 cup nonfat plain Greek yogurt
1 small Kirby cucumber, finely
  chopped
1 teaspoon dried fines herbes
1 teaspoon red wine vinegar
⅛ teaspoon white pepper
2 tablespoons chopped fresh dill,
  or 2 teaspoons dried dill and
  2 tablespoons chopped fresh
  parsley

3 sprigs fresh dill for garnish

1. Place bundles of asparagus in spokelike fashion in center of 12- to 14-inch platter. Leave room in the center for a bowl of sauce.

2. Fill spaces between spokes with radishes, corn, and green onions.

3. Arrange the tomatoes, onions, and endive around perimeter of the platter.

4. *To make the dill sauce:* Process all the remaining ingredients but the dill sprigs in a food processor or blender.

5. Pour the sauce into a footed bowl, garnish with sprigs of fresh dill, and place the bowl in the center of the platter.

Per serving: 10 mg cholesterol, 1.61 gm saturated fat, 3 gm total fat, 3.5 gm fiber, 77 mg sodium, 154 calories, 0 gm trans fat

Sliced Fresh Pineapple with Blueberries
♦ Salmon Hash ♦
Sliced Tomato   Steamed Broccoli
Assorted Pumpernickel, Rye, or Whole Wheat Bagel
with Nonfat Whipped Cream Cheese

Salmon Hash

Serves: 4 to 6

This delicious dish will allow you to reap the health benefits of omega-3 fatty acids in the salmon.

1 small onion, chopped

1 small green pepper, seeded and chopped

1 small red pepper, seeded and chopped, or 2 ounces canned chopped pimiento, drained

2 teaspoons canola or cold-pressed safflower oil

4 cups diced cooked potato or leftover baked potato

Freshly ground pepper

8 ounces poached fresh salmon, drained (save liquid) and flaked, or 1 7½-ounce can red salmon, drained (save juice), skin and bones removed, and flaked

1 tablespoon fresh lemon juice

⅔ cup defatted organic vegetable broth combined with drained salmon liquid to equal 1 cup

2 teaspoons grated Parmesan cheese mixed with ½ cup dry bread crumbs

Chopped fresh dill or parsley for garnish

1. Sauté the onion and peppers in oil in a nonstick skillet until limp.

2. Add the potatoes, sprinkle with pepper, and heat briefly.

3. Sprinkle the flaked salmon with lemon juice, add to the potato mixture with the salmon juice and broth, and mix lightly with a fork.

4. Coat a 10-inch glass pie plate with olive oil–flavored nonstick spray and heat in 400° oven for 3 minutes.

5. Spoon the salmon mixture into the heated pie plate. Sprinkle with the bread-crumb mixture and bake in the upper third of a preheated 400° oven for 20 to 25 minutes or until browned.

6. Sprinkle with fresh dill before serving.

Variation: Poach 4 extra-large egg whites or 4 Eggland's Best eggs and place them on top of the hash before sprinkling with dill.

Per serving: 31 mg cholesterol, 0.96 gm saturated fat, 5.6 gm total fat,1.2 gm fiber, 156 mg sodium, 295 calories, 0 gm trans fat

---

The American Heart Association recommends eating at least 2 to 3 fish meals a week—broiled, not fried— for heart protection.

Melon Wedges with Fresh Strawberries
♦ Pasta and Vegetable Casserole ♦
Four-Leaf Salad with Black-Eyed Peas
Whole Grain Toast

Pasta and Vegetable Casserole

Serves: 8

1 shallot, minced
2 large cloves garlic, minced
½ red pepper, seeded and diced
½ green pepper, seeded and diced
2 small zucchini, thinly sliced
1 tablespoon extra-virgin olive oil
½ pound fresh mushrooms, cleaned and sliced
½ pound eggplant, diced
2 crookneck squash, diced
½ cup sliced okra
5 extra-large egg whites, lightly beaten

1 cup 1%-fat cottage cheese, blended in food processor until smooth
2 cups low-fat soy milk
Freshly ground pepper
2 teaspoons Italian herb blend, crushed
8 ounces whole wheat or spelt linguine, cooked al dente°
1 tablespoon grated Parmesan cheese

2 Italian plum tomatoes, diced, and 2 green onions, sliced, for garnish

1. Sauté the shallot, garlic, peppers, and zucchini slices in oil in a non-stick skillet for 2 to 3 minutes. Remove zucchini slices.

2. Add the mushrooms and sauté 3 minutes. Add the eggplant, diced crookneck squash and okra and sauté 3 minutes.

3. Combine the egg whites, cottage cheese, milk, pepper, and herb seasoning. Blend until smooth.

4. Add the sauce and the cooked pasta to the vegetable mixture. Blend thoroughly.

5. Spoon the mixture into a 3-quart rectangular casserole coated with nonstick spray. Arrange a line of zucchini slices down the center of the casserole and sprinkle with Parmesan cheese. Bake in a preheated 350° oven for 35 to 40 minutes.

To Serve: Sprinkle with tomatoes and green onions as garnish.

Per serving: 3 mg cholesterol, 0.65 gm saturated fat, 3.9 gm total fat, 3.6 gm fiber, 113 mg sodium, 220 calories, 0 gm trans fat

°Whole wheat linguine must be slightly undercooked because it will continue cooking in the casserole when baking in the oven.

♦ Cheese Bread Soufflé ♦
Vegetarian Sausage
Marinated Three-Bean Salad
Poached Pears with Fresh Strawberry Sauce (page 318)

Cheese Bread Soufflé

Serves: 6

6 slices day-old whole wheat bread
4 leeks, white part only, split, washed, and sliced
2 teaspoons extra-virgin olive oil
5 extra-large egg whites
2 cups 1% milk or soy milk
2 teaspoons Worcestershire sauce
¼ teaspoon ground white pepper
2 teaspoons salt-free vegetable seasoning
1 teaspoon dried thyme, crushed, or 1 tablespoon fresh thyme, chopped
½ teaspoon garlic powder
3 ounces sliced tofu cheese
1 cup 1%-fat cottage cheese, blended in food processor until smooth
1 tablespoon Parmesan cheese (optional)

1. Cut the bread into 1-inch cubes and place in a 2-quart rectangular baking dish sprayed with butter-flavored nonstick spray.
2. In a nonstick skillet, sauté the leeks 3 to 5 minutes or until wilted in olive oil.
3. Beat the egg whites with a whisk until foamy. Add the milk, Worcestershire sauce, pepper, thyme, and garlic powder and combine.
4. Add the cheeses and leeks to the egg white mixture; blend well with a fork.
5. Pour the mixture over the bread and let stand 30 minutes or overnight. If desired, sprinkle with Parmesan cheese.
6. Bake in a preheated 325° oven for 25 to 30 minutes.

Variation: Slice 3 vegetarian sausages and brown slightly. Add with cheese and leeks to egg whites mixture.

Per serving: 16 mg cholesterol, 2.4 gm saturated fat, 5.1 gm total fat, 2.5 gm fiber, 300 mg sodium, 195 calories, 0 gm trans fat

♦ Frittata Loaf ♦
Mixed Greens Salad
with Balsamic Lite Vinaigrette
Assorted Sliced Fruits

Frittata Loaf ⓠ

Serves: 8

A meal in one for lunch, brunch, or supper.

1 10-inch round loaf whole wheat,
  pumpernickel, or rye bread
3 tablespoons Dijon mustard
3 large ripe tomatoes, sliced to
  ½-inch
3 slices red onion, ¼-inch (optional)
1 roasted red pepper, peeled and
  sliced
2 whole eggs and 7 egg whites,
  beaten

2 tablespoons Parmesan cheese
½ tablespoon olive oil
2 cloves garlic, minced
3 green onions, sliced
2 small zucchini, sliced
1 cup sliced fresh mushrooms
3 tablespoons chopped fresh basil
1 cup fresh bean sprouts

1. Halve the loaf of bread and remove the soft center, leaving ½-inch-thick shell.

2. Spread mustard or reduced-fat mayonnaise on bottom surface of bread, arrange tomato, red onion, and pepper slices on top of bread. Reassemble and wrap in foil.

3. Sauté green onion, garlic, zucchini, and mushrooms in oil, in 10-inch nonstick skillet, for several minutes. Add bean sprouts and basil.

4. Beat eggs with 1 tablespoon Parmesan cheese.

5. Add sautéed vegetables to beaten eggs and blend.

6. Pour mixture into heated skillet coated with nonstick olive-oil spray and cook until nearly firm.

7. Sprinkle with 1 tablespoon cheese and place under broiler until top is lightly browned.

8. Slide frittata onto bread. Set top half of bread in place, rewrap in foil, and keep warm until serving time.

9. Reheat in 300° oven until warm, place on platter and cut into pie-shaped pieces to serve.

Per serving: 53.98 mg cholesterol, 0.78 gm saturated fat, 4.02 gm total fat, 9.11 gm fiber, 349.15 calories, 62.43 gm carbohydrate, 5.79 gm sugar, 0 gm trans fat

Papaya and Mango Slices with Fresh Raspberries
♦ Breakfast Burritos ♦
Café con Leche

Breakfast Burritos Ⓠ

Yield: 2 burritos (1 burrito = 1 serving)

Instead of huevos rancheros for breakfast or brunch, how about a breakfast burrito? Its beans are high in cholesterol-lowering soluble fiber and it contains *no* saturated fat or cholesterol.

2 corn or whole wheat tortillas
⅔ cup canned *vegetarian* fat-free refried beans, or cooked pinto and/or red beans (page 131) mashed with 1 teaspoon canola oil
1 tablespoon chopped red onion
¼ cup chopped fresh Italian plum tomatoes

2 slices Galaxy tofu cheese, diced (optional)
¼ cup Fresh Salsa (page 185) or canned Newman's Own salsa

2 tablespoons plain nonfat yogurt and 1 tablespoon chopped fresh cilantro, for garnish

1. Microwave the tortillas between two sheets of slightly dampened white paper towels on high for about 15 seconds.
2. Mix the beans with the onion and tomatoes. Divide the mixture between the two tortillas. Sprinkle with cheese.
3. Fold each tortilla to enclose filling. Place on a microwave-safe serving dish and spoon salsa over each burrito.
4. Microwave on high for about 15 seconds.

To Serve: Top each burrito with yogurt and sprinkle with chopped cilantro.

Per serving: 0 mg cholesterol, 0.33 gm saturated fat, 3.8 gm total fat, 2.9 gm fiber, 69 mg sodium, 187 calories, 0 gm trans fat

One of my clients chose this for a vegetarian dinner. He started with a salad, then had burritos with fresh broccoli and steamed brown rice, and fruit for dessert. By the way, he lowered his cholesterol from 239 to 166 in just six weeks—a 30 percent reduction!

Lunch or Supper

The menus for lunch and supper can be used interchangeably since both are meals that require less preparation time than the main meal and tend to be rather simple—generally some combination of soup, salad, sandwich, casserole, or stir-fry.

Remember, if you choose to eat animal protein for lunch or supper, select a pasta dish or vegetarian entrée for your main meal—or at the very most, a dish that uses only a minimal amount of fish, poultry, or meat—an Oriental stir-fry recipe, with cubed tofu for example, or a casserole in which animal protein is used just as a flavoring ingredient.

I have included basic directions for preparing dried peas, beans, lentils, and grains since they are frequently used in many of the dishes.

RECIPES

Some Basics (beginning on page 129)

Chicken Broth in the Microwave
Basic Directions for Preparing Dried Peas, Beans, and Lentils
Basic Directions for Preparing Grains

Soups (beginning on page 134)

Old-Fashioned Vegetarian Bean Soup
Hearty Eight-Bean Soup
Daal (Indian Yellow Split Pea Soup)
Bean Curd and Spinach Soup
Last-Minute Soup
Hot Cabbage Borscht

Sandwiches (beginning on page 140)

Tuna Melt
Open-Faced Eggplant and Cheese Sandwiches
Stuffed French Toast
Salmon Burgers

Healthy Burgers
Spicy Pita Rolls
Pesto, Cheese, and Tomato Sandwich
Chopped Vegetable Spread

Salads (beginning on page 148)

Tostada
Pasta and Vegetable Salad with Fresh Salsa
Turkey Chef's Salad with Green Goddess Dressing (2 recipes)
Pasta Salad with Seafood
Warm New Potato and Green Bean Salad
Layered Luncheon Salad
Marinated Mixed Vegetable Salad
Fresh Vegetable Salad with Japanese Noodles
Italian Bean and Tuna Salad

Casseroles and One-Dish Meals (beginning on page 158)

Pastel de Calabacitas (Zucchini Pie) with Salsa
Skillet Supper
Spinach Frittata
Chili Beans
Black Bean Chili

Some Basics

Making Chicken Broth

Chicken broth is essential for low-cholesterol cooking. Not only is it the basis for many soups and sauces, but it is an essential cooking liquid in a great variety of dishes, can be used instead of fat in sautéeing and stir-frying, and is also used as a seasoning.

In the recipes in this book, when I call for chicken broth, I mean either defatted, sodium-reduced homemade broth or defatted canned broth. Canned sodium-reduced chicken broth is more costly than the regular. I would like to think that this is because the food processor has to use better quality ingredients to develop flavor in salt-free broth than in salted. To defat canned broth, chill first and then spoon the globules off the top.

Making your own broth is really not a chore, especially if you prepare it in a microwave oven. You can make it with chicken parts, and freeze the meat for future sandwiches, salads, or casserole dishes. Or you can buy chicken wings, necks, and backs to use as the basis of your stock. Collect leftover bones and scraps in your freezer and add them to the stockpot as well.

It is extremely important to defat your homemade broth before using or storing. The easiest way is to chill the broth in the refrigerator or freezer: the fat will rise to the top and solidify and then can easily be removed with a spoon. If you need to use the broth right away, you can either pour the fat off with a special pitcher called a "gravy strain" or pour the broth through a large paper coffee filter.

The basic recipe for microwave (with instructions for stove top preparation) appears below.

Chicken Broth in the Microwave Ⓜ

Yield: about 8 cups (1 cup = 1 serving)

3-pound chicken (remove giblets), cut into 8 pieces, fat removed, or 3 pounds halved chicken breasts
1 medium onion, coarsely chopped
3 stalks celery with leaves, coarsely chopped
3 carrots, coarsely chopped
1 whole leek, washed and sliced

1 parsnip, quartered
Bouquet garni (Italian parsley, bay leaf, fresh dill, peppercorns, and thyme)
1 cup cold water
7 additional cups cold water
Kosher salt (optional)°
White pepper to taste

1. Place the first eight ingredients in a large 5-quart microwave casserole, cover, and cook on high for 5 minutes.

2. Stir, add the 7 cups cold water, cover, and continue cooking on high for 40 minutes. Stir once during cooking.

3. Remove chicken, cool slightly; skin, bone, and refrigerate or freeze the meat for future use.

4. Strain, chill, and defat the broth. It can be stored in the refrigerator for several days (no more than 3), or frozen for future use.

Variation: To make Chicken in the Pot, skin the chicken but leave the bones in. Return the chicken and vegetables to the strained and defatted broth and add a bit of salt* and white pepper and cooked brown rice.

To Freeze Broth: Divide it among several small airtight containers (1 cup is a useful size), leaving an inch of head space for expansion, and cover tightly.

On the Stove: Place chicken and 8 cups cold water in a 5-quart saucepan. Bring to a boil; remove scum. Add remaining ingredients and simmer for 2 hours, partially covered. Proceed as in steps 3 and 4 above.

Per serving: 0 mg cholesterol, 0 gm saturated fat, 0 gm total fat, 0 gm fiber, 5 mg sodium, 34 calories, 0 gm trans fat

*Remember, each teaspoon of salt contains about 2,000 milligrams of sodium.

Basic Directions for Preparing Dried Peas, Beans, and Lentils

Rich in protein, iron, complex carbohydrates, soluble fiber, and other nutrients, dried beans were one of the earliest foods to be cultivated. You can cut way down on the preparation time if you use a microwave.

In the Microwave

To Soak:

1. Place 1 to 2 cups beans in 2-quart casserole with 2 cups water.
2. Cover tightly with microwave plastic wrap and cook on high for 15 minutes. Remove from oven.
3. Let stand 5 minutes, uncover, and add 2 cups *hot* water.
4. Re-cover and let stand 1 hour. Drain.

To Cook:

1. Place presoaked beans in a microwave casserole.
2. Add 4 cups water, cover tightly with 2 sheets microwave plastic wrap, and microwave on high for about 35 minutes.
3. Let stand 20 minutes before using.

NOTE: Navy beans and white beans require 40 minutes of cooking time and 30 minutes of standing time.

On the Stove:

To Soak:

1. Rinse beans in cold water thoroughly and drain. (Small lima beans, lentils, or split peas do not require soaking before cooking.)
2. Bring about 2½ quarts water to a boil in a 5-quart casserole or saucepan, add the beans, and bring to a boil. Remove from heat, cover, and let stand 1 hour.
3. Pour off the soaking water and drain.°

To Cook:

1. Return the beans to the soaking pan and cover with water two to three times their volume.
2. Bring to a boil; reduce to a slow simmer, and cook until just tender, referring to the chart below for cooking time.

NOTE: Cool, drain, and freeze those beans not to be used in a few days in airtight plastic bags.

°It seems that flatulence is less of a problem if soaking water is not used to cook beans.

COOKING TIMES FOR DRIED PEAS, BEANS, AND LENTILS°

1 LB. DRIED BEANS	COOKING TIME AFTER SOAKING
Soybeans	3 to 3½ hours
Chickpeas (garbanzo beans)	2 to 3 hours
Black beans or turtle beans	1½ to 2 hours
Kidney or pinto beans	1½ to 2 hours
Black-eyed peas	1½ hours
Northern beans or navy beans	1½ hours
Small lima beans (do not soak)	45 minutes to 1½ hours
Split peas or lentils (do not soak)	45 minutes

°1⅓ cups uncooked dried beans, or 8 ounces = about 3 cups cooked beans.

Basic Directions for Preparing Grains

Cereal grains today comprise the principal source of food for most of the world's people. Rice is the main food for half of the world's population. Grains are easily digested and rich in complex carbohydrates, B-complex vitamins, and iron. They are low in fat and of course contain no cholesterol.

1. Rinse the uncooked grain in cold water; drain.
2. Refer to the chart below for the amount of cooking water needed. Bring the water to a boil in a saucepan over medium-high heat.
3. Add the grain and stir. Return to a boil, reduce heat to low, cover, and cook according to the time on the chart.
4. Fluff with a fork and serve or use in your favorite recipe. (If grain is not soft enough, add a small amount of hot water and cook a little longer. If liquid remains and grain is tender, remove lid and continue cooking until liquid evaporates.)

COOKING TIMES AND MEASURES FOR GRAINS*

GRAIN	NUMBER OF SERVINGS	UNCOOKED AMOUNT	AMOUNT OF WATER	COOKING TIME	COOKED AMOUNT
Barley	4	½ cup (4 oz.)	3 cups	50–60 minutes	2 cups
Buckwheat	4	⅔ cup (4 oz.)	1⅓ cups	8–10 minutes	2 cups
Bulgur	4	¾ cup (4 oz.)	1½ cups	15–20 minutes	2 cups
Brown rice (quick cooking— cooks in 15 minutes)	4	⅔ cup (4 oz.)	1⅔ cups	50 minutes	2 cups
Converted rice	4	⅔ cup (4 oz.)	1⅔ cups	20 minutes	2 cups
Quinoa†	5	1 cup (6 oz.)	2 cups	10–15 minutes	2½ cups

*These weights and measures are approximate.
†A milletlike seed, with twice the protein of rice.

Soups

♦ Old-Fashioned Bean Soup ♦
Corn Bread
Apple and Pear Waldorf Salad

Old-Fashioned Vegetarian Bean Soup

Yield: about 30 cups (1¼ cups = 1 serving)

This hearty soup is newly recognized for its cholesterol-lowering qualities. Half a cup of cooked navy beans contains about 3.8 grams of soluble fiber. This soup freezes beautifully and tastes even better the next day.

1 pound navy beans, washed
1 large onion, peeled and quartered
5 quarts cold water°
2 whole carrots, sliced in 1-inch pieces
3 stalks celery with leaves, sliced in 1-inch pieces
1 leek, split, sliced, and washed

Bouquet garni†
1 cup chopped onion
1 tablespoon extra-virgin olive oil
½ cup unbleached white flour
1 16-ounce can diced San Marzano tomatoes with juice
1 16-ounce package frozen mixed vegetables (carrots, corn, beans, and peas)

1. Cover the beans with cold water, bring to a boil, cover, and let stand 1 to 2 hours off heat (or microwave on high for about 10 minutes and let stand). Drain.

2. Place quartered onion on a shallow baking pan and brown about 15 minutes in the upper third of a preheated 450° oven.

3. Cover the beans with 5 quarts cold water. Add onions, and the carrots, celery, leek, and bouquet garni. Bring to a boil and simmer 1½ hours or until beans are tender.

4. In a nonstick skillet, sauté 1 cup chopped onion in 1 tablespoon extra-virgin olive oil until barely colored.

5. Add the flour and brown lightly. Stir the flour mixture into the soup and cook 30 minutes.

6. Add the tomatoes and frozen vegetables and cook 15 minutes more. Taste and adjust seasonings. Like most soups, it tastes even better the next day!

Per serving: 0 mg cholesterol, 0.17 gm saturated fat, 1 gm total fat, 2.8 gm fiber, 49 mg sodium, 99 calories, 0 gm trans fat

°32 ounces of organic vegetable broth may be substituted for 1 quart water.
†*Bouquet garni:* Fresh Italian parsley, thyme, bay leaf, and red pepper flakes tied in cheese-cloth or tea caddy.

◆ Hearty Eight-Bean Soup ◆
Mixed Green and Red Cabbage Salad
Sourdough Rolls
Seasonal Fresh Fruit

Hearty Eight-Bean Soup

Yield: 16 cups (1½ cups = 1 serving as an entrée)

This soup is a meal in itself; all these beans and legumes are high in soluble fiber, which helps to lower cholesterol. Since the recipe makes a lot, freeze some for future use. Don't be concerned about having to buy all these different beans, for they can be stored dry or prepared and frozen for use in casseroles, salads, and other soups.

⅓ cup each dried lima beans, black beans, white Northern beans, kidney beans, and black-eyed peas
½ cup each lentils, barley, yellow split peas, and green split peas
4 quarts cold water
1 large onion, chopped
3 large carrots, chopped

3 stalks celery with leaves, chopped
1 bay leaf
Few grains crushed red pepper
1 28-ounce can San Marzano tomatoes with juice, chopped
2 tablespoons fresh basil, chopped, or 1½ teaspoons dried basil, crushed

1. Wash all the dried beans and lentils thoroughly. Place in a large bowl, cover with cold water, and soak 1 to 2 hours or overnight, or soak and cook in microwave (page 131).

2. Place the drained beans and all the other ingredients except the basil in an 8-quart saucepan.

3. Bring to a boil over high heat; reduce to simmer, and cook for 2½ to 3 hours. Add the basil just before serving; taste and adjust seasonings.

Variation: Any combination of your favorite beans or lentils may be used in preparing this soup as long as you have a total of about 3⅔ cups of the mixture.

Per serving: 0 mg cholesterol, 0.19 gm saturated fat, 1 gm total fat, 7.5 gm fiber, 151 mg sodium, 260 calories, 0 gm trans fat

◆ Daal ◆
Marinated Cucumber and Yogurt Salad
Whole Wheat Pita Bread
Lemon-Lime Yogurt Pie (page 240)

Daal (Indian Yellow Split Pea Soup)

Yield: 18 cups (1¼ cups = 1 serving)

The Indian seasonings give this hearty yellow split pea soup a very different taste from the traditional green split pea soup that we're accustomed to. Once again, you can freeze the leftovers for future use.

1 pound yellow split peas, soaked in cold water overnight (or microwaved on high for 10 minutes) and drained
4 large cloves garlic, chopped
3 celery stalks, chopped
4 carrots, chopped
3 red onions, chopped
3 leeks, chopped
1½ red peppers, seeded and chopped
1½ green peppers, seeded and chopped
2 tablespoons extra-virgin olive oil or canola oil

1 16-ounce can peeled, diced San Marzano tomatoes
1⅓ tablespoons tumeric
1⅓ tablespoons cumin
1 teaspoon coriander
¼ teaspoon freshly ground nutmeg
3½ quarts organic vegetable broth or water
Juice of 2 limes

Chopped fresh cilantro, for garnish

1. In a large soup pot, sauté the garlic, celery, carrots, onion, leeks, and peppers in the oil for 2 to 3 minutes.

2. Add the tomatoes, spices, and yellow split peas, and sauté for 2 minutes.

3. Add the broth and lime juice. Bring to a boil and simmer for about 1 hour, uncovered.

4. Remove from the heat, taste, and adjust seasonings as needed.

To Serve: Spoon into heated soup bowls and garnish with chopped cilantro.

Per serving: 0 mg cholesterol, 0.73 gm saturated fat, 4 gm total fat, 2.9 gm fiber, 75 mg sodium, 184 calories, 0 gm trans fat

♦ Bean Curd and Spinach Soup ♦
Salmon Salad Sandwich
Crudités: Radish, Green Pepper, Carrot, and Cucumber
Seasonal Fresh Fruit

Bean Curd and Spinach Soup ⓠ

Serves: 6 (¾ cup = 1 serving)

4 cups defatted, sodium-reduced chicken broth
⅔ cup cubed bean curd (tofu)
1 teaspoon sodium-reduced soy sauce
Freshly ground pepper

1½ cups raw spinach leaves, washed and shredded
2 whole green onions, finely chopped
½ cup cooked bay shrimp (optional)

1. Place the chicken broth, bean curd, soy sauce, and pepper into a saucepan. Bring to a boil and cook for 1 minute.

2. Add the spinach, turn off heat, and stir.

3. Add the green onions and serve immediately.

Per serving: 0 mg cholesterol, 0.2 gm saturated fat, 1.4 gm total fat, 0.7 gm fiber, 43 mg sodium, 49 calories, 0 gm trans fat

♦ Last-Minute Soup ♦
Grilled Cheese Sandwich on Whole Grain Bread
Baked Apple with Nonfat Milk

Last-Minute Soup ⓠ

Serves: 4 (1 cup = 1 serving)

When a hearty hot soup seems to be in order, try this one instead of a canned soup that is high in fat and sodium.

3 cups organic vegetable or
   chicken broth
1 stalk celery, thinly sliced
2 carrots, thinly sliced
4 fresh mushroom caps, thinly
   sliced

⅛ teaspoon white pepper
3–4 tablespoons orzo
4 tablespoons frozen peas
2 tablespoons chopped Italian
   parsley

1. Combine the chicken broth, celery, carrots, mushrooms, and pepper in a saucepan.
2. Bring to a boil, reduce heat to simmer, cover, and cook 10 minutes.
3. Add the orzo and cook 10 minutes.
4. Add the peas and parsley, cook 3 minutes.

Per serving: 0 mg cholesterol, 0.02 gm saturated fat, 0.2 gm total fat, 1.1 gm fiber, 24 mg sodium, 54 calories, 0 gm trans fat

---

Fiber keeps us regular, prevents colon cancer, and lowers cholesterol. We need 25 to 30 grams of fiber per day. Check page 396 in the Appendix for further information.

♦ Hot Cabbage Borscht ♦
with
Nonfat Plain Yogurt and Freshly Chopped Dill
Hearty Pumpernickel Bread
Fresh Fruit Cup

Hot Cabbage Borscht Ⓠ Ⓜ

Yield: 16 to 18 cups (1½ cups = 1 serving as an entrée)

1 tablespoon canola oil
2 large onions, coarsely chopped
5 large cloves garlic, minced
4 leeks (white part only), washed and thinly sliced
3 stalks celery with leaves, coarsely chopped
½ cup chopped Italian parsley
2 cups canned diced San Marzano tomatoes
3 cups crushed San Marzano plum tomatoes, in puree
1 1-pound head green cabbage, cut into 1-inch cubes
1 carton Wolfgang Puck's organic vegetable broth

1 quart cold water
2 bay leaves
2 teaspoons dried thyme, crushed
½ teaspoon dried oregano
1 teaspoon crushed red pepper flakes
2 cups fresh green beans, cut into 2-inch pieces (optional)
1 cup Cascadian Farms sauerkraut (optional)

Nonfat plain yogurt and chopped fresh dill, for garnish

1. In a 6-quart nonstick saucepan, heat the oil; add the onions and garlic and sauté until wilted. Add the leek and cook 5 minutes, stirring occasionally.

2. Add the celery, parsley, tomatoes, cabbage, broth, water, bay leaves, thyme, oregano, and pepper flakes. Bring to a boil, reduce heat, cover, and simmer 1½ hours.

3. Add the green beans and continue to simmer for 1 hour more.

To Serve: Place the soup in heated bowls and garnish with a dollop of nonfat plain yogurt and a sprinkle of dill. Remove bay leaves.

Variation: Sometimes I brown 3 tablespoons of unbleached white flour in a 6-inch nonstick skillet and add it to soup with the water. This gives the soup a wonderful flavor, rather like a roux without fat.

Per serving: 0 mg cholesterol, 0.23 gm saturated fat, 1.9 gm total fat, 2.6 gm fiber, 219 mg sodium, 81 calories, 0 gm trans fat

Sandwiches

Low-Sodium V-8 Juice
♦ Tuna Melt ♦
Crudités: Radishes, Carrot, and Zucchini Sticks
Seasonal Fresh Fruit

Tuna Melt Ⓠ

Yield: 4 sandwiches (1 sandwich = 1 serving)

1 6½-ounce can white-meat
   or light-meat tuna in water,
   drained
1 teaspoon sweet pickle relish,
   drained
1 green onion, sliced

¼ red pepper, finely diced
3 tablespoons low-fat mayonnaise
8 slices whole grain bread (rye,
   whole wheat, or pumpernickel)
4 slices Galaxy Veggie cheese

1. Flake the tuna in a bowl with a fork.
2. Add the relish, onion, pepper, and low-fat mayonnaise and blend thoroughly.
3. Divide the tuna mixture onto four slices of bread, spread evenly, and top with one slice of cheese each and remaining four slices of bread.
4. Place the sandwiches on a heated, nonstick griddle or skillet sprayed with olive-oil-flavored nonstick spray and heat until browned.
5. Turn over and brown the remaining side.

To Serve: Cut the hot sandwiches in half and place on a serving plate garnished with fresh vegetable crudités.

Per serving: 24 mg cholesterol, 0.92 gm saturated fat, 3.2 gm total fat, 4.4 gm fiber, 457 mg sodium, 195 calories, 0 gm trans fat

Fresh Vegetable Soup (page 278)
♦ Open-Faced Eggplant and Cheese Sandwiches ♦
Carrot and Pepper Sticks
Fresh Apples

Open-Faced Eggplant and Cheese Sandwiches Ⓠ Ⓜ

Yield: 8½ English Muffins (two muffin halves = 1 serving)

1 1-pound eggplant, peeled and sliced about ½ inch thick (8 slices)

1–2 large, ripe tomatoes, cut into ½-inch-thick slices (8 slices)

1 teaspoon dried Italian herb blend, crushed

8 slices Galaxy mozzarella or pepper jack cheese

4 whole grain Thomas' English Muffins, toasted

Fresh basil sprigs, for garnish

1. Arrange the eggplant in a single layer in a microwave dish. Coat with olive oil spray. Cover tightly with microwave plastic wrap and microwave on high for about 1 to 2 minutes.

2. Remove the plastic and drain juice.

3. Top each eggplant slice with one slice of tomato, sprinkle with the herbs and 1 cheese slice, and microwave on medium for 45 seconds to 1 minute to just melt the cheese.

4. Place one eggplant slice on ½ English muffin toasted, garnish with basil, and serve immediately.

Per serving: 7 mg cholesterol, 2.24 gm saturated fat, 8.5 gm total fat, 3 gm fiber, 343 mg sodium, 270 calories, 0 gm trans fat

---

One serving of avocado contains 12 grams of fiber.

Tomato Bouillon (page 95)
♦ Stuffed French Toast ♦
Date Waldorf Salad (page 289)

Stuffed French Toast Ⓠ

Yield: 4 sandwiches (1 sandwich = 1 serving)

8 slices whole wheat or raisin
   bread

Filling:
1¼ cups 1%-fat cottage cheese,
   blended until smooth
1 tablespoon sugar-free apricot or
   peach preserves
1 teaspoon grated lemon zest
1 teaspoon cinnamon

Batter:
⅔ cup 1% milk or low-fat soy milk
2 extra-large egg whites, slightly
   beaten or Eggbeaters
1 teaspoon pure vanilla extract

1. Blend the filling ingredients.
2. Spread the mixture onto four slices of bread and top with the remaining slices.
3. Combine the batter ingredients in shallow pan.
4. Dip the sandwiches into batter, coating both sides.
5. Brown sandwiches on both sides in a nonstick skillet or griddle sprayed with butter-flavored nonstick spray.
6. Cut the browned sandwich in half and serve immediately.

Per serving: 7 mg cholesterol, 0.3 gm saturated fat, 1.8 gm total fat, 4.3 gm fiber, 328 mg sodium, 202 calories, 0 trans fat

---

1 or 2 teaspoons of cinnamon daily sprinkled over your morning cereal or oatmeal has been shown to lower blood sugar, triglycerides, and cholesterol.

Celery Soup (page 274)
♦ Salmon Burgers with Tartar Sauce ♦
on Whole Wheat Buns
Lettuce and Tomato Slices
Pears

Salmon Burgers Ⓠ

Yield: 4 burgers (1 burger with about 2 ounces cooked fish = 1 serving)

This recipe provides a way to serve a fast food without the red meat or frying usually associated with fast foods. It also gives you one of your three fish meals for the week.

¼ cup Panko or dry bread crumbs for coating patties

4 whole wheat buns, or English muffins, toasted

Burgers:

1 7½-ounce can salmon, skinned, boned, drained, and flaked

2 whole green onions, thinly sliced

2 tablespoons chopped celery

5 ounces frozen chopped spinach, thawed and squeezed dry

1 teaspoon Worcestershire sauce

½ cup nonfat plain yogurt or low-fat mayonnaise

1 tablespoon chopped fresh dill

2 tablespoons lemon juice

Freshly ground pepper

¼ cup Panko crumbs mixed with 3 tablespoons oat bran

Tartar Sauce:

2 tablespoons nonfat plain yogurt mixed with 1 tablespoon low-fat mayonnaise

1 teaspoon grated onion

1 teaspoon sweet pickle relish

1. Place all the burger ingredients in a mixing bowl, blend thoroughly with a fork, and shape into four patties.

2. Coat the patties on both sides with bread crumbs.

3. Place the patties on a nonstick baking sheet sprayed with canola oil spray and bake in the upper third of a *preheated* 425° oven for 10 minutes; turn and bake 10 to 15 minutes more.

4. *To make the tartar sauce*, combine the four ingredients thoroughly.

To Serve: Place each warm burger on a toasted whole wheat bun and top with a dollop of tartar sauce. Serve with leaves of romaine and slices of tomato.

Per serving: 23 mg cholesterol, 1.01 gm saturated fat, 4.3 gm total fat, 2.3 gm fiber, 292 mg sodium, 181 calories, 0 gm trans fat

Fresh Vegetable Soup (page 278)
♦ Healthy Burgers on Whole Wheat Buns ♦
Tomato Slices and Romaine Lettuce
Cole Slaw with Parsley
Seasonal Grapes

Healthy Burgers Ⓠ

Yield: 5 burgers (1 burger with about 2½ ounces cooked turkey = 1 serving)

Actually, this menu is hearty enough to be used for dinner. When using ground turkey, it's better to buy a raw turkey breast and have it skinned, boned, and ground. Three ounces of skinned turkey breast contains less than 2 grams of saturated fat, whereas a 3-ounce patty of packaged already-ground turkey may contain as much as 9 grams.

1 pound ground raw turkey breast
1 extra-large egg white
½ small onion, chopped
½ red pepper, seeded and chopped
1 carrot, grated
¼ cup sodium-reduced vegetable juice, or ½ cup vegetarian broth, with 1 teaspoon fresh lemon juice

½ cup dry bread crumbs
1 tablespoon Worcestershire sauce
¼ teaspoon dried thyme, crushed
Freshly ground pepper and salt to taste
5 whole wheat buns, toasted

1. Combine all the burger ingredients in a mixing bowl, stirring with a fork. Do not overmix.
2. Shape into five round patties.
3. Heat a nonstick skillet coated with nonstick spray and grill patties 4 to 5 minutes on each side. Serve immediately.

To Serve: Place each warm burger on a toasted whole wheat bun with a slice of tomato, romaine lettuce, and Dijon mustard or Chopped Vegetable Spread (page 147). Grilled or raw red onion slices may be added.

NOTE: Unused patties may be wrapped in plastic wrap, placed in freezer bags, and frozen for future use. To serve, microwave the frozen patty in microwave plastic wrap on high for about 3 minutes, turning over halfway through cooking. If you do not have a microwave, defrost and reheat in a hot nonstick skillet.

Per serving: 47 mg cholesterol, 0.81 gm saturated fat, 2.7 gm total fat, 0.4 gm fiber, 160 mg sodium, 163 calories, 0 gm trans fat

Mixed Green Salad
Daal with Croutons (page 136)
♦ Spicy Pita Rolls ♦
Fresh Fruit Cup

Spicy Pita Rolls ⓠ

Yield: 5 pita rolls (1 roll = 1 serving)

Whether you are six or sixty, you'll love these easy, piquant pita rolls. Leftovers can be frozen for future use.

½ pound ground raw turkey breast (see page 144)
1 teaspoon spicy salt-free vegetable seasoning
About ⅓ cup green chili salsa
1 clove garlic, minced
2 whole green onions, sliced

5 romaine leaves, washed and crisped
5 6-inch whole wheat pita breads, warmed in the oven or microwave and split
4 tablespoons diced green chilies
5 Galaxy Veggie slices

1. Crumble the turkey into a hot nonstick skillet coated with nonstick spray and sprinkle with the vegetable seasoning.
2. Cook several minutes over medium-high heat, stirring constantly. If it sticks, add a bit of the salsa. Add the garlic and stir.
3. Add the green onion and salsa and stir.
4. Place one fifth of the turkey mixture on top of romaine on a warmed pita, layer with 1 scant tablespoon chilis and 1 slice veggie cheese. Roll up tightly and serve.

NOTE: Wrap leftovers tightly in plastic wrap and refrigerate or freeze. To serve frozen rolls, heat on high in microwave for about 2 minutes (without romaine).

Per serving: 26 mg cholesterol, 1.04 gm saturated fat, 3 gm total fat, 4.8 gm fiber, 145 mg sodium, 199 calories, 0 gm trans fat

Vegetarian Lentil Soup (page 87)
♦ Pesto, Cheese, and Tomato Sandwich ♦
Crudités: Green Pepper, Radish, and Carrot
Fresh Pear

Pesto, Cheese, and Tomato Sandwich Ⓠ

Serves: 1

In Italy, this is called a panino, but to Americans it's just a sandwich. It's always a popular lunch or quick supper.

1 5-inch section whole wheat baguette, halved
1 tablespoon Pesto Sauce (page 250) or Chopped Vegetable Spread (page 147)

1 slice Galaxy Veggie cheese
1 fresh Italian plum tomato, sliced
4 fresh basil leaves

1. Spread pesto on both halves of the baguette.
2. Layer the cheese, tomato, and basil on half of the baguette; top with remaining half.

To Serve: Cut the sandwich in half and garnish with crudités.

Variation: May be grilled as a panino.

Per serving: 10 mg cholesterol, 1.85 gm saturated fat, 3.8 gm total fat, 2.2 gm fiber, 380 mg sodium, 231 calories, 0 gm trans fat

---

Don't buy any packaged foods that list trans fats or partially hydrogenated oils in the ingredient list.

Spicy Cold Tomato Soup (page 88)
Sliced Turkey Breast with
♦ Chopped Vegetable Spread ♦
on
Whole Grain Bread
Carrot Sticks
Seasonal Fresh Fruit

Chopped Vegetable Spread ⓠ

Yield: about 2½ cups (1 tablespoon = 1 serving)

This vegetable spread is great to use by itself on a sandwich, or instead of mayonnaise or mustard on a turkey or chicken sandwich. It also blends well with steamed rice. Try 1½ cups of vegetable spread mixed with 2 cups hot cooked rice.

2 medium fresh mushrooms
3 canned artichoke hearts, well
drained and quartered
½ small red pepper, cored,
seeded, and quartered
1 small zucchini, quartered
1 small summer squash, quartered
1 carrot, quartered

2 to 3 pepperoncini peppers,
drained
8 fresh basil leaves and 1 teaspoon
extra-virgin olive oil, or 1
tablespoon Pesto Sauce (page
250) or commercial pesto sauce
1 Italian plum tomato, quartered
(optional)

1. Place all the ingredients in the food processor and process only until finely chopped. *Do not puree.*

2. Pack into a container and cover tightly. This will keep nicely in the refrigerator for five to six days. Drain and stir before each use.

Per serving: 0 mg cholesterol, 0.02 gm saturated fat, 0.1 gm total fat, 0.2 gm fiber, 6 mg sodium, 7 calories, 0 gm trans fat

Salads

Vegetarian Lentil Soup
♦ Tostada ♦
Mango Fruited Mousse (page 322)

Tostada ⓠ

Serves: 4

A Mexican salad served as an appetizer. To serve as a main dish add shredded chicken or turkey breast.

4 corn tortillas
garlic powder to taste
1 cup nonfat, canned, vegetarian refried beans*
⅔ cup Newman's Own salsa
4 cups assorted vegetables, such as shredded romaine, cucumber, radish, green onion, tomato, green or red pepper, or jicama

½ avocado, diced

yogurt or low-fat sour cream, if desired

1. Place tortilla on nonstick skillet and season with garlic powder and paprika. Heat until crisp.
2. Combine beans and ⅓ cup chili salsa.
3. Spread ¼ cup mixture on tostada shell, top with ⅔ cup assorted vegetables, additional salsa, and a dollop of yogurt or low-fat sour cream.

Per serving: 0 mg cholesterol, 1.5 gm total fat, 7.8 gm fiber, 442 mg sodium, 143 calories, 0 gm trans fat

*For spicier bean spread, add chopped green chilies.

Trans fats in foods lower HDL cholesterol levels
and raise LDL cholesterol levels.

♦ Pasta and Vegetable Salad with Fresh Salsa ♦
Whole Wheat Bread Sticks
Sliced Peaches with Nonfat Vanilla Yogurt

Pasta and Vegetable Salad with Fresh Salsa Ⓠ

Serves: 4 (as an antrée)

This pasta salad may be served cold or heated briefly in a microwave oven or saucepan before serving.

8 ounces whole wheat fusilli, cooked al dente and well drained
½ red pepper, seeded and thinly sliced
1 10-ounce package frozen white peg corn
1 cup frozen peas, defrosted
1 cup canned black beans or kidney beans, drained and rinsed, or 1 cup cooked beans (page 131)

1½ cups fresh broccoli, chopped and steamed, or 1 10-ounce package frozen broccoli florets, defrosted
2 cups Fresh Salsa (page 185) or Newman's Own salsa
1 tablespoon grated Parmesan cheese

1. Combine the pasta with the peppers, peas, beans, and broccoli. Toss lightly.
2. Add the salsa and mix with two forks.
3. Sprinkle with the cheese, toss lightly, and chill in refrigerator for 20 minutes before serving.

Variation: Shredded leftover bits of roast turkey or chicken may be added as additional protein for a heartier salad.

Per serving: 1 mg cholesterol, 0.43 gm saturated fat, 1.8 gm total fat, 6 gm fiber, 86 mg sodium, 304 calories, 0 gm fat

Per 1 tablespoon serving of salsa: 0 mg cholesterol, 0.004 gm saturated fat, 0.03 gm total fat, 1 gm fiber, 1.4 mg sodium, 4 calories, 0 gm trans fat

♦ Turkey Chef's Salad
with
Green Goddess Dressing ♦
Pita Chips
Café au Lait Custard (page 323)

Turkey Chef's Salad with Green Goddess Dressing Ⓠ

Serves: 4

8 cups torn or chopped mixed
  salad greens: romaine, butter
  lettuce, endive, red leaf lettuce,
  radicchio, or red cabbage
½ pound cooked turkey breast, cut
  into thin strips
1 cup cooked, sliced green beans
1 small red pepper, seeded and
  cut into thin strips

½ cup Green Goddess Dressing
  (page 151; save the rest of the
  dressing for a salad to be served
  in the next few days)

Halved cherry tomatoes, sliced
  beets, radishes, and cucumber
  and carrot strips, for garnish.

1. Place the greens, turkey, beans, and pepper in a large salad bowl.
2. Add the salad dressing and toss lightly with two forks.
3. Arrange the desired garnishes on top of salad in the bowl and serve immediately.

Variations: Arrange the greens, turkey, peppers, and garnishes on individual salad plates and serve the dressing on the side.

You may prefer to use Russian Dressing (page 268) or low-calorie vinaigrette instead of Green Goddess.

Per serving: 41 mg cholesterol, 0.82 gm saturated fat, 3.2 gm total fat, 1.3 gm fiber, 86 mg sodium, 137 calories, 0 gm trans fat

Green Goddess Dressing Ⓠ

Yield: about 1¼ cups (1 tablespoon = 1 serving)

1 tablespoon light-style
   mayonnaise
1 cup buttermilk, strained
1 clove garlic, minced
1 tablespoon chopped fresh
   tarragon, or 1 teaspoon dried
   tarragon, crushed

2 tablespoons chopped fresh
   parsley
1 tablespoon fresh lemon juice
½ teaspoon Dijon mustard
Pinch of white pepper
2 tablespoons mashed ripe
   avocado (optional)

1. Stir the mayonnaise in a small bowl until smooth. Add the buttermilk
gradually while mixing.
2. Add the remaining ingredients and blend thoroughly.
3. Place in a tightly covered container and store in the refrigerator until
ready to use. It will keep for several weeks.

Per serving: 1 mg cholesterol, 0.09 gm saturated fat, 0.5 gm total fat, 0 gm fiber,
19 mg sodium, 10 calories, 0 gm trans fat

---

*Americans spend about **15 cents** out of every food dollar
on fruits and vegetables.*

♦

*Americans spend about **19 cents** out of every food dollar
on candy, gum, soda pop, and bakery items.*

♦ Pasta Salad with Seafood ♦
Whole Wheat Rolls
Mixed Melon Cubes

Pasta Salad with Seafood Ⓠ

Serves: 6

The complex carbohydrates supplied by the pasta and vegetables in this salad means you can use a smaller amount of seafood, limiting your intake of animal protein and cholesterol.

3 cups cooked soba or whole
   wheat fusilli, cooked al dente
   and well drained
8 ounces cooked bay shrimp
8 ounces bay scallops, poached in
   ⅓ cup white wine until opaque
½ green pepper, seeded and diced
½ red pepper, seeded and diced
1 cup sliced celery
1 cup unpeeled diced English
   cucumber
1 large carrot, shredded

1 cup frozen petit peas, defrosted
   under cold running water
3 fresh plum tomatoes, diced
¾ cup low-calorie oil-free
   vinaigrette mixed with 1
   tablespoon raspberry vinegar,
   1 teaspoon extra-virgin olive
   oil, or Green Goddess Dressing
   (page 151)
8 cups mixed shredded romaine
   and red cabbage

1. In a salad bowl, combine all the ingredients *except* the romaine and cabbage and the dressing. Sprinkle with freshly ground pepper and toss lightly.

2. Drizzle with salad dressing and toss lightly to combine.

3. Refrigerate 30 minutes or longer before serving.

To Serve: Arrange the shredded cabbage and romaine on a large serving platter, mound the pasta and seafood mixture on top.

NOTE: If you can find vegetable pasta made without egg yolks, it makes an even more attractive presentation.

Per serving: 70 mg cholesterol, 0.28 gm saturated fat, 1.8 gm total fat, 3.6 gm fiber, 395 mg sodium, 243 calories, 0 gm trans fat

♦ Warm New Potato and Green Bean Salad ♦
Sliced Turkey Breast
Pumpernickel Bread
Crudités: Carrots, Green Pepper, Cucumber,
Radishes, and Tomato
Watermelon

Warm New Potato and Green Bean Salad Ⓠ Ⓜ

Serves: 6 to 8

2 pounds unpeeled small red new or Yukon Gold potatoes, quartered
4 cloves garlic, chopped
2 tablespoons extra-virgin olive oil
1 small red onion or mild-flavored white onion thinly sliced or chopped
3 tablespoons dry white wine
2 tablespoons defatted sodium-reduced chicken broth

1 tablespoon Worcestershire sauce
2 teaspoons each Dijon and coarse-grain mustard
¼ cup chopped fresh parsley
1 tablespoon chopped fresh thyme or 1 teaspoon dried thyme
½ pound fresh green beans, cut into 2-inch lengths and steamed

1. Microwave the potatoes, garlic, and 1 tablespoon of oil for 5 minutes on high in a shallow baking dish covered with microwave plastic wrap. Add onions, stir, cover, and microwave on high for 5 to 6 minutes.

2. While the potatoes are cooking, combine the remaining tablespoon of oil, wine, broth, Worcestershire sauce, mustard, parsley, and thyme in a small jar. Shake well.

3. Place the warm potatoes, garlic, and onion in a large bowl, add the beans, sprinkle with the salad dressing, and toss gently so that liquid may be absorbed.

To Cook on Stove:

1. Steam whole potatoes and quarter them.

2. Sauté garlic and onions in oil for 2 to 3 minutes, then proceed as in Step 2 above.

Per serving: 0 mg cholesterol, 0.71 gm saturated fat, 5 gm total fat, 1.6 gm fiber, 59 mg sodium, 205 calories, 0 trans fat

Spicy Gazpacho with Croutons (page 261)
♦ Layered Luncheon Salad ♦
Whole Wheat Rolls
Papaya with Blueberries

Layered Luncheon Salad Ⓠ

Serves: 6

This is a lovely salad that can be prepared hours ahead of time and just topped with its salad dressing so that it does not wilt. It makes a great dish for a buffet or to take to a potluck supper.

4 cups shredded romaine and red
   leaf lettuce
1 cup canned kidney beans,
   drained and rinsed, or 1 cup
   cooked beans (page 131)
1 cup canned corn
1 cup peeled, diced jicama, red
   radishes, or water chestnuts
1 cup defrosted frozen peas
¼ cup finely chopped red onion
3 chopped, hard-cooked, extra-
   large egg whites (*no yolks*)
1 cup thinly sliced celery
3 tablespoons chopped red pepper
   or pimiento

6 halved cherry tomatoes and
   1 tablespoon chopped fresh
   thyme or parsley, for garnish

Dressing:
1 tablespoon light sour cream
3 tablespoons light-style
   mayonnaise
1 tablespoon salt-free ketchup
2 teaspoons sweet relish, drained
⅛ teaspoon white pepper
2 tablespoons mashed avocado
   (optional)

1. Place the shredded lettuce on the bottom of a 3-quart glass soufflé dish or salad bowl and sprinkle separate layers of beans, corn, jicama, peas, red onion, egg whites, celery, and red pepper or pimiento over the top.

2. Mix together the dressing ingredients and spread salad dressing mixture on top of salad.

3. Garnish with tomato halves and thyme and chill in refrigerator until serving time.

To Serve: Gently toss salad until mixture is coated lightly with dressing.

NOTE: Jicama is a brown-skinned tuberous root vegetable with crisp white flesh. It is best served raw as a crudité or in salads.

Per serving: 1 mg cholesterol, 0.11 gm saturated fat, 1.4 gm total fat, 3.1 gm fiber, 132 mg sodium, 134 calories, 0 gm trans fat

♦ Marinated Mixed Vegetable Salad ♦
Oysters or Clams* on the Half Shell with
Cocktail Sauce and/or Lime
Whole Grain Crackers
Corn on the Cob
Cantaloupe

Marinated Mixed Vegetable Salad Ⓠ Ⓜ

Serves: 4

An easy supper for a warm summer evening.

4 cups mixed fresh vegetables (for example: cauliflower, broccoli, carrots, corn, and red peppers), coarsely chopped
1 cup canned kidney beans, drained and rinsed, or cooked kidney beans (page 131)
⅓ cup low-calorie oil-free vinaigrette

1 teaspoon Dijon mustard
1 teaspoon finely chopped shallot or red onion
½ teaspoon dried fines herbs
1 teaspoon balsamic vinegar
4 cups shredded salad greens

1. Place the vegetables in a microwave-safe bowl, cover, and cook on high for 3 minutes or steam until just crisp. Add the beans and combine.

2. Mix the salad dressing with remaining ingredients and pour over vegetable-bean mixture. Toss lightly and let marinate 20 minutes or overnight in the refrigerator before serving.

To Serve: Place 1 cup of greens on each plate and top with ¼ of marinated vegetable mixture.

Per serving: 0 mg cholesterol, 0.11 gm saturated fat, 0.8 gm total fat, 4.1 gm fiber, 260 mg sodium, 114 calories, 0 gm trans fat

*Four large shrimp may be substituted for oysters or clams.

Bean Curd and Spinach Soup (page 137)
♦ Fresh Vegetable Salad with Japanese Noodles ♦
Brown Rice Cakes with Oat Bran
Fresh Plums or Pluots

Fresh Vegetable Salad with Japanese Noodles Ⓠ

Serves: 4 to 6

Most whole wheat pasta cannot be cooked al dente; the Japanese pasta called soba is an exception.

4 stalks bok choy, thinly sliced
1 medium zucchini, thinly sliced
1 crookneck squash, coarsely shredded
1 small red pepper, seeded and thinly sliced
1 carrot, thinly sliced
1 cup diced eggplant
3 whole green onions, thinly sliced
6 ounces soba noodles, cooked al dente, drained, rinsed in cold water, and drained again.

1 cup fresh or frozen snow peas, defrosted, washed, and cut into lengthwise strips, for garnish

Dressing:
2 teaspoons sesame oil
⅓ cup defatted sodium-reduced chicken broth or vegetable broth
2 cloves garlic, minced
½ teaspoon fresh ginger, peeled and grated
1 teaspoon Chinese five-spice seasoning
2 teaspoons sodium-reduced soy sauce
2 tablespoons frozen unsweetened apple juice concentrate
¼ cup Japanese rice vinegar
1 tablespoon rice wine or sherry
2 teaspoons Dijon mustard

1. Place the first seven ingredients in a salad bowl; toss lightly to combine.

2. Mix the dressing ingredients together, drizzle over the vegetables, and toss lightly.

3. Let stand 15 minutes at room temperature; then add the pasta and toss.

To Serve: Mound the mixture on a serving plate and sprinkle with snow pea strips. Serve at room temperature.

Per serving: 0 mg cholesterol, 0.71 gm saturated fat, 4.9 gm total fat, 6.9 gm fiber, 143 mg sodium, 257 calories, 0 gm trans fat

Tabatchnik Vegetable Soup
♦ Cannellini Bean and Tuna Salad ♦
Carrot Sticks
Whole Wheat Baguette
Kiwi and Strawberries

Italian Bean and Tuna Salad Ⓠ

Serves: 4

2 cups cooked cannellini beans
(page 131), or 1 16-ounce can,
drained and rinsed
1 small red onion, finely chopped
1 tablespoon red wine or balsamic
vinegar
2 tablespoons low-calorie oil-free
Italian dressing
1 tablespoon lemon juice
1 teaspoon Dijon mustard
1 garlic clove, minced
Freshly ground pepper

2 tablespoons chopped fresh basil
or 2 teaspoons dried basil,
crushed
¼ cup chopped fresh parsley
3 cups shredded romaine and
radicchio
1 6½-ounce can light-meat tuna in
oil, drained and flaked

2 large carrots, cut into strips, for
garnish

1. Place the beans and onion in a mixing bowl.
2. Combine the vinegar, dressing, lemon juice, mustard, garlic, pepper, basil, and parsley. Sprinkle over beans and toss lightly. Marinate for 15 minutes at room temperature.
3. Place the romaine and radicchio on a serving dish. Arrange the tuna on top of greens. Spoon the beans over the tuna and garnish with carrot sticks.

Per serving: 18 mg cholesterol, 0.48 gm saturated fat, 3.3 gm total fat, 4.8 gm fiber, 268 mg sodium, 236 calories, 0 gm trans fat

*People of Latino or African-American origin are at very
high risk for developing diabetes.*

Casseroles and One-Dish Meals

Mixed Green Salad with Pinto Beans
♦ Pastel de Calabacitas with Salsa ♦
Pumpernickel Garlic Toast (page 331)
Melon Slices

Pastel de Calabacitas (Zucchini Pie) with Salsa

Serves: 6 to 8

The original recipe, which came from Lillian, a student studying at the University of Mexico, used chayote squash instead of zucchini. After several translations, the following recipe has become a hit with my family.

2 teaspoons canola or corn oil
2 large onions, coarsely chopped
3 cloves garlic, minced
1 tablespoon chopped fresh oregano
Freshly ground pepper
2 teaspoons salt-free vegetable seasoning
4 large zucchini, coarsely chopped
3 extra-large egg whites, slightly beaten
1 teaspoon dried dill, or 1 tablespoon chopped fresh dill
1 cup 1%-fat cottage cheese, blended until smooth, or nonfat ricotta cheese

1 teaspoon baking powder
½ cup yellow cornmeal
2 tablespoons finely shredded part-skim mozzarella cheese
1 tablespoon finely shredded Parmesan cheese

2 tablespoons chopped fresh cilantro for garnish and warm Fresh Salsa (page 185) or Newman's Own salsa

1. Put the oil in a 10-inch nonstick skillet; add the onions and garlic. Sprinkle with oregano, pepper, and vegetable seasoning, and sauté until the onions are wilted.

2. Add the zucchini and stir-fry 3 minutes. Remove from heat.

3. Blend the egg whites, dill, cottage cheese, and baking powder in a blender or food processor. Add to the zucchini mixture and mix.

4. Add the cornmeal and mozzarella cheese to the zucchini mixture and blend.

5. Pour into a 10-inch glass pie plate or quiche pan coated with nonstick corn oil cooking spray. Sprinkle with 1 tablespoon Parmesan cheese.

6. Bake in a preheated 350° oven for 40 to 45 minutes or until golden brown. Cool slightly and cut into wedges.

To Serve: Sprinkle with chopped cilantro and serve warm with heated salsa.

Per serving: 15 mg cholesterol, 2.7 gm saturated fat, 5.9 gm total fat, 2.2 gm fiber, 157 mg sodium, 166 calories, 0 gm trans fat

Skillet Supper Ⓠ

Serves: 4 (2 ounces cooked turkey = 1 serving)

This one-dish meal is easy to prepare and requires minimal clean-up afterward. While the skillet dish is cooking, you can prepare the salad and bake the apples in your microwave.

¾ **pound ground turkey or chicken breast**
1 **large onion, chopped**
2 **large cloves garlic, minced**
1 **green pepper, cut into 1-inch chunks**
1¾ **cups water**
1 **16-ounce can San Marzano tomatoes, chopped**
3 **tablespoons tomato paste**
1 **cup converted or brown rice**

⅓ **cup seeded dark raisins**
1 **tablespoon red wine vinegar**
½ **teaspoon ground cinnamon**
Freshly ground pepper
4 **½-inch-thick slices beefsteak tomato**
2 **teaspoons shredded Parmesan cheese**

2 **sliced green onions, for garnish**

1. In a large nonstick or iron skillet, heat the turkey until no longer pink. Add the onions and garlic and sauté 5 minutes.

2. Add all the remaining ingredients except the tomato slices and Parmesan cheese, cover, and simmer 20 minutes or until the rice is tender and liquid absorbed.

3. Arrange the tomato slices on top of the mixture, sprinkle with Par-

mesan cheese, and place under the broiler a few minutes, until lightly browned.

4. Sprinkle with green onions and serve.

Per serving: 16 mg cholesterol, 0.58 gm saturated fat, 2.1 gm total fat, 2.5 gm fiber, 44 mg sodium, 326 calories, 0 gm trans fat

Tofu and Corn Soup (page 277)
♦ Spinach Frittata ♦
Snow Peas and Carrots
Orange Slices and a Chocolate Cookie (page 342)

Spinach Frittata ⓠ

Serves: 1

½ 10-ounce package frozen chopped spinach, defrosted and squeezed dry

2 green onions, thinly sliced

1 fresh Italian plum tomato, diced

1 teaspoon fresh thyme or Italian parsley, chopped

Freshly ground pepper

3 extra-large egg whites, slightly beaten with 1 tablespoon nonfat milk or 4 ounces Eggbeaters

1 teaspoon shredded Parmesan cheese

½ slice Milton's whole wheat or rye bread, cut into ½-inch cubes

1. Place the drained spinach, onions, tomato, seasonings, egg-white mixture, and cheese in a bowl and stir well with a fork.

2. Coat an 8-inch nonstick skillet with nonstick cooking spray. Heat the skillet, sprinkle the cubed bread over the bottom of pan, and sauté on medium heat for 1 minute until lightly toasted.

3. Pour the egg mixture over the bread and smooth the mixture.

4. Cook over medium heat until bottom of frittata is lightly browned. Turn and cook until lightly browned on second side.

To Serve: Flip frittata, bread side up, onto a serving plate and serve hot.

Per serving: 1 mg cholesterol, 0.81 gm saturated fat, 3.9 gm total fat, 6.9 gm fiber, 361 mg sodium, 176 calories, 0 gm trans fat

♦ Chili Beans ♦
Brown Rice Pilaf
Zucchini, Corn, and Red Peppers
Fresh Fruit Compote (page 322)

Chili Beans Ⓠ Ⓜ

Serves: 12 as a side dish (½ cup = 1 serving) or 6 as an entrée (1 cup = 1 serving)

2 15-ounce cans kidney, pinto,
  or black beans, drained and
  rinsed, or 4 cups cooked beans
  (page 131)
1 14-ounce can tomatoes, chopped
1 cup sodium-reduced vegetable
  broth
1 large onion, chopped

1 4-ounce can chopped green
  chilies, drained
½ teaspoon ground coriander
½ teaspoon garlic powder
1–2 tablespoons chili powder
Chopped Maui, Walla Walla,
  or Vidalia onion, as topping
  (optional)

1. Combine all the ingredients in a 3-quart saucepan; mix well.
2. Bring to a simmer, cover, and cook 30 to 40 minutes. (Or cover with microwave plastic wrap and microwave on high for 5 minutes; reduce to medium and cook 5 minutes, stirring occasionally.)
3. Taste and adjust seasonings before serving.

Per serving: 0 mg cholesterol, 0.24 gm saturated fat, 1.3 gm total fat, 5.6 gm fiber, 26 mg sodium, 190 calories, 0 gm trans fat

Remember to move more and eat less!

Chilled Mixed Green Salad
♦ Black Bean Chili ♦
Corn Tortillas
Kiwi Slices with Mango Puree

Black Bean Chili

Serves: 12 (1 cup = 1 serving)

1 large onion, chopped
6 garlic cloves, minced
2 large carrots, chopped
1 green pepper, seeded and
   chopped
1 red pepper, seeded and chopped
2 teaspoons canola oil
1 cup sliced fresh mushrooms
1 pound ground turkey breast (see
   page 144)
2 teaspoons dried oregano,
   crushed
1 teaspoon ground cumin

1 to 2 tablespoons chili powder
Freshly ground pepper
2 28-ounce cans crushed San
   Marzano tomatoes in puree
2 15-ounce cans black beans,
   drained and rinsed, or 4 cups
   cooked beans (page 131)
1 teaspoon hot red pepper sauce

Fresh salsa (page 185) or
   Newman's Own salsa and nonfat
   plain yogurt, for garnish

1. Sauté the vegetables for 3 minutes in the oil in a large nonstick saucepan.

2. Add the mushrooms and cook 3 minutes.

3. Add the turkey and all the seasonings and sauté until the meat is no longer pink.

4. Add the remaining ingredients, stir, and simmer over low heat for 30 minutes, stirring occasionally. Taste and adjust seasonings.

To Serve: Serve hot in warm bowls; pass the nonfat plain yogurt and fresh salsa as toppings.

Per serving: 19 mg cholesterol, 0.56 gm saturated fat, 2.7 gm total fat, 5.5 gm fiber, 253 mg sodium, 193 calories, 0 gm trans fat

Dinner

In North America, dinner, the largest meal, is generally served at the end of the workday, usually between six and eight o'clock. In many European and South American countries, however, the largest meal is served at noon, with enough time off to enjoy the food, relax, and even take a siesta. There is a real advantage to this custom, for when dinner is eaten at midday there is ample time to work off the added calories. Certainly, if you are concerned about weight control, it is better to eat a lighter meal in the evening, with the larger meal at noon. Although for most of us this is not always practical, when it is, I recommend it—for example, the "business lunch" can be your main meal instead of getting a double dose of calories by later having dinner at home.

In the low-cholesterol menus that follow, you will notice that many meals start with a salad or light soup. When you fill up a bit on these items, you cut your need for a large entrée. Most of the entrées offer small portions of animal protein with larger servings of vegetables and complex carbohydrates. Simple fresh fruit desserts round out the meals, with an occasional dessert that may be a bit more caloric but is still low in cholesterol, saturated fat, and trans fat.

RECIPES

Fish (beginning on page 166)

Sea Bass or Branzino with Microwaved Vegetables
Savory Sole Provençal
Red Snapper with Curry Sauce
Salmon Loaf with Creole Sauce
Brochettes of Scallops and Scrod
Fish Curry with Condiments
Microwave-Poached Whitefish with Mustard Sauce in Lime Shells
Salmon Mousse with Dill
Trout Stuffed with Veggies
Seafood Jambalaya
Capellini with Clams in Red Sauce
Salmon Tetrazzini
Turbot with Spanish Sauce
Piquant Broiled Mahimahi with Mango Salsa

Tuna-Stuffed Mushrooms with Creole Sauce
Stir-Fried Scallops with Garlic, Mushrooms, and Snow Peas
Grilled Red Snapper and Tomato
Broiled Swordfish Paillard with Fresh Salsa
Mediterranean Fish Soup
Salmon, Spinach, and Rice Casserole
Grilled Salmon Scallops on Mixed Greens with Assorted Salsas
Cajun Blackened Redfish
Flounder with Creole Sauce
Perfect Petrale Sole
Helen's Orange Roughy with a Vegetable Mélange

Poultry (beginning on page 194)

Chunky Turkey Chili
Turkey Roulades Stuffed with Asparagus, Carrots, and Red Pepper
Mini Turkey Loaves with Piquant Salsa
Stuffed Peppers in the Pot
Turkey Ragout
Italian Turkey Sausage
Ever-Ready Rotisserie Chicken
Turkey Chow Mein
Roast Chicken with Tomatillo Sauce
Poached Chicken with Braised Endive and Carrots
Citrus Chicken Breasts
Hearty Chicken Wrap
Rosemary Chicken Breasts with Garlic and Lemon
Grilled Chicken Breasts with Apples Calvados
Chicken Enchiladas
Hot Cajun Chicken and Black Bean Salad
Orange-Glazed Cornish Hens

Pastas (beginning on page 216)

Whole Wheat Fusilli with Broccoli Florets, Garlic, and Hot Red
    Pepper Flakes
Vegetarian Lasagna Rolls
Sweet Pepper Pasta
Linguini with Red Clam Sauce

Lillian's Quick and Easy Manicotti
Pasta Shells with Mushrooms
Fresh Tomato, Basil, and Mozzarella Pasta

Vegetarian Dishes (beginning on page 224)

Eggplant Lasagna
Stir-Fry Vegetables with Tofu
Tuscan Minestrone
Vegetable Lo Mein
Celery Root, Red Cabbage, and Orange Salad
Angela's Herbed Squash Medley
Lentil Vegetable Salad with Low-Calorie Tarragon Vinaigrette
Vegetarian Paella
Stanford Moroccan Vegetable Stew with Couscous and Spicy Red
    Pepper Sauce (2 recipes)
Ratatouille

Desserts (beginning on page 236)

Papaya Ambrosia
Fresh White Nectarine Scallop
Baked Alaska Pears
Lemon-Lime Yogurt Pie
Chocolate Zucchini Cupcakes
Orange Baked Alaska

Fish

Hearts of Romaine with Mustard-Yogurt Dressing
♦ Sea Bass with Microwaved Vegetables ♦
Slim Asparagus Spears
Steamed Baby New Potatoes
Pineapple Wedges with Fresh Sliced Strawberries

Sea Bass with Microwaved Vegetables Ⓠ Ⓜ

Serves: 4 (3 ounces cooked fish = 1 serving)

If you are lucky enough to find branzino, use it; otherwise, sea bass or cod will do. This is one of our family favorites.

1 pound fillet of sea bass or cod, cut into 4 equal pieces
2 teaspoons extra-virgin olive oil
2 small onions, thinly sliced
2 cups fresh mixed carrots, cauliflower, and zucchini, coarsely chopped, or ½ 16-ounce package frozen mixed vegetables
1 teaspoon dried thyme, crushed

Freshly ground pepper
1 tablespoon sodium-reduced soy sauce
Juice of ½ lemon
1 teaspoon salt-free vegetable seasoning
1 large plum tomato, diced
½ pound fresh pencil-thin asparagus

1. Wash the fish in cold water, drain, and dry with paper towel.
2. Place the olive oil and onion slices in a 9-inch microwave dish, cover with microwave plastic wrap, and cook on high for 2 minutes.
3. Add the vegetables, thyme, pepper, and soy sauce. Stir, cover, and microwave on high 1 minute.
4. Place the fish in a microwave dish and sprinkle with the lemon juice and vegetable seasoning.
5. Spoon the vegetable mixture over the fish, sprinkle with the diced tomato, and lay the asparagus on the center of the fish. Cover with microwave plastic wrap and cook on high for 5 minutes, or until fish flakes with fork.

Per serving: 58 mg cholesterol, 1.14 gm saturated fat, 5.9 gm total fat, 2.4 gm fiber, 210 mg sodium, 186 calories, 0 gm trans fat

Orange and Red Cabbage Slaw
♦ Savory Sole Provençal ♦
Brown and Wild Rice Pilaf
Steamed Carrots and Peas
Chocoholic's Chocolate Cake (page 344)

Savory Sole Provençal Ⓠ Ⓜ

Serves: 4 (4 ounces cooked fish = 1 serving)

Sole and flounder are low-fat, mild fishes that lend themselves beautifully to this savory sauce.

4 5-ounce fillets of sole or flounder
Juice of ½ lemon (about 2 tablespoons)
Ground pepper
2 large cloves garlic, minced
½ red pepper, diced

½ green pepper, diced
1 cup diced Italian plum tomatoes
1 teaspoon olive oil

6 tablespoons chopped green onion, for garnish

1. Season the fish with the lemon juice and pepper, and place in a shallow microwave dish.
2. Mix the garlic, green pepper, and tomato with the olive oil and spoon the mixture over the fish.
3. Cover tightly with microwave plastic wrap and microwave on high for 5 minutes, or until fish flakes with fork.

To Serve: Place the fish on a serving plate and top with sauce and vegetables. Sprinkle with green onions.

Per serving: 54 mg cholesterol, 0.49 gm saturated fat, 2.6 gm total fat, 0.6 gm fiber, 97 mg sodium, 132 calories, 0 gm trans fat

Chinese Cabbage and Sliced Radish Slaw
♦ Red Snapper with Curry Sauce ♦
Brown Rice (page 133)
Steamed Zucchini Spears and Red Peppers
Mango Slices with Blueberries

Red Snapper with Curry Sauce Ⓠ

Serves: 4 (4 ounces cooked fish = 1 serving)

Red snapper is a low-fat, delicate-flavored fish that is made even more appealing with this flavorful sauce.

4 5-ounce red snapper fillets
Juice of ½ lemon
½ teaspoon onion powder
1 teaspoon salt-free vegetable
**   seasoning**

2 green onions, sliced, for garnish

Curry Sauce:
2 teaspoons minced shallot
1 teaspoon sesame oil
½ cup nonfat plain yogurt
1–2 teaspoons curry powder
½ ripe banana, mashed

1. Sprinkle the fish with the lemon juice and seasonings and broil 5 minutes or until the fish flakes.

2. *To make the curry sauce,* in a 6-inch nonstick skillet, sauté the shallots in sesame oil 2 to 3 minutes. Do not brown. Remove the skillet from the heat, add the yogurt, 1 teaspoon curry powder, and banana. Blend well and taste. If desired, add more curry.

To Serve: Place the fish on a warm platter, top with curry sauce, and sprinkle with green onion slices.

Per serving: 43 mg cholesterol, 0.55 gm saturated fat, 2.9 gm total fat, 0.6 gm fiber, 96 mg sodium, 157 calories, 0 gm trans fat

---

*Red-skinned Delicious apples are higher in antioxidants—
wash before eating the peel.*

Mixed Greens with Kidney Beans
♦ Salmon Loaf with Creole Sauce ♦
Baked Potato
Steamed Broccoli Spears
Fresh Melon with Lime Wedge

Salmon Loaf with Creole Sauce

Serves: 8 (1 slice = 1 serving)

Using salmon, egg whites, whole grain bread, vegetables, and even oat bran, the cholesterol content is just 28 milligrams.

½ onion, quartered
1 carrot, quartered
1 small zucchini, quartered
½ green or red pepper, seeded and quartered
3 slices rye bread, crumbled and soaked in ¾ cup light soy milk
¼ cup oat bran
2 extra-large egg whites (egg substitutes may be used)
3 tablespoons lemon juice
2 teaspoons Worcestershire sauce

1 15½-ounce can pink salmon, drained, bones and skin removed
2 teaspoons baking powder

Creole Sauce:

1 15-ounce can sodium-reduced stewed or diced tomatoes, chopped
¼ green pepper, slivered
¼ red pepper, slivered
1 tablespoon cornstarch

1. Process the onion, carrot, zucchini, and pepper in a food processor until minced.
2. Add the soaked bread, oat bran, egg whites, lemon juice, and Worcestershire sauce. Blend well.
3. Add the salmon and baking powder and process just until combined.
4. Coat a 9 × 5-inch glass loaf pan with nonstick spray, press the salmon mixture into the pan, and bake in a preheated 425° oven for 45 minutes or until loaf is firm and browned.
5. *To make the creole sauce,* combine all the ingredients and heat in a 1-quart saucepan until shiny, stirring constantly.

To Serve: Allow the loaf to stand 10 minutes, then unmold on a heated platter, top with creole sauce, and surround with broccoli spears.

Variation: Layer 1½ cups chopped mixed vegetables (broccoli, carrots, and peas) in the center of the loaf mixture and bake as directed.

Per serving: 28 mg cholesterol, 0.95 gm saturated fat, 4.1 gm total fat, 2.3 gm fiber, 175 mg sodium, 149 calories, 0 gm trans fat

◆ Brochettes of Scallops and Scrod ◆
Bulgur Wheat Pilaf (page 315)
Steamed Broccoli
Kiwi and Orange Slices

Brochettes of Scallops and Scrod

Serves: 4 (1 brochette, 3 ounces cooked fish = 1 serving)

Since scallops are one of the shellfish relatively low in cholesterol (see chart page 19), this delectable dish may be served and enjoyed without worry.

8 1-ounce sea scallops, rinsed
8 ounces scrod, sea bass, or
  halibut, cut into 8 equal pieces
½ small green pepper, seeded and
  quartered
½ small red pepper, seeded and
  quartered
4 small wedges mild onion
1 small zucchini, cut into 4 chunks
8 mushroom caps, cleaned
4 fresh water chestnuts, rinsed,
  scrubbed, and peeled or 4
  canned whole water chestnuts
  (optional)

4 bamboo skewers (soaked for 10
  minutes in cold water)

Marinade:
2 tablespoons sodium-reduced soy
  sauce
3 tablespoons frozen unsweetened
  pineapple juice concentrate
1 teaspoon grated fresh ginger
½ teaspoon finely minced garlic
¼ teaspoon sesame oil
Few grains crushed red pepper
  flakes
¼ cup plum wine or sake

1. Combine all marinade ingredients in a plastic bag.
2. Wash all seafood under cold tap water, dry thoroughly with paper towels, and add the vegetables to the plastic bag. Marinate several hours

in the refrigerator. Add fish and marinate 15 minutes more. Remove 30 minutes before preparing.

3. Thread a mushroom, a scallop, an onion, a zucchini chunk, scrod, red pepper, another scallop, green pepper, scrod, and another mushroom onto a skewer. Repeat on the remaining three skewers.

4. Broil or barbecue 3 to 4 inches from high heat for 5 to 7 minutes, turning frequently. Brush with the remaining marinade while cooking. Do not overcook; marinated fish cooks more rapidly.

To Serve: Arrange the brochettes on a bed of wheat pilaf and surround with broccoli spears.

Per serving: 45 mg cholesterol, 0.28 gm saturated fat, 2 gm total fat, 0.8 gm fiber, 125 mg sodium, 135 calories, 0 gm trans fat

Tomato Bouillon (page 95) with Whole Wheat Bread Sticks
♦ Fish Curry with Condiments ♦
in a Ring of Steamed Brown Rice (page 133)
Steamed Cauliflower and Broccoli Florets
Mango Sorbet

Fish Curry with Condiments Ⓠ

Serves: 6 (1¼ cups = 1 serving)

1½ pounds sea bass, cod, and/or monkfish, cut into 1-inch cubes
Juice of ½ lemon
Freshly ground white pepper
2 teaspoons salt-free vegetable seasoning
1 large onion, finely chopped
1 clove garlic, finely chopped
2 celery stalks, thinly sliced
3 tablespoons dry white wine
½ pound fresh mushrooms, sliced
½ green pepper, seeded and cut into 1-inch squares

½ red pepper, seeded and cut into 1-inch squares
1½ teaspoons curry powder, or to taste
1½ cups organic vegetable broth
1½ tablespoons cornstarch mixed with ¼ cup vegetable broth

Condiments:
Sliced green onion, plumped dark raisins,° toasted almond slivers, unsweetened banana flakes, and chutney

1. Sprinkle the fish with the lemon juice, white pepper, and vegetable seasoning.

2. Sauté the onion, garlic, and celery in the white wine until transparent.

3. Add the mushrooms, peppers, and curry; stir to combine. Add the broth and continue to cook about 5 minutes.

4. Add the seasoned fish, bring to a simmer, and cook 5 minutes.

5. Stir in the cornstarch mixture and simmer until the sauce is shiny and coats the spoon. Taste and adjust seasonings.

To Serve: Spoon a ring of steamed brown rice onto a warm serving platter. Place the curried fish in the center, surround with cauliflower and broccoli florets, and accompany with condiments served in small separate bowls.

Per serving: 49 mg cholesterol, 0.2 gm saturated fat, 1.2 gm total fat, 0.9 gm fiber, 79 mg sodium, 145 calories, 0 gm trans fat

*To plump raisins, place 1 cup of raisins in a single layer on a plate and sprinkle with 2 tablespoons of fresh orange juice or apple juice. Cover tightly with microwave plastic wrap and cook on high for 1 minute.

Make smarter food choices, not needless sacrifices.

◆

One small apple with skin has five grams of fiber.

Watercress and Shredded Carrot Salad with
Low-Calorie Orange Vinaigrette
♦ Microwave-Poached Whitefish
with
Mustard Sauce in Lime Shells ♦
French-Cut Green Beans
Roasted Sliced Beets
Parsleyed New Potatoes
Mixed Berry Crisp

Microwave-Poached Whitefish with Mustard Sauce in Lime Shells Ⓠ Ⓜ

Serves: 4 (4 ounces cooked fish = 1 serving)

4 5-ounce whitefish or salmon
  fillets, skinned
Freshly ground white pepper
½ teaspoon dried thyme, or 1½
  teaspoons fresh thyme
1 small onion, coarsely chopped
1 carrot, coarsely chopped
1 stalk celery with leaves, coarsely
  chopped

Few sprigs fresh parsley
½ cup dry white wine

Mustard Sauce
½ cup nonfat plain yogurt
½ teaspoon fines herbes
1 teaspoon Dijon mustard
2 limes, halved and juiced (save
  the juice for future use)

1. Place the fish in a 9- or 10-inch round glass baking dish (a pie plate will do nicely) and sprinkle with the pepper, thyme, and vegetables.

2. Pour the wine over the fish. Cover tightly with microwave plastic wrap and microwave on high for 5 minutes. Let stand in poaching liquid for 2 to 3 minutes before serving.

3. *To make the mustard sauce*, combine the first three ingredients and mix thoroughly. Cut a slice from the bottom of each lime half (so that they do not tip) and spoon sauce into the half-lime shells.

To Serve: Remove fish with vegetables from the liquid and place on a heated platter. Surround with bundles of green beans, steamed new potatoes, and sliced beets. Garnish with mustard-sauce-filled lime shells.

Per serving: 64 mg cholesterol, 0.21 gm saturated fat, 5.2 gm total fat, 0.8 gm fiber, 116 mg sodium, 115 calories, 0 gm trans fat

♦ Salmon Mousse with Dill ♦
Steamed Asparagus Spears
Pickled Beets, Hearts of Palm, and Corn Salad
Pumpernickel Bread
Fresh Fruit Compote (page 322)

Salmon Mousse with Dill

Serves: 6 as an entrée or 16 as an appetizer

1 15½-ounce can salmon, skinned, boned, and drained (save juice), or 1¼-pound salmon fillets, poached (page 173), save the liquid

1½ tablespoons plain gelatin

⅔ cup hot, organic vegetable broth

½ cup Fage plain yogurt

3 tablespoons light-style mayonnaise

1 tablespoon sweet relish

1 tablespoon white horseradish, drained

1 tablespoon lemon juice

2 tablespoons tarragon vinegar

2 tablespoons grated onion

1 teaspoon Worcestershire sauce

½ cup diced red pepper, or 1 2-ounce jar chopped pimientos, drained

¼ cup finely diced celery

2 tablespoons chopped fresh dill

2 bunches fresh dill, for garnish

1 bunch Belgian endive, 2 tablespoons nonfat plain yogurt, and 1 tablespoon chopped black olives, for garnish (optional)

1. Flake the salmon in a mixing bowl with a fork.
2. Soften the gelatin in the salmon juice or ½ cup poaching liquid; add the hot vegetable broth and stir until liquefied.
3. Add the remaining ingredients to the salmon and blend.
4. Add the liquefied gelatin and mix thoroughly.
5. Turn the salmon mixture into a 3-cup fish mold coated with nonstick spray, cover with plastic wrap, and chill in the refrigerator for 5 to 6 hours until firm, or overnight.

To Unmold and Serve: Loosen the edges of the mousse with a metal spatula, invert the mold on a platter, and shake gently until mousse is unmolded. Garnish with bunches of fresh dill. Surround the mousse with leaves of Belgian endive that have a dollop of yogurt and a dab of chopped black olives if you like.

Per serving as an entrée: 43 mg cholesterol, 0.46 gm saturated fat, 5 gm total fat, 0.3 gm fiber, 146 mg sodium, 141 calories, 0 gm trans fat

Per serving as an appetizer: 16 mg cholesterol, 0.17 gm saturated fat, 1.9 gm total fat, 0.1 gm fiber, 55 mg sodium, 53 calories, 0 gm trans fat

Lettuce Wedges with Herbed Yogurt Dressing
♦ Trout Stuffed with Veggies ♦
Steamed Quinoa (page 133)
Julienned Green Beans with Toasted Almonds
Blueberry Meringue Cobbler (page 347)

Trout Stuffed With Veggies Ⓠ

Serves: 1

The freshest and odor-free fish should be used. It should have fresh eyes and slippery skin. Stiff fish is indicative of poor quality. Remember, the fresher the trout the more delicious the dish.

**1 10-ounce whole trout, boned
with the head and tail remaining**

Stuffing:
1 tablespoon olive oil
¼ cup onion, minced
¼ cup celery, minced
¼ cup carrots, minced

½ cup mushrooms, chopped
**½ teaspoon fresh thyme or Herbes
de Provence**
1 tablespoon bread crumbs
2 ounces bay shrimp or crab
Pepper to taste
½ lemon

1. Mince vegetables in food processor.
2. Place oil in small saucepan. Add veggies, Herbes de Provence, pepper, and mix.
3. Cover pan and steam until soft.
4. Remove from heat and add shellfish. Mix thoroughly.
5. Season cavity of fish with a bit of lemon juice, salt, and pepper.

6. Stuff fish with vegetables and place on a baking dish coated with olive-oil spray.

7. Coat the fish with olive-oil spray.

8. Place in preheated 450° oven and bake for 12 to 18 minutes or until fish flakes.

9. Brown lightly under broiler.

To Serve: Serve on heated plate with lemon wedges.

Per serving: 167.25 mg cholesterol, 6.41 gm saturated fat, 29.48 gm total fat, 2.57 gm fiber, 612.54 calories, 0 gm trans fat, 14.69 gm carbs, 5.42 gm sugar

Hearts of Romaine and Hearts of Palm with
Chopped Red Pepper Vinaigrette
♦ Seafood Jambalaya ♦
Spinach
Pitted Bing Cherries with Brandy

Seafood Jambalaya

Serves: 6 to 8 (2 ounces cooked fish = 1 serving)

1 tablespoon unbleached white flour
2 teaspoons extra-virgin olive oil
2 medium onions, chopped
3 cloves garlic, minced
2 cups defatted sodium-reduced chicken broth or clam juice
1 28-ounce can chopped San Marzano tomatoes with juice
1 cup sodium-reduced vegetable juice
1 cup diced celery with leaves
1 green pepper, seeded and chopped

1 bay leaf
2 teaspoons dried thyme, crushed
Few grains crushed red pepper flakes
1 teaspoon hot pepper sauce or Tabasco
2 tablespoons Worcestershire sauce
⅓ cup chopped fresh Italian parsley
1 cup converted or brown rice
8 ounces monkfish or sea bass, cut into 1-inch cubes
8 ounces fresh or canned lump crab meat

1. Brown the flour in the oil in a 5-quart nonstick saucepan. Add onions and garlic and stir 5 minutes or until wilted.

2. Add the broth, stir, and cook until slightly thickened.

3. Add the tomatoes, vegetable juice, celery, green pepper, seasonings, and parsley, and mix well. Simmer for 30 minutes.

4. Add the rice, cover, and simmer for 20 minutes (15 minutes for quick brown rice).

5. Stir in the fish and cook about 10 minutes.

6. Add the crab meat, stir, heat, and adjust seasonings (remove bay leaf).

To Serve: Spoon into warm soup plates.

Variation: Jambalaya may be cooked without the rice, and served over steamed rice.

Per serving: 35 mg cholesterol, 0.61 gm saturated fat, 3.4 gm total fat, 1.8 gm fiber, 493 mg sodium, 201 calories, 0 gm trans fat

---

Dry-roasted edamame (soy bean) is one of the oldest and most healthful snack foods—¼ cup has 14 grams of protein and 8 grams of fiber.

♦

To reduce or control diabetes: lose weight, exercise, and follow a carbohydrate-reduced diet prescribed by a dietician, nutritionist, or diabetes educator.

Roasted Pepper & Red Onion Salad
♦ Capellini with Clams in Red Sauce ♦
Braised Escarole or Rapini
Hot Crusty Sourdough Bread
Ribière Grapes

Capellini with Clams in Red Sauce Ⓠ

Serves: 8

The good news is that clams and mussels are both low in cholesterol as well as saturated fat. The flavor is delicious; save some bread and enjoy the soup.

1 tablespoon extra-virgin olive oil
2 shallots, finely chopped
3 large cloves garlic, finely minced
2 carrots, thinly sliced
½ teaspoon crushed red pepper flakes
¾ cup clam juice
¾ cup dry white wine
16 ounces crushed San Marzano tomatoes
⅔ cup chopped fresh Italian parsley
4 dozen clams and/or mussels, well scrubbed under cold running water

2 tablespoons fresh oregano, finely chopped, or 1 tablespoon dried oregano, crushed
10 ounces capellini (angel hair pasta), cooked al dente and drained
2 tablespoons fresh basil, finely chopped, or 1 tablespoon dried basil, crushed
Freshly ground pepper
1 tablespoon shredded Parmesan cheese, optional

1. Combine the olive oil, shallots, garlic, carrots, and red pepper flakes in a 4-quart nonstick saucepan or casserole and cook over medium heat until onions are soft, not browned. Add clam juice, wine, and tomatoes. Cook 5 minutes.

2. Add the clams, ½ cup of the parsley, and the oregano and stir to coat clams. Cover, bring to a boil, lower heat, and cook until clams are open (about 8 minutes). *Discard the clams that do not open.*

3. Add the drained pasta, basil, pepper, and mix lightly.

To Serve: Divide the pasta mixture with liquid among four deep heated soup bowls. Surround with *open* clams, sprinkle with the remaining chopped parsley, and serve immediately with hot crusty bread.

Per serving: 55 mg cholesterol, 0.75 gm saturated fat, 4.9 gm total fat, 2.5 gm fiber, 121 mg sodium, 326 calories, 0 gm trans fat

Marinated Tomato and Cucumber Salad
♦ Salmon Tetrazzini ♦
Steamed Brussels Sprouts
Cinnamon Baked Apple

Salmon Tetrazzini Ⓠ Ⓜ

Serves: 8 (2 ounces cooked fish = 1 serving)

2 teaspoons canola or cold-pressed safflower oil
1 medium onion, chopped
2 large cloves garlic, minced
¼ teaspoon white pepper
⅓ cup unbleached white flour
1 teaspoon salt-free vegetable seasoning
¼ teaspoon freshly ground nutmeg
4 cups nonfat or 1% milk (including drained salmon liquid, if canned salmon is used)
2 teaspoons Worcestershire sauce
1 bay leaf
2 stalks celery, diced
1 small green pepper, seeded and diced
1 small red pepper, seeded and diced

1½ cups sliced fresh mushroom caps
2 tablespoons grated Parmesan cheese
8 ounces spaghettini, soba noodles, or linguine, cooked al dente
1 15½-ounce can salmon, drained (save liquid), skinned, and boned, or 1¼-pound salmon, poached (page 173, save the liquid)
1 tablespoon grated Parmesan cheese mixed with 2 tablespoons dry bread crumbs

3 tablespoons chopped fresh dill, for garnish

1. Heat the oil in a 3-quart nonstick saucepan with the onion, garlic, and pepper. Sauté 3 minutes.
2. Add the flour and seasonings; stir to combine.

3. Add the milk, Worcestershire sauce, bay leaf, celery, peppers, mushrooms, and cheese and stir over medium heat until sauce coats the spoon. Remove the bay leaf.

4. Combine half the sauce with the cooked pasta and place in the bottom of a 3-quart shallow casserole.

5. Flake the salmon, stir into remaining sauce, and pour over pasta.

6. Sprinkle with the cheese mixture and bake in a preheated 350° oven for 25 to 30 minutes until bubbly, or microwave on high for 12 minutes.

To Serve: Sprinkle with chopped dill and serve hot.

Per serving: 33 mg cholesterol, 1.01 gm saturated fat, 4.6 gm total fat, 1.4 gm fiber, 172 mg sodium, 275 calories, 0 gm trans fat

Red and White Cabbage Slaw
♦ Turbot with Spanish Sauce ♦
Corn on the Cob
Snow Peas and Carrot Slices
Stewed Prunes with Fresh Pineapple Chunks

Turbot with Spanish Sauce Ⓠ Ⓜ

Serves: 6 (3½ ounces cooked fish = 1 serving)

1¾ pounds turbot, haddock, or
   cod, cut into 6 portions
Juice of 1 lime
2 teaspoons extra-virgin olive oil
1 small onion, chopped
2 large cloves garlic, minced
2½ cups chopped San Marzano
   tomatoes, canned
½ green pepper, seeded and thinly
   sliced

2 tablespoons tomato paste
¼ cup chopped fresh Italian
   parsley
½ teaspoon Italian herb blend,
   crushed
1 bay leaf
¼ cup dry white wine

1. Sprinkle the fish with the lime juice and set aside for 10 minutes.

2. Place the oil, onions, and garlic in a round shallow glass dish, cover tightly with microwave plastic wrap, and microwave on high for 2 minutes.

3. Add the remaining ingredients except the fish, stir, and cover with plastic. Cook on high for 6 minutes, stirring one time during cooking.

4. Remove the bay leaf and add the fish to the sauce. Cover with plastic and microwave on high for about 6 minutes, or until fish flakes with fork.

To Serve: Arrange fish with sauce on heated platter and surround with pea pods and carrots.

Per serving: 47 mg cholesterol, 0.39 gm saturated fat, 2.6 gm total fat, 1.1 gm fiber, 78 mg sodium, 138 calories, 0 gm trans fat

Marinated Mushroom Salad
♦ Piquant Broiled Mahimahi with Mango Salsa ♦
Baked Sweet Potato (Yam)
Brussel Sprouts
Angel Food Cake (page 327) with Sliced Fresh Strawberries

Piquant Broiled Mahimahi with Mango Salsa Ⓠ

Serves: 4 (3 ounces cooked fish = 1 serving)

This flavorful fish comes from the dolphin family (but not Flipper). It is delicious grilled, sautéed, or baked.

2 teaspoons Worcestershire sauce
2 tablespoons white wine
1 garlic clove, minced
¼ teaspoon onion powder
½ teaspoon Dijon mustard

Juice of 1 lime
Freshly ground pepper
1 pound mahimahi or sea bass, cut into 4 pieces
Mango Salsa (page 329)

1. Combine the first seven ingredients in a small jar or custard cup and blend thoroughly.

2. Brush the fish on one side with the sauce and broil or barbecue 4 inches from heat for 3 minutes.

3. Turn the fish and cook, basting frequently with sauce, until fish flakes with fork. (Total cooking time about 8 to 9 minutes per inch of thickness.)

To Serve: Place fish on platter, spoon salsa onto fish, and surround with potatoes and brussels sprouts.

Per serving: 43 mg cholesterol, 1.2 gm saturated fat, 4.4 gm total fat, 0 gm fiber, 132 mg sodium, 137 calories, 0 gm trans fat

Three-Bean Salad Vinaigrette
♦ Tuna-Stuffed Mushrooms with Creole Sauce ♦
Bulgur Wheat (page 133) with Peas
Persimmon Freeze (page 323)

Tuna-Stuffed Mushrooms with Creole Sauce ⓠ

Serves: 4 as an entrée (3 stuffed mushrooms = 1 serving)

or 1 as an appetizer (1 stuffed mushroom = 1 serving)

1 small onion, quartered
½ red pepper, seeded and
  quartered
1 stalk celery, quartered
1 large clove garlic
16 large cremini mushrooms,
  cleaned and stemmed (save
  stems for vegetable mixture)
2 teaspoons extra-virgin olive oil
½ teaspoon dried Italian herb
  blend
2 ounces chopped pimiento,
  drained
½ cup soft whole wheat bread
  crumbs

2 tablespoons mashed tofu
1 teaspoon Worcestershire sauce
1 6½-ounce can salt-reduced
  light-meat tuna in water, flaked,
  or 6½ ounces fresh or canned
  lump crab meat
1 tablespoon light mayonnaise
Freshly ground pepper
1½ tablespoons shredded
  Parmesan cheese

Creole Sauce:
1½ cups salt-reduced stewed
  tomatoes, chopped
1 teaspoon cornstarch

1. Chop the onion, red pepper, celery, garlic, and mushroom stems in the food processor.
2. Sauté the vegetable mixture in oil in a nonstick skillet for 5 minutes.
3. Add the herb blend, pimiento, bread crumbs, egg whites, Worcestershire sauce, tuna, mayonnaise, and pepper. Mix well with a fork.

4. Mound the mixture lightly into the mushroom caps and sprinkle with the cheese. Place in a shallow baking pan and bake in a preheated 400° oven 7 minutes or·until lightly browned.

5. *To prepare the creole sauce:* Combine the tomatoes and cornstarch in a 1-quart saucepan and mix thoroughly. Stir over medium heat until shiny.

To Serve: Place the mushrooms on a serving platter, and spoon hot sauce over them.

Per serving: 13 mg cholesterol, 0.83 gm saturated fat, 3.9 gm total fat, 1.1 gm fiber, 191 mg sodium, 180 calories, 0 gm trans fat

Belgian Endive and Shredded Beet Salad
♦ Stir-Fried Scallops with Garlic, Mushrooms, and Snow Peas ♦
Steamed Wild Rice
Asparagus
Orange Baked Alaska (page 243)

Stir-Fried Scallops with Garlic, Mushrooms, and Snow Peas ⓠ

Serves: 4 (3 ounces cooked scallops = 1 serving)

2 teaspoons extra-virgin olive oil
1 ounce dried shiitake mushrooms
   (soaked 20 minutes in warm
   water, drained, stems removed,
   and sliced)
4 whole green onions, sliced
1 tablespoon lemon juice
1 tablespoon sodium-reduced soy
   sauce

Freshly ground pepper
3 cloves garlic, minced
1 pound bay scallops, thoroughly
   rinsed and drained
⅓ cup dry white wine mixed with 2
   teaspoons cornstarch
1 cup fresh or frozen snow peas,
   halved lengthwise

1. Place the oil in a nonstick skillet and add the mushrooms and green onions; sprinkle with the lemon juice, soy sauce, and pepper and stir-fry 2 to 3 minutes.

2. Add the garlic and sauté 1 minute.

3. Add the scallops and stir-fry until opaque.

4. Add the wine and snow peas and cook for several minutes.

To Serve: Place a mound of rice on a warm serving platter, spoon the scallop mixture on top.

Per serving: 37 mg cholesterol, 0.43 gm saturated fat, 3.3 gm total fat, 1.7 gm fiber, 310 mg sodium, 182 calories, 0 gm trans fat

Salad of Radicchio, Corn, and Hearts of Palm
♦ Grilled Red Snapper and Tomato ♦
Parsleyed Potatoes
Seasoned Green Beans
Cantaloupe with Strawberry Sauce

Grilled Red Snapper and Tomato Ⓠ

Serves: 4 (3 ounces cooked fish = 1 serving)

4 4-ounce fillets red snapper,
 halibut, or Spanish mackerel
¼ cup low-calorie oil-free Italian
 dressing
Freshly ground pepper
1½ teaspoons dried oregano,
 crushed

1 tablespoon freshly grated
 Parmesan cheese
2 ripe medium tomatoes, cut in
 half

Watercress sprigs, for garnish

1. Brush the fish with half of the salad dressing and sprinkle with pepper, oregano, and Parmesan cheese.

2. Arrange fish seasoned-side-down on a heated nonstick griddle or sauté pan and cook 3 minutes.

3. Brush the fish with the remaining salad dressing and turn. Place the tomato halves cut-side-down alongside the fish and continue grilling for 2 to 3 minutes or until fish flakes when tested with a fork. *Do not overcook.*

To Serve: Place the red snapper and tomato halves on a heated serving plate and garnish with watercress.

Variation: Halibut, tuna, or salmon fillets may be substituted for the red snapper and served as a salad on shredded romaine with the grilled tomato and dilled steamed green beans.

Per serving: 41 mg cholesterol, 0.58 gm saturated fat, 2 gm total fat, 0.5 gm fiber, 237 mg sodium, 134 calories, 0 gm trans fat

Salad of Julienne Carrots and Jicama with Romaine
♦ Broiled Swordfish Paillard with Fresh Salsa ♦
Peas and Artichoke Hearts
Warm Corn Tortillas
Fresh Raspberries with Mango Puree

Broiled Swordfish Paillard with Fresh Salsa Ⓠ

Serves: 4 (3 ounces cooked fish = 1 serving)

Paillard refers to a thin slice of fish, poultry, or meat. It need be broiled on only one side. I serve swordfish very infrequently because it is believed to have excessive levels of methylmercury.

4 4-ounce swordfish, ocean perch, or Spanish mackerel fillets, cut ½-inch thick
1½ tablespoons lime juice or balsamic vinegar
Garlic powder
Freshly ground pepper

Fresh Salsa:
2 medium tomatoes, chopped
½ small onion, finely chopped
2 tablespoons canned chilies, chopped, or 1 fresh jalapeño pepper, chopped
1–2 tablespoons lime juice
3 tablespoons fresh chopped parsley or cilantro

1. Preheat the broiler. Brush the fish with the lime juice and sprinkle with garlic powder and pepper.
2. Place the fish in a broiler pan and broil for 3 to 4 minutes on one side only. *Do not overcook.*

3. *To make the fresh salsa:* Combine all the ingredients in a bowl and blend with a fork.

To Serve: Place the fish on a platter and pass the salsa.

NOTE: Fresh Salsa is also wonderful served with warm corn tortillas as an appetizer or as a topping for broiled chicken or baked potatoes.

Per Serving: 43 mg cholesterol, 1.23 gm saturated fat, 4.6 gm total fat, 0.8 gm fiber, 107 mg sodium, 155 calories, 0 gm trans fat

Marinated Broccoli Rapini and Red Pepper Salad
♦ Mediterranean Fish Soup ♦
Crusty Whole Wheat Baguette
Mixed Berries and Oat Nut Slices (page 350)

Mediterranean Fish Soup ℚ

Serves: 6 to 8 (1½ cups = 1 serving)

Yield: about 9 to 10 cups

This easy-to-make dish can be partially prepared the day before. It is a wonderful choice for informal entertaining. Like most soups, this one tastes even better the next day.

3 shallots or 1 small onion, minced
4 cloves garlic, minced
2 teaspoons extra-virgin olive oil
1 28-ounce can crushed San Marzano tomatoes with juice
1 teaspoon chopped fresh oregano, or ½ teaspoon dried oregano
1 teaspoon chopped fresh thyme, or ½ teaspoon dried thyme
Few grains crushed red pepper

1 bay leaf
1½ cups organic vegetable broth
½ cup dry red or white wine
6 ounces frozen okra, sliced
3 tablespoons chopped Italian parsley
½ pound sea bass or red snapper, in 1-inch cubes
½ pound monkfish, in 1-inch cubes
½ pound small shrimp or bay scallops

1. In a large saucepan, sauté the shallots and garlic in the oil until lightly colored.

2. Add all the remaining ingredients except the fish, okra, and parsley and simmer uncovered about 20 minutes. This dish may be prepared ahead to this point and refrigerated until the next day.

3. Add the okra, parsley, and fish, cover, and cook about 6-8 minutes. Taste and adjust seasoning.

To Serve: Spoon into shallow heated soup bowls and serve with lots of crusty whole wheat bread.

Per serving: 42 mg cholesterol, 0.61 gm saturated fat, 3.5 gm total fat, 2.2 gm fiber, 267 mg sodium, 163 calories, 0 gm trans fat

Shredded Carrot and Zucchini Slaw
♦ Salmon, Spinach, and Rice Casserole ♦
Broiled Tomato Halves
Broccoli Spears
Seasonal Fresh Fruit

Salmon, Spinach, and Rice Casserole Ⓠ Ⓜ

Serves: 4

Casseroles always provide an easy, convenient method of serving because they can be prepared well ahead of time.

2 teaspoons canola oil or cold-pressed safflower oil
½ cup chopped onion
1 10-ounce package frozen chopped spinach, defrosted and drained
Freshly ground nutmeg
1 7½-ounce can salmon, drained (save liquid), bones removed, and flaked
2 cups cooked brown rice (page 133)
2 tablespoons lemon juice
½ cup chopped celery with leaves

½ cup chopped red pepper
½ cup chopped zucchini
2 whole green onions, sliced
2 teaspoons dried dill
2 extra-large egg whites, slightly beaten
½ cup part-skim ricotta cheese mixed with ¾ cup nonfat milk, drained salmon liquid, and 1 teaspoon dry or Dijon mustard
2 tablespoons dry bread crumbs mixed with 1 tablespoon grated Parmesan cheese

1. Microwave the oil and onions on high in a 10-inch glass pie plate or quiche pan for 2 minutes (or sauté in nonstick skillet until wilted and place in pie plate). Top with spinach and sprinkle with nutmeg.

2. Combine the salmon, rice, lemon juice, celery, red pepper, zucchini, green onion, dill, egg whites, and ricotta cheese mixture in a bowl. Stir lightly with a fork to blend; spoon on top of the spinach.

3. Sprinkle with the bread-crumb and cheese mixture.

4. Cook uncovered in a microwave oven on high for 12 to 15 minutes or in a preheated 400° oven for 35 minutes.

Per serving: 34 mg cholesterol, 2.92 gm saturated fat, 7.5 gm total fat, 5.1 gm fiber, 252 mg sodium, 306 calories, 0 gm trans fat

Tofu and Corn Soup (page 277)
Whole Wheat Bread Sticks
♦ Grilled Salmon Scallops on Mixed Greens ♦
with
Dijon Mustard, Chili Pepper, and Yogurt Sauce
Fresh Tomato and Green Pepper Salsa
Jicama and Orange Relish
Boysenberries with Vanilla Yogurt

Grilled Salmon Scallops on Mixed Greens with Assorted Salsas Ⓠ

Serves: 4 (3 ounces cooked fish = 1 serving)

8 cups torn assorted greens
½ cup low-calorie oil-free
    vinaigrette mixed with 1
    teaspoon extra-virgin olive oil
12 small leaves radicchio
16-ounce salmon fillet, sliced into
    12 thin scallops
Juice of ½ lemon

Dijon Mustard, Chili Pepper,
and Yogurt Sauce:
¼ cup nonfat plain yogurt mixed
    with 2 tablespoons finely
    diced jalapeño peppers and 2
    teaspoons Dijon mustard

*Fresh Tomato and Green
Pepper Salsa:*
**3 diced Italian plum tomatoes
mixed with ¼ finely diced green
pepper, ¼ finely diced medium
white onion, and 1 tablespoon
lime juice**

Jicama and Orange Relish:
**1 large navel orange, peeled and
diced, mixed with ⅔ cup finely
diced jicama or water chestnuts**

1. Prepare the salsas.
2. Toss the greens lightly with the vinaigrette and divide among four serving plates. Place three small radicchio leaves around the greens on each plate and fill each leaf with a quarter of the prepared salsas.
3. Season the salmon scallops with the lemon juice and sear in a hot nonstick skillet 1 minute on each side.
4. Place the hot salmon scallops on top of the dressed greens and serve.

Per serving: 45 mg cholesterol, 0.75 gm saturated fat, 4.9 gm total fat, 3.7 gm fiber, 131 mg sodium, 204 calories

---

*Smaller portion sizes, good nutrition, and regular
exercise are still the most important parts of
maintaining a healthy lifestyle.*

♦

"To lengthen thy life, lessen thy meals."
—Benjamin Franklin

◆ Cajun Blackened Redfish ◆
Roast Potatoes with Basil (page 311)
Sautéed Broccoli with Garlic
Dilled Cucumber and Sliced Onion Salad
Lemony Ricotta Cheesecake

Cajun Blackened Redfish ⓠ

Serves: 4 (3½ ounces cooked fish = 1 serving)

Cajun food lovers should avoid catfish, even "farmed catfish," these days. The Center for Science in the Public Interest cautions us to avoid catfish and carp "since they are bottom feeders and are particularly vulnerable to contamination from tainted sediments." However, red snapper, pompano, or redfish are good substitutes.

4 5-ounce red snapper, pompano, or redfish fillets (about ½-inch thick)
Juice of ½ lemon
2 teaspoons spicy Hungarian paprika°

½ teaspoon each white pepper, freshly ground black pepper, cayenne pepper, celery seed, and garlic and onion powders°
1 teaspoon dried thyme, crushed°

1. Wash the fish in cold water. Sprinkle with lemon juice.
2. Blend the spices together, place on waxed paper, and press into both sides of each piece of fish.
3. Heat a heavy iron skillet coated with nonstick spray over high heat, add fish, and grill 3 to 4 minutes on each side, depending upon thickness of fish. Fish may also be cooked on the oiled grill of a barbecue. Serve immediately.

Per serving: 47 mg cholesterol, 0.41 gm saturated fat, 2 gm total fat, 0.5 gm fiber, 58 mg sodium, 137 calories

°Substitute 2 or 3 teaspoons salt-free commercial Cajun seasoning for all the spices listed if you like.

Caesar Salad (page 91)
♦ Flounder with Creole Sauce ♦
French Green Beans
Pureed Rutabaga
Fresh Fruit Cup with Mint

Flounder with Creole Sauce Ⓠ

Serves: 4 (3 ounces cooked fish = 1 serving)

2 teaspoons extra-virgin olive oil
½ small onion, finely chopped
2 cloves garlic, minced
½ small green pepper, seeded and diced
1 cup sliced fresh mushrooms
⅓ cup dry white wine
3 fresh plum tomatoes, finely chopped
Few grains crushed red pepper flakes

1½ teaspoons Hungarian paprika
4 4-ounce flounder, sturgeon, or sea bass fillets
½ lemon
1 teaspoon salt-free vegetable seasoning
½ cup nonfat plain yogurt mixed with 1 teaspoon cornstarch
2 tablespoons chopped fresh parsley

1. Heat the oil in a nonstick saucepan. Add the onion, garlic, pepper, and mushrooms and sauté 2 minutes.

2. Add the wine, tomatoes, pepper flakes, and paprika and simmer 15 minutes to reduce. Remove from heat.

3. Sprinkle the flounder with the lemon juice and vegetable seasoning. Grill in a hot nonstick skillet (or broil) 3 to 4 minutes on each side.

4. Just after turning the fish, add the yogurt mixture and parsley to the tomato mixture and warm briefly. *Do not bring to a boil.*

To Serve: Spoon a quarter of the warm sauce onto each of four dinner plates and top with the hot fish.

Per serving: 58 mg cholesterol, 0.7 gm saturated fat, 4 gm total fat, 1.2 gm fiber, 122 mg sodium, 172 calories, 0 gm trans fat

Pickled Beet Salad
♦ Perfect Petrale Sole ♦
Baked Potato with Chives
Steamed Asparagus Spears
Stewed Rhubarb and Strawberries

Perfect Petrale Sole ℚ

Serves: 4 (3 ounces cooked fish = 1 serving)

½ cup nonfat plain yogurt
½ teaspoon salt-free vegetable
seasoning
½ teaspoon onion powder
¼ teaspoon garlic powder
⅛ teaspoon white pepper
1 pound petrale sole or flounder,
cut in 4 portions

⅔ cup dry bread crumbs mixed with
1 teaspoon salt-free vegetable
seasoning, 3 tablespoons
chopped parsley, and 2 teaspoons
grated Parmesan cheese

Lemon juice, lemon slices, and 1½
tablespoons rinsed capers, for
garnish (optional)

1. Combine the yogurt with the seasonings and coat the petrale sole on both sides with the mixture. Then dip the sole into the bread crumb mixture.

2. Place the sole on a rack coated with olive oil spray on a nonstick baking sheet and bake in a preheated 450° oven for 12 to 15 minutes or until golden brown.

To Serve: Place the sole on a warm serving platter, surround with asparagus spears, and sprinkle with lemon juice, lemon slices, and capers.

Per serving: 62 mg cholesterol, 0.65 gm saturated fat, 2.2 gm total fat, 0.1 gm fiber, 224 mg sodium, 174 calories, 0 gm trans fat

Celery Soup (page 274)
♦ Helen's Orange Roughy with a Vegetable Mélange ♦
Steamed Zucchini Spears
Poached Pears and Prunes (page 320)

Helen's Orange Roughy with a Vegetable Mélange Ⓠ Ⓜ

Serves: 4 (4 ounces cooked fish = 1 serving)

1 large onion, thinly sliced
½ green pepper, seeded and sliced
½ red pepper, seeded and sliced
1¼ pounds orange roughy,
   flounder, or cod, cut into 4
   portions
¼ teaspoon white pepper

½ teaspoon garlic powder
2 tablespoons dry vermouth
2 tablespoons fresh orange juice
8 mushroom caps, thinly sliced
8 slices dehydrated tomatoes, or 4
   cherry tomatoes, halved

1. Place the sliced onion in a 9-inch baking dish coated with nonstick cooking spray. Cover with microwave plastic wrap and microwave on high for 2 minutes.

2. Add the green and red pepper slices, cover, and microwave on high for 1 minute.

3. Season the fish with the white pepper and garlic powder and arrange fish over the onions, moving the pepper slices to top fish.

4. Pour the vermouth and orange juice over the fish; add the sliced mushrooms and tomatoes.

5. Cover and microwave on high for 4 minutes or until fish flakes with a fork.

Per serving: 35 mg cholesterol, 0.2 gm saturated fat, 8.1 gm total fat, 1 gm fiber, 74 mg sodium, 178 calories, 0 gm trans fat

---

"Eat breakfast like a king, lunch like a prince, but eat dinner like a pauper."—Adele Davis

Poultry

Crisp Green Salad with Shredded Red Cabbage
with Low-Calorie Ranch Dressing
♦ Chunky Turkey Chili ♦
Sourdough Rolls
Bowl of Red and Green Grapes

Chunky Turkey Chili ⓠ

Serves: 8 (1¼ cups = 1 serving)

Chili is always a favorite of mine for informal menus. This chili is particularly great not only because it tastes terrific, but also because the beans, high in soluble fiber, help to lower cholesterol. In this case the traditional ground beef is replaced by low-cholesterol low-fat turkey with no sacrifice in flavor.

1 small onion, quartered
3 garlic cloves
3 stalks celery, quartered
1 green pepper, quartered
2 teaspoons canola oil
8 ounces turkey breast fillet
 (cooked or raw), diced
¼ cup dry white or red wine
1–2 tablespoons chili seasoning
1 teaspoon dried thyme, crushed
1 teaspoon dried oregano, crushed

1 teaspoon spicy salt-free
 vegetable seasoning
1 28-ounce can crushed San
 Marzano tomatoes, in puree
1 15½-ounce can kidney beans,
 drained and rinsed, or 2 cups
 cooked beans, (page 131)
1 15½-ounce can garbanzo beans,
 pinto beans, or black beans,
 drained and rinsed, or 2 cups
 cooked beans (page 131)

1. Coarsely chop the onion, garlic, celery, and green pepper in the food processor or blender; then sauté for 3 minutes in the oil in nonstick 2-quart saucepan.

2. Add the diced turkey and sauté for 5 minutes, stirring constantly.

3. Add the remaining ingredients, cover, and bring to a simmer for 20 minutes, stirring occasionally. Taste and adjust seasonings.

4. Serve with toppings—chopped red onion, light sour cream, and diced Galaxy Veggie cheese slices.

Variation: To make *vegetarian chili*, substitute 1½ cups chopped carrots and 1½ cups chopped zucchini or 3 cups chopped eggplant for the turkey.

Per serving: 20 mg cholesterol, 0.59 gm saturated fat, 3.8 gm total fat, 4.4 gm fiber, 208 mg sodium, 216 calories

Tomato Bisque
♦ Turkey Roulades Stuffed with
Asparagus, Carrots, and Red Pepper ♦
Steamed Green Beans with Water Chestnuts
Barley Pilaf
Pineapple Chunks with Fresh Strawberry Sauce (page 319)

Turkey Roulades Stuffed with Asparagus, Carrots, and Red Pepper Ⓠ Ⓜ

Serves: 4 (2 roulades = 1 serving)

Ordinary raw turkey slices, sold in packages at your market (your butcher may also have turkey breast slices available), can be transformed into an extraordinary dinner for guests.

8 2-ounce slices raw turkey breast,
  ½ inch thick
Juice of ½ lemon
2 teaspoons salt-free vegetable
  seasoning
Freshly ground pepper
1 teaspoon extra-virgin olive oil
1 shallot, minced
½ 10-ounce package frozen
  chopped spinach, defrosted and
  drained
3 tablespoons part-skim ricotta
  cheese
1 tablespoon grated Parmesan
  cheese

Freshly ground nutmeg
Freshly ground pepper
16 thin asparagus spears
2 small carrots, quartered
  lengthwise
½ small red pepper, seeded and
  cut into 8 strips
⅓ cup crushed oat bran flake
  cereal mixed with 2 tablespoons
  oat bran, 1 tablespoon each
  dried parsley flakes and onion
  flakes, and ½ teaspoon each
  garlic powder and salt-free
  vegetable seasoning
Hungarian paprika

1. Flatten the turkey slices between sheets of plastic wrap to ¼-inch thickness. Remove the plastic and season the turkey with the lemon juice, vegetable seasoning, and pepper.

2. Microwave the oil and shallot on high in a 10-inch glass pie plate or quiche pan for 30 seconds.

3. Combine the shallot with the spinach, cheeses, nutmeg, and pepper and mix thoroughly.

4. Spread each turkey slice with about 1 tablespoon of the spinach mixture. Place two asparagus spears, one carrot stick, and one pepper strip crosswise on each fillet. Roll up and coat the roll with the oat mixture. Secure with a toothpick.

5. Arrange the roulades in a pie plate in spokelike fashion, sprinkle with paprika, cover tightly with microwave plastic wrap, and microwave on high for 6 minutes.

To Serve: Spoon hot barley pilaf onto serving platter, arrange roulades on top of barley, and surround with green beans and water chestnuts.

Per serving: 63 mg cholesterol, 1.93 gm saturated fat, 5.9 gm total fat, 3.5 gm fiber, 166 mg sodium, 244 calories, 0 gm trans fat

---

"The more you eat, the less flavor; the less you eat, the more flavor."—Chinese Proverb

---

♦

Lean meat has as much cholesterol as fatty meat.

Hearts of Romaine with Nancy's Light Blue Cheese Dressing
♦ Mini Turkey Loaves with Piquant Salsa ♦
Sweet Potato Chips (page 270)
Steamed Cauliflower, Carrots, and Corn
Cherry Meringue Cobbler (page 347)

Mini Turkey Loaves with Piquant Salsa

Yield: 6 loaves (1 miniloaf = 1 serving)

In this recipe, I have replaced ground beef with ground turkey breast, since white meat of turkey is the lowest in saturated fat of all meats.

1 small onion, chopped
½ small green pepper, seeded and
    chopped
1 large carrot, chopped
1 stalk celery with leaves, diced
1 large clove garlic, minced
2 teaspoons canola oil
Freshly ground pepper
1 pound ground turkey breast
½ cup rolled oats, soaked in ½ cup
    nonfat milk or defatted sodium-
    reduced chicken broth
¼ cup oat bran
2 extra-large egg whites, slightly
    beaten

1 tablespoon Worcestershire sauce
2 teaspoons Dijon mustard
1 teaspoon fines herbes or thyme
Hungarian paprika

Watercress, for garnish

Piquant Salsa:
1 8-ounce jar Newman's Own salsa
    or 1 cup Fresh Salsa (page 185)
1 teaspoon cornstarch
3 tablespoons fresh cilantro,
    chopped, optional

1. Place the onion, green pepper, carrot, celery, garlic, and oil in a nonstick skillet. Sauté 5 minutes; sprinkle with pepper.

2. In a large mixing bowl, combine the turkey, the onion mixture, and the soaked oats, oat bran, egg whites, Worcestershire sauce, mustard, and fines herbes. Mix lightly with a fork until well blended.

3. Shape into six miniloaves and place in a shallow nonstick baking pan. Sprinkle lightly with paprika.

4. Bake in the upper third of a preheated 375° oven for 25 minutes.

5. *To prepare the salsa:* Place the salsa and cornstarch in a saucepan and

blend. Heat 2 to 3 minutes, stirring constantly, until shiny and thickened. Add the cilantro and mix.

To Serve: Arrange the hot turkey loaves on a serving platter, top with hot salsa, and garnish with watercress.

Per serving: 46 mg cholesterol, 0.97 gm saturated fat, 4.7 gm total fat, 2.4 fiber, 129 mg sodium, 210 calories, 0 gm trans fat

Two-Pea Salad (200)
♦ Stuffed Peppers in the Pot ♦
Hearth Whole Grain Bread
Apple Crisp (page 318)

Stuffed Peppers in the Pot

Serves: 6 (1 pepper with 1⅓ ounces turkey = 1 serving)

A refreshing pea salad, a soup with peppers stuffed with brown rice, vegetables, and a small amount of ground turkey, whole grain bread, and apples—all high-fiber, low-fat foods perfect for your low-cholesterol lifestyle. The stuffed peppers are even more delicious prepared the day before.

2 teaspoons extra-virgin olive oil
1 small onion, chopped
1 large carrot, chopped
1 stalk celery with leaves, chopped
1 zucchini, chopped
2 large cloves garlic, minced
1 teaspoon dried oregano
Freshly ground pepper
1 cup ground turkey or chicken
   breast
2 teaspoons salt-free vegetable
   seasoning
1 tablespoon sodium-reduced soy
   sauce
¼ cup chopped fresh Italian parsley
1½ cups cooked brown rice (page
   133)

3 each small green and red
   peppers, tops removed and
   cleaned inside
3 tablespoons unbleached white
   flour
1 28-ounce can crushed San
   Marzano tomatoes, in puree
3 cups water or defatted vegetable
   broth
1 teaspoon crushed red pepper
   flakes
1 bay leaf
1 teaspoon dried thyme, crushed,
   or 1 tablespoon chopped fresh
   thyme

1. Heat the oil in a 6-inch nonstick skillet. Add the onion, carrot, celery, zucchini, garlic, oregano, and pepper and sauté around 5 minutes.

2. Place the turkey, corn, vegetable seasoning, soy sauce, parsley, cooked rice, and onion mixture into a mixing bowl and blend with a fork.

3. Fill the hollowed peppers with the turkey mixture.

4. Brown the flour in a 10-inch sauté pan or casserole until golden brown, stirring constantly. Add the tomatoes and water, stirring to blend in the flour. Bring to a boil.

5. Add the stuffed peppers, red pepper flakes, bay leaf, and thyme. Reduce heat, cover, and simmer 1½ to 2 hours over low heat, basting the peppers occasionally.

6. Taste and adjust seasonings before serving. Remove bay leaf.

To Serve: Spoon into shallow heated soup plates, allowing one pepper for each serving, and serve immediately. If using a casserole, serve directly at the table. Additional rice may be served and added to the soup plates at the table.

Per serving: 16 mg cholesterol, 0.73 gm saturated fat, 3.9 gm total fat, 4.3 gm fiber, 333 mg sodium, 211 calories

Two-Pea Salad ⓠ

Serves: 6 (1 cup = 1 serving)

This two-pea salad takes just about two minutes to prepare!

⅓ cup reduced-fat mayonnaise
2 tablespoons plain nonfat yogurt
½ cup chopped fresh dill
Freshly ground pepper
2 10-ounce packages frozen petits pois, defrosted, or 4 cups fresh peas, steamed and chilled
1 cup fresh pea pods or sugar snap peas, stem and strings removed

¼ cup chopped fresh chives or green onions
2 hard-cooked eggs (use whites only), diced
1 2-ounce jar chopped pimiento

Drained, crisp romaine lettuce leaves for serving

1. Combine mayonnaise, yogurt, dill, and freshly ground pepper in bowl.

2. Add peas, pea pods, green onions, egg whites, and pimiento. Mix lightly with a fork and sprinkle with chives.

3. Cover with plastic wrap and chill in refrigerator for 15 minutes before serving.

To Serve: Serve in a glass bowl lined with crisp romaine lettuce leaves or radicchio.

Per serving: 0 mg cholesterol, 0.01 gm saturated fat, 3.31 gm total fat, 4.75 gm fiber, 124.67 calories, 0 gm trans fat

Red Pepper and Corn Salad
♦ Turkey Ragout ♦
Braised Red Cabbage
Zucchini Circles
Raisin and Pear Bread Pudding (page 324)

Turkey Ragout ⓠ

Serves: 8 (3 ounces cooked turkey = 1 serving)

We usually think of red meat in stews; however, this hearty peasant-style turkey ragout provides wonderful flavor without excess saturated fat and cholesterol. This recipe may be prepared a day ahead and reheated, or frozen for future use.

¼ cup flour mixed with 2 teaspoons onion powder and 2 teaspoons Hungarian paprika
2 pounds boned raw turkey thigh or chicken thigh, cut into 1-inch cubes
1 tablespoon extra-virgin olive oil
2 cloves garlic, minced
1 bay leaf
6 canned or peeled fresh Italian plum tomatoes, chopped
6 fresh mushrooms, quartered
1 red pepper, seeded and cut into chunks
½ green pepper, seeded and cut into chunks

1 cup small whole fresh or frozen onions
1 teaspoon dried tarragon, or 1 tablespoon chopped fresh tarragon
½ cup defatted sodium-reduced chicken broth
½ cup dry white wine
1 tablespoon Worcestershire sauce
Freshly ground pepper
1 strip orange zest

3 tablespoons chopped fresh tarragon, for garnish

1. Place the seasoned flour in a plastic or paper bag, add the turkey pieces, and shake to coat with flour.

2. Heat the oil in a nonstick pan and sauté the turkey to a golden brown.

3. Add the remaining ingredients, cover, and cook over low heat, stirring occasionally, for about 20 minutes or until tender (chicken will cook faster than turkey). Remove the bay leaf and orange zest.

To Serve: Place in a warmed casserole and sprinkle lightly with fresh tarragon.

Per serving: 68 mg cholesterol, 0.85 gm saturated fat, 3.8 gm total fat, 0.9 fiber, 143 mg sodium, 188 calories, 0 gm trans fat

Last-Minute Soup (page 138)
Arugula, Red Cabbage, and Orange Salad with
Oil-Free Vinaigrette
♦ Italian Turkey Sausage ♦
Sliced Tomatoes
Larry's Scalloped Potatoes and Onions (page 308)
Pinkberry Topped with Strawberry Slices

Italian Turkey Sausage Ⓠ

Serves: 4 (1 patty = 1 serving)

Fennel and garlic give these sausages their Italian flavor. You may increase or eliminate any of the spices in the recipe to suit your palate.

1 pound ground turkey breast (see page 144) or lean veal (or a combination of the two)
1 extra-large egg white
¼ cup oat bran, soaked in ⅓ cup dry white wine or defatted sodium-reduced chicken broth
1 shallot, finely minced
1 teaspoon onion powder

1 teaspoon crushed fennel seeds
½ teaspoon ground sage
½ teaspoon dried oregano
3 cloves garlic, minced
½ teaspoon crushed red pepper flakes
¼ cup chopped fresh Italian parsley
¼ teaspoon salt (optional)

1. Place all the ingredients in a bowl, mix thoroughly with a fork, and chill for several hours to allow flavors to blend.

2. Shape into four patties.

3. Heat a nonstick skillet coated with nonstick cooking spray and sear the patties until browned, about 5 to 6 minutes on each side.

NOTE: These may be frozen for future use and reheated in your microwave oven.

Per serving: 59 mg cholesterol, 0.89 gm saturated fat, 3.4 gm total fat, 1.6 gm fiber, 69 mg sodium, 169 calories, 0 gm trans fat

Radicchio and Romaine Caesar Salad (page 91)
♦ Ever-Ready Rotisserie Chicken ♦
Microwaved White Corn on the Cob
Sliced White Peaches with Blueberries
Cranberry Oatmeal Cookies (page 349)

Ever-Ready Rotisserie Chicken ⓠ

Serves: 2 (3–4 ounces cooked meat = 1 serving)

On that hot summer day when cooking just seems like too much effort, stop by your local market and pick up a two-pound rotisserie broiler, white corn on the cob (shucked), a box of grape tomatoes, a bag of cut romaine, a head of radicchio, and a few white peaches and blueberries. If you're really lucky, you'll have some chocolate or oatmeal cookies (page 342 and 349) in the freezer to top it off and enough energy left to enjoy your evening.

1 2-pound broiler, skinned and quartered

Newman's Own salsa to taste (optional)

1. Serve chicken cold with corn on the cob and salsa.
2. Store the remainder of chicken in a Ziploc bag.
3. Refrigerate to use in salad or sandwich the next day.

Per serving: 100.93 mg cholesterol, 2.31 gm saturated fat, 8.4 gm total fat, 0 gm fiber, 97.52 mg sodium, 215.46 calories, 0 gm trans fat

Tomato Boullion
♦ Turkey Chow Mein ♦
Steamed Brown Rice (page 133)
Steamed Broccoli Florets
Persimmon Freeze (page 323)

Turkey Chow Mein Ⓠ

Serves: 4 to 6 (3 ounces cooked turkey = 1 serving)

2 teaspoons canola oil
1 large onion, thinly sliced and
  separated
2 cloves garlic, minced
2 stalks celery, cut into ½-inch
  diagonal slices
½ red pepper, seeded and cut into
  ¼-inch strips
½ green pepper, seeded and cut
  into ¼-inch strips
1 cup mushrooms, thinly sliced
1 6½-ounce can water chestnuts,
  drained and thinly sliced
3 stalks bok choy, cut into ½-inch
  slices or 2 cups frozen French-
  cut green beans

2 cups fresh bean sprouts
1 teaspoon Chinese five-spice
  seasoning
2 cups cooked turkey, cut into
  ¾-inch chunks, or 1 pound
  packaged raw turkey breast
  slices, cut into ½-inch strips
2 tablespoons sodium-reduced soy
  sauce
1 cup defatted sodium-reduced
  chicken broth
2 to 3 tablespoons cornstarch

3 tablespoons slivered toasted
  almonds, for garnish

1. Heat the oil in a 10-inch nonstick skillet or wok. Add the onions and garlic and sauté 3 to 4 minutes; then add celery and sauté 3 minutes.

2. Add the peppers, mushrooms, water chestnuts, bok choy, and bean sprouts, stirring after each addition. Sprinkle with Chinese five-spice seasoning, add the turkey, cover and cook 5 to 7 minutes.

3. Combine the soy sauce, broth, and cornstarch and pour over the turkey mixture.

4. Bring to a simmer while stirring constantly and cook until mixture is shiny.

To Serve: Serve over steamed brown rice and sprinkle with almonds.

Variation: To make this a vegetarian meal, substitute ½ pound eggplant, cut into strips, and 1 cup diced tofu for the turkey.

Per serving: 32 mg cholesterol, 0.62 gm saturated fat, 3.4 gm total fat, 1.3 gm fiber, 237 mg sodium, 151 calories, 0 gm trans fat

Shredded Carrot and Fresh Pineapple Salad
♦ Roast Chicken with Tomatillo Sauce ♦
Brown Rice Pilaf with Chopped Tomatoes
Crookneck Squash
Café au Lait Custard (page 323)

Roast Chicken with Tomatillo Sauce Ⓠ Ⓜ

Serves: 4 (4 ounces cooked chicken = 1 serving)

½ **pound fresh tomatillos, husks removed and quartered**
4 **cloves garlic, minced**
2 **ounces diced green chilies**
½ **bunch fresh cilantro, chopped**
1 **small onion, chopped**

Freshly ground pepper
2 **whole chicken breasts (about 14–16 ounces each), halved, skin and fat removed**
4 **red pepper rings**

1. Puree the first six ingredients. Place in a 9-inch quiche pan or pie plate, cover with microwave plastic wrap, and microwave on high for 5 minutes. To cook on top of stove: place pureed ingredients in saucepan and simmer for 20 minutes.

2. Place the chicken in the sauce, flesh side up, with the thick side toward the outside of the dish. Baste with the sauce mixture.

3. Cover tightly with double plastic wrap and cook on high for 7 minutes. Uncover and cook on high for 2 minutes. Place a pepper ring on each piece of chicken, return to the oven, and microwave on high for 2 minutes more.

To Serve: Place the chicken on a bed of rice pilaf and coat with sauce.

To Bake in Oven: Spoon the sauce over the chicken, cover, and bake in a preheated 350° oven for 35 to 40 minutes.

Per serving: 85 mg cholesterol, 1.37 gm saturated fat, 4.9 gm total fat, 1.6 gm fiber, 97 mg sodium, 219 calories, 0 gm trans fat

Green Pea and Red Pepper Salad with
Red Onion-Yogurt Dressing
♦ Poached Chicken with Braised Endive and Carrots ♦
Barley Pilaf
Whole Wheat Baguette
Fresh Pineapple with Spiced Honey Tea Loaf (page 343)

Poached Chicken with Braised Endive and Carrots

Serves: 4 (3 ounces cooked meat = 1 portion)

4 chicken legs (1½ pounds), skin
 and fat removed
Freshly ground pepper
1 teaspoon dried thyme, crushed
2 cloves garlic, minced
1 shallot, minced
1 cup vermouth or dry white wine
½ teaspoon celery seed
1 medium onion, peeled, halved,
 and thinly sliced

2 stalks celery with leaves,
 diagonally sliced ¾-inch thick
1 bay leaf
1¾ cups defatted sodium-reduced
 chicken broth
½ pound slim fresh carrots, peeled
 and cut in 4 pieces
2 heads fresh Belgian endive,
 halved lengthwise

1. Sprinkle the chicken with the pepper and thyme.
2. Place the garlic, shallot, and vermouth in a sauté pan or casserole;
bring to a boil.
3. Add the seasoned chicken and sprinkle with the celery.seed, onion,
celery slices, and bay leaf. Cover with the chicken broth, bring to a boil,
reduce to a simmer, and cook 15 minutes.
4. Baste the chicken with juices, add the carrots and endive, covering
with liquid, and cook covered for 15 minutes, or until the juices in the
chicken run clear.
5. Remove the vegetables and chicken to a heated platter and cover
with foil.
6. Reduce the remaining broth to about half.

To Serve: Pour the hot sauce over the chicken and vegetables.

Per serving: 79 mg cholesterol, 2.49 gm saturated fat, 8.6 gm total fat, 1.8 gm fiber,
143 mg sodium, 252 calories, 0 gm trans fat

Radicchio, Romaine, and Mushroom Salad
♦ Citrus Chicken Breasts ♦
Couscous
Snow Peas and Petit Peas
Pineapple and Strawberry Slices

Citrus Chicken Breasts Ⓠ Ⓜ

Serves: 4 (4 ounces cooked chicken = 1 serving)

3 tablespoons lemon juice
⅔ cup fresh orange juice
½ cup chopped green onions
2 tablespoons dry vermouth
1 tablespoon sodium-reduced soy
    sauce
2 teaspoons grated orange and
    lemon zest
1 teaspoon garlic powder
1 teaspoon dried thyme

2 teaspoons freshly grated ginger
Freshly ground pepper
2 whole chicken breasts (about
    14–16 ounces each), halved,
    skin and fat removed

8 peeled orange slices, 4 lemon
    slices, and watercress for
    garnish

1. Combine all the ingredients except the chicken breasts in a plastic bag.

2. Add the chicken and marinate in the refrigerator for an hour, turning occasionally.

3. Place the chicken with marinade in a shallow microwave dish with the thick portion toward the outside of the dish. Cover with wax paper and microwave on high for 7 minutes.

4. Remove the chicken to bake uncovered in a 375° oven for about 35 minutes more. Baste occasionally.

5. Remove chicken and microwave the sauce on high until reduced by one-third, about 3 minutes.

To Serve: Pour the sauce over the chicken, and garnish with watercress, and fresh orange and lemon slices.

Per serving: 84 mg cholesterol, 1.27 gm saturated fat, 4.7 gm total fat, 0.3 gm fiber, 200 mg sodium, 207 calories, 0 gm trans fat

♦ 2-Squash "Coleslaw" ♦
Poached Chicken Breasts
Steamed Asparagus Spears
Bulgur Wheat Pilaf
Dark Chocolate–Dipped Fresh Strawberries

2-Squash "Coleslaw" ⓠ

Serves: 6 (½ cup = 1 serving)

The term "coleslaw" means cabbage salad; however, many other vegetable combinations can be used for a similar salad, such as zucchini or broccoli.

3 crookneck and/or zucchini squash, scrubbed, trimmed, and coarsely shredded
1 clove garlic, minced
2 tablespoons grated onion
3 carrots, thinly sliced
Freshly ground pepper
3 tablespoons water
2 tablespoons canola oil

2 tablespoons lemon juice or rice vinegar
2 teaspoons Splenda
1 shallot, finely minced
½ teaspoon each thyme, chervil, and basil, crushed
½ teaspoon Dijon mustard (optional)

1. Place shredded squash on paper towels. Pat gently to remove moisture.

2. Turn squash into salad bowl with minced garlic, onions, carrots, and ground pepper. Toss to blend.

3. To make vinaigrette, combine water, oil, vinegar or lemon juice, shallot, thyme, chervil, basil, and mustard in screw-top jar. Shake vigorously.

4. Add dressing to squash mixture and blend well.

5. Cover and chill in refrigerator for several hours.

To Serve: Place in a chilled bowl or on a bed of greens with a garnish of crisp red button radishes or grape tomatoes.

Per serving: 0 mg cholesterol, 0.36 gm saturated fat, 4.73 gm total fat, 1.62 gm fiber, 2.85 gm sugar, 0 gm sodium, 65.04 calories, 0.01 gm trans fat

Black Bean and Corn Salad (page 282)
Tofu Dill Dip with Baked Blue Corn Chips
♦ Hearty Chicken Wrap ♦
Fresh Fruit Compote (page 322)

Hearty Chicken Wrap Ⓠ

Serves: 6

The FDA has currently ruled that 1½ tablespoons of canola oil per day *may* reduce the risk of coronary heart disease when used *in place of saturated fats.*

2 tablespoons canola oil
2 tablespoons lime juice
3 cloves garlic, minced
½ teaspoon ground cumin
2 teaspoons ground fennel
1 tablespoon grated lime zest
2 tablespoons chopped fresh
   cilantro or Italian parsley

3 8-ounce skinless, boneless chicken
   breasts, cut into ½-inch strips
6 whole wheat tortilla wraps
6 small Roma tomatoes
½ red bell pepper, diced
4 green onions, chopped
½ English cucumber, diced
Nonfat sour cream

1. In a large bowl, combine canola oil, lime juice, garlic, cumin, fennel, lime zest, and cilantro. Add chicken to bowl and toss to coat with mixture. Let stand for 20 minutes.

2. In large, nonstick frying pan, cook the chicken mixture over medium-high heat for 6 to 8 minutes or until chicken is cooked through and the juices run clear.

3. Place chicken on wraps. Add tomato, green onion, cucumber, and a dollop of sour cream. Fold and serve immediately.

Per serving: 66.01 mg cholesterol, 1.72 gm saturated fat, 10.54 gm total fat, 4.79 gm fiber, 0 gm sodium, 369.59 calories, 0.04 gm trans fat

---

The glycemic index is the speed with which sugar in foods is absorbed by the body.

Tofu Dill Dip Ⓠ

Yield: 1½ cups (12 tablespoons = 1 serving)

Soybeans provide the most nearly complete nutritional balance of any vegetable. A reliable way for your body to get the most beneficial advantages of soy is by adding 20 to 40 grams of a soy isolate powder to a shake each day. (Isoflavens, including genistein, are believed to slow prostate cancer progression.) Healthy soy foods, such as tofu, vary with each crop and how it is processed; however, tofu is still considered a source of healthy protein.

1 10½-ounce package Mori Nu Silken Low-Fat Tofu	¼ teaspoon ground white pepper
½ English cucumber, cut into eighths	2 tablespoons chopped fresh dill
	2 tablespoons red pepper, seeded, and diced fine
2 large cloves garlic, smashed and peeled	
2 slices onion	Additional chopped fresh dill for garnish

1. Combine the tofu, cucumber, garlic, ground white pepper, and dill in a food processor or blender. Process until smooth.

2. Pour into a bowl and mix in the diced bell pepper. Sprinkle with chopped dill, cover, and chill in the refrigerator at least 1 hour before serving.

To Serve: Place the bowl in the center of a large salad basket or platter. Surround with mounds of fresh vegetables such as carrots, celery, Belgian endive, zucchini spears; red, yellow, or green bell pepper slices; cherry tomatoes, sliced peeled black radish, red radishes; scallions; sliced rutabaga, turnip, or fennel; sugar snap peas or snow peas; slim asparagus; broccoli and cauliflower florets, or any vegetable that you enjoy. Baked corn chips, bagel chips, Stacy's Pita Chips, or whole wheat matzo crackers can also be offered.

Harriet's Hint—Unused portions of tofu should be stored in the refrigerator in cold water to cover. The water should be changed every day.

Per Serving: 0 mg cholesterol, 0.01 gm saturated fat, 0.17 gm total fat, 0.16 gm fiber, 0 gm sodium, 13.04 calories, 0 gm trans fat

Tomato Salad with Chopped Red Onion, Green Beans,
and Balsamic Vinegar
♦ Rosemary Chicken Breasts with Garlic and Lemon ♦
Brown and Wild Rice
Broccoli Puree and Carrot Coins
Poached Pears with Natural Juices

Rosemary Chicken Breasts with Garlic and Lemon

Serves: 4 (3 ounces cooked chicken = 1 serving)

Chicken is a popular and relatively inexpensive entrée to serve. The following is a delicious recipe that is quick and easy even though you do not use a microwave.

2 whole chicken breasts (about 14–16 ounces each), halved, boned, skin and fat removed
2 teaspoons extra-virgin olive oil
1 tablespoon dry rosemary, crushed
4 cloves garlic, minced
3 tablespoons lemon juice
1 teaspoon grated lemon zest

½ cup dry white wine or vermouth
1½ cups defatted sodium-reduced chicken broth
2 teaspoons arrowroot mixed with 3 tablespoons defatted sodium-reduced chicken broth

Rosemary or watercress, for garnish

1. Marinate the chicken breasts in the olive oil, rosemary, garlic, lemon juice, and zest in the refrigerator for 3 to 4 hours.
2. Heat an oven-proof skillet coated with butter-flavored nonstick spray and brown the breasts lightly on both sides. Add any remaining marinade.
3. Bake uncovered in a preheated 350° oven for 12 to 15 minutes.
4. Remove the chicken from the skillet and keep warm. Add the wine and broth to the skillet and simmer for 5 minutes.
5. Add the arrowroot mixture and thicken the sauce. Return the chicken to the sauce and heat for 5 minutes.

To Serve: Place the chicken breasts on a bed of rice, top with sauce, and garnish with watercress or rosemary.

Per serving: 72 mg cholesterol, 1.38 gm saturated fat, 6.2 gm total fat, 0.2 gm fiber, 70 mg sodium, 200 calories, 0 gm trans fat

COMPANY DINNER

Steamed Artichoke with Lemon
♦ Grilled Chicken Breasts with Apples Calvados ♦
Seasonal Vegetable Brochette
Polenta
Today's Coffee Cake (page 340)
Fresh Fruit with Sorbet

Grilled Chicken Breasts with Apples Calvados ⓠ

Serves: 4 (3 ounces cooked chicken = 1 serving)

4 4-ounce boned, skinned, and
defatted chicken breasts
Juice of ½ lemon
1 teaspoon salt-free vegetable
seasoning
1 teaspoon onion powder
2 teaspoons canola or cold-pressed
safflower oil
2 tablespoons Calvados

2 cups peeled apples (Golden
Delicious or McIntosh), sliced ⅔
inch thick
¼ cup frozen unsweetened apple
juice concentrate, defrosted
1 tablespoon cornstarch

Watercress, for garnish

1. Season the chicken breasts with lemon juice, vegetable seasoning, and onion powder.

2. Place the oil in a 10-inch nonstick skillet and heat; add the chicken breasts and grill 3 minutes on each side.

3. Sprinkle the Calvados over the chicken and heat 2 minutes.

4. Arrange the apple slices over the chicken, pour the apple juice over the chicken and apples, and partially cover.

5. Cook 12 to 15 minutes or until chicken is tender. Baste halfway through cooking.

6. Remove the chicken and apples to a heated platter and keep warm. Add the cornstarch to the remaining liquid and stir over heat until shiny.

To Serve: Spoon the sauce over the chicken breasts and garnish with watercress.

Variation: Pears may be substituted for the apples and pear liqueur substituted for the Calvados.

Per serving: 72 mg cholesterol, 1.23 gm saturated fat, 6.3 gm total fat, 1.7 gm fiber, 68 mg sodium, 241 calories, 0 mg trans fat

Sopa de Ajo (page 275)
Mixed Green Salad with Pico de Gallo
♦ Chicken Enchiladas ♦
Vegetarian Black Beans
Steamed Brown Rice (page 133)
Papaya with Lime

Chicken Enchiladas Ⓠ Ⓜ

Serves: 4 (2 enchiladas = 1 serving)

1 medium onion, chopped
3 cloves garlic or green garlic, minced
2 teaspoons canola oil
1 stalk celery, chopped
6 green tomatillos, husked and finely chopped
½ cup defatted sodium-reduced chicken broth
½ cup chopped fresh cilantro
1¼ pound boned, skinned, and defatted chicken breast, poached, or about 3 cups shredded leftover cooked chicken or turkey

2 tablespoons nonfat plain yogurt
8 corn tortillas, warmed in microwave oven for 10 seconds
1½ to 2 cups canned red or green enchilada sauce
3 tablespoons finely shredded part-skim mozzarella cheese

⅔ cup nonfat plain yogurt mixed with 2 tablespoons light-style sour cream, and chopped green onions, for garnish

1. Sauté the onion and garlic in the oil in a one-quart nonstick saucepan for 3 minutes. Add the celery, tomatillos, chicken broth, and cilantro and simmer 10 minutes.

2. Shred the chicken breasts and add with the yogurt to the tomatillo sauce.

3. Lay a tortilla flat and place a scant ½ cup of the chicken mixture along the center. Fold over the ends to cover the mixture and place seam-

side-down in a 13 × 9 x 2-inch casserole that has a thin layer of enchilada sauce on the bottom. Repeat with the remaining tortillas.

4. Cover with enchilada sauce. Sprinkle with shredded mozzarella cheese° and bake in a preheated 350° oven for 20 to 25 minutes or until bubbly, or in microwave on high for 12 minutes.

To Serve: Garnish with the yogurt mixture topped with chopped green onions.

Per serving: 47 mg cholesterol, 1.22 gm saturated fat, 5.4 gm total fat, 1 gm fiber, 127 mg sodium, 218 calories

°At this point, the enchiladas may be wrapped and frozen for future use.

♦ Hot Cajun Chicken and Black Bean Salad ♦
Warm Corn Tortillas
Papaya Filled with Raspberries and
a Dollop of Yogurt

Hot Cajun Chicken and Black Bean Salad

Serves: 4 (3 ounces cooked chicken = 1 serving)

1 tablespoon chopped onion
1 large clove garlic, minced
1 teaspoon olive oil
½ cup dried black beans, soaked overnight and drained°
1½ cups defatted sodium-reduced chicken broth
1 tablespoon chopped canned green chilies
¼ cup fresh cilantro or parsley, chopped
4 6-ounce chicken breasts, skinned, boned, and flattened

Juice of 1 lemon
2 teaspoons Cajun spice seasoning or spicy vegetable seasoning

8 cups shredded red leaf or romaince lettuce
1 cup diced tomato
1 cup fresh white or sodium-reduced canned kernel corn
1 cup salt-free canned salsa

1. In a nonstick saucepan, sauté the onion and garlic in oil until wilted.
2. Add the beans and sauté 1 minute.

3. Add the chicken broth, bring to a boil, reduce heat, cover, and simmer 45 minutes or until very tender. Add chilies and cilantro and set aside.

4. Season the chicken with the lemon juice and spicy seasoning. Grill on a hot nonstick skillet until browned on both sides. Cut each breast into six slices.

To Serve: Mound 2 cups of greens on each of four dinner plates. Pour a quarter of the hot black beans over the lettuce. Sprinkle with a quarter of the chopped tomatoes and corn. Top with hot chicken slices and serve with salsa on the side.

Per serving: 72 mg cholesterol, 1.48 gm saturated fat, 6.4 gm total fat, 5.9 gm fiber, 103 mg sodium, 333 calories

°One can of black beans or 2 cups cooked beans (page 131) may be substituted for the dry beans. In this case, reduce the amount of chicken broth to ⅔ cup and cook uncovered 20 minutes. Then proceed as in recipe.

. Watercress, Endive, and Mushroom Salad
♦ Orange-Glazed Cornish Hens ♦
Bulgar Wheat Pilaf (page 315)
Succotash
Marbled Angel Food Cake (page 327)

Orange-Glazed Cornish Hens

Serves: 4 (4 ounces cooked meat = 1 serving)

2 1-pound Cornish game hens,
    halved, skin and fat removed
Juice of ½ lemon
2 teaspoons salt-free vegetable
    seasoning
1 teaspoon onion powder
Freshly ground pepper
1 medium onion, chopped

1 6-ounce can frozen unsweetened
    orange juice or pineapple-
    orange juice (not reconstituted)

8 orange wedges and 1 large
    bunch grapes, for garnish
    (optional)

1. Season both sides of the hens with lemon juice, vegetable seasoning, onion powder, and pepper.

2. Sprinkle the chopped onion over the bottom of an 8 × 11-inch glass

baking dish coated with nonstick cooking spray. Place the hens flesh-side-down on top of the onions.

3. Spoon 1 tablespoon of the orange juice over each half.

4. Bake uncovered in a preheated 350° oven for 15 minutes. Turn the hens over and cover with the remaining juice.

5. Continue to bake for 30 minutes or until nicely browned and tender. If the juice dries out during cooking, add a bit of chicken broth or water to the pan.

To Serve: Mound pilaf on a serving platter and spoon the onions and sauce over it. Arrange the hens on top and garnish with orange wedges and grapes.

Per serving: 101 mg cholesterol, 4.0 gm saturated fat, 8.6 gm total fat, 0.4 gm fiber, 102 mg sodium, 305 calories, 0 gm trans fat

---

Larger plates and bowls lend to more eating!

Pastas

Artichoke Heart, Tomato, and Onion Salad with
Low-Calorie Balsamic Vinaigrette
♦ Fusilli with Broccoli Florets,
Garlic, and Hot Red Pepper Flakes ♦
Fresh Figs and Yogurt

Whole Wheat Fusilli with Broccoli Florets, Garlic, and Hot Red Pepper Flakes

Serves: 4

Here's a recipe that combines complex carbohydrates with high fiber vegetables in a delicious and colorful mixture.

1 tablespoon extra-virgin olive oil
3 large cloves garlic, minced
4 cups chopped broccoli florets,
   steamed until barely tender, or
   microwaved 3 minutes on high
Few grains crushed red pepper
   flakes

8 ounces whole wheat fusilli,
   cooked al dente and drained
1 tablespoon shredded Parmesan
   cheese

1. Heat the oil in a 10-inch nonstick skillet, add the garlic, and cook 2 minutes; do not brown. Add the broccoli and heat 2 minutes over medium heat.

2. Add the red pepper flakes and hot cooked pasta; stir with a wooden fork 2 to 3 minutes or until heated through.°

To Serve: Spoon onto a heated platter and sprinkle with Parmesan cheese. Pass more crushed hot red pepper flakes for heartier souls.

Per serving: 1 mg cholesterol, 0.85 gm saturated fat, 4.8 gm total fat, 2.7 gm fiber, 49 mg sodium, 273 calories, 0 gm trans fat

°If the pasta mixture is not as moist as you like, add a bit of chicken broth.

Chilled Greens with Corn and Black Beans
♦ Vegetarian Lasagna Rolls ♦
Garlic Toast (page 331)
Steamed Fresh Asparagus
Sorbet with Fresh Berries

Vegetarian Lasagna Rolls Ⓠ Ⓜ

Serves: 8 (2 rolls = 1 serving)

1 small onion, finely chopped
2 cloves garlic, minced
½ red pepper, seeded and finely chopped
2 teaspoons salt-free vegetable seasoning
1 teaspoon dried Italian herb blend, crushed
2 teaspoons extra-virgin olive oil
1 cup coarsely shredded carrot
1 cup thinly sliced zucchini
1 cup thinly sliced fresh mushrooms
1 10-ounce package frozen chopped spinach, defrosted and squeezed dry

1 cup part-skim ricotta cheese
2 extra-large egg whites, slightly beaten
8 lasagna noodles (7 to 8 ounces), cooked, drained, rinsed, drained, and halved lengthwise
2½ cups marinara sauce, tomato sauce, or Garden Vegetable Marinara Sauce (page 291)
3 fresh Italian plum tomatoes, sliced crosswise (16 slices)
3 tablespoons shredded Galaxy soy mozzarella cheese (optional)
Fresh basil leaves, for garnish

1. Sauté the onion, garlic, red pepper, and seasonings in the olive oil in a nonstick skillet for about 2 to 3 minutes.

2. Add the carrot, zucchini, and mushrooms and sauté 3 minutes.

3. Remove from heat and add the spinach, ricotta cheese, and egg whites. Blend well.

4. Spread one sixteenth of the mixture on each lasagna strip and roll up in jelly roll fashion.

5. Place the rolls (filled-side-up) into a shallow baking dish (13 × 9 × 2 inches). Spoon the marinara sauce over the rolls.

6. Top each roll with a tomato slice and sprinkle with mozzarella cheese if desired.

7. Bake uncovered on high in a microwave oven for about 15 minutes, or covered in a preheated 350° oven for 30 to 35 minutes.

To Serve: Garnish with leaves of fresh basil and serve hot.

Per serving: 10 mg cholesterol, 1.76 gm saturated fat, 4.2 gm total fat, 3 gm fiber, 105 mg sodium, 206 calories, 0 gm trans fat

Cannellini Bean, Tomato, and Red Onion Salad Vinaigrette
♦ Sweet Pepper Pasta ♦
Whole Wheat Baguette
Apple Crisp (page 318)

Sweet Pepper Pasta Ⓠ

Serves: 4

1 tablespoon extra-virgin olive oil
½ small onion, thinly sliced
4 large cloves garlic, chopped fine
1 small red pepper, seeded and
    cut into ½-inch strips
1 small yellow pepper, seeded and
    cut into ½-inch strips
1 small green pepper, seeded and
    cut into ½-inch strips
1 small orange pepper, seeded and
    cut into ½-inch strips (optional)
1 teaspoon Italian herb blend
½ cup dry white wine or vermouth
⅔ cup defatted sodium-reduced
    chicken broth

1 tablespoon sodium-reduced soy
    sauce
1 teaspoon grated peeled fresh
    ginger
⅛ teaspoon crushed red pepper
    flakes or freshly ground pepper
    to taste
½ teaspoon sesame oil
8 ounces soba or spaghettini pasta,
    cooked 3 or 4 minutes, or al
    dente, and drained

2 tablespoons grated Parmesan
    cheese, for garnish

1. Coat a nonstick skillet with nonstick spray; add the olive oil and heat over medium heat.

2. Separate the onion slices, add to the pan, and sauté quickly about 3 minutes. Add the garlic and sauté quickly about 1 minute, stirring constantly.

3. Add the peppers and herb blend and sauté 1 more minute.

4. Stir in the wine, chicken broth, soy sauce, ginger, and pepper flakes. Bring the mixture to a boil, reduce the heat, cover, and simmer 3 minutes.

5. Uncover and continue cooking over high heat about 3 minutes. Sprinkle with sesame oil.

6. Combine the pepper mixture with the hot cooked pasta.

To Serve: Mound the hot pasta mixture onto a warm serving platter and sprinkle with Parmesan cheese.

Variation: Three fresh shiitake or oyster mushrooms may be added with the peppers.

Per serving: 0 mg cholesterol, 0.69 gm saturated fat, 5 gm total fat, 2.4 gm fiber, 128 mg sodium, 286 calories, 0 gm trans fat

Mixed Greens and Fennel with
Balsamic Vinaigrette
♦ Linguini with Red Clam Sauce ♦
Crisp Whole Wheat Bread Sticks
Poached Pears and Prunes (page 320)
Biscotti

Linguini with Red Clam Sauce ⓠ

Serves: 6

The sauce in this recipe may be prepared earlier in the day, or you may use 3½ cups of the Garden Vegetable Marinara Sauce on page 291.

12 ounces whole wheat linguine, cooked al dente and drained

Red Clam Sauce:
6 cloves garlic, minced
½ small onion, minced
2 teaspoons extra-virgin olive oil
1 28-ounce can crushed San Marzano tomatoes
½ cup dry red wine
⅔ cup chopped celery
1 strip orange zest
1 teaspoon dried oregano, crushed, or 1 tablespoon fresh oregano, chopped

1 teaspoon dried thyme, crushed, or 1 tablespoon fresh thyme, chopped
Freshly ground pepper
½ teaspoon crushed red pepper flakes
¼ cup chopped fresh Italian parsley leaves
4 dozen fresh clams, *well scrubbed and washed* under cold running water

1. Sauté the garlic and onion in the oil in a 4-quart saucepan until wilted.

2. Add all the remaining sauce ingredients except the parsley and clams. Bring to a boil, reduce heat, and simmer for 20 minutes, stirring occasionally.

3. Add the clams and parsley and steam, covered, over medium heat, shaking the pan occasionally, for 5 to 7 minutes or until the shells are opened. *Discard any unopened clams* and remove the orange zest.

To Serve: Place the drained linguini in a large serving bowl and spoon the sauce and clams over the pasta. Serve immediately.

Per serving: 54 mg cholesterol, 0.63 gm saturated fat, 4.9 gm total fat, 2.9 gm fiber, 321 mg sodium, 336 calories, 0 gm trans fat

Three-Bean Salad
♦ Lillian's Quick and Easy Manicotti ♦
Steamed Zucchini Spears
Lemon Sorbet with Raspberry Sauce

Lillian's Quick and Easy Manicotti Ⓜ

Serves: 6 (2 manicotti = 1 serving)

15 ounces part-skim ricotta cheese
1 10-ounce package frozen chopped spinach, defrosted and drained
2 whole green onions, sliced
2 extra-large egg whites, or ¼ cup egg substitute

1 tablespoon dried dill, or 2 tablespoons chopped fresh dill
¼ teaspoon freshly ground nutmeg
About 8 ounces uncooked egg-free manicotti shells (12)
3 cups marinara sauce

1. Combine the ricotta cheese, drained spinach, onions, egg whites, dill, and nutmeg. Mix thoroughly.

2. Stuff the *uncooked* manicotti shells with the mixture.

3. Coat an 11 × 14 × 2-inch glass baking pan with olive-oil cooking spray.

4. Cover the bottom of the pan with a layer of marinara sauce. Arrange the stuffed manicotti shells next to each other in the pan and cover with the remaining sauce.

5. Cover the pan tightly with aluminum foil. Bake in a preheated 350° oven for 1 hour.

NOTE: This dish may be prepared ahead or frozen for future use. To serve if frozen, place in a cold oven and bake 1½ hours at 350°.

To Microwave:

1. Spread half of the *heated* sauce on the bottom of a baking dish.

2. Lay filled shells over sauce and top with remaining sauce.

3. Cover dish tightly with plastic wrap and microwave on high for 10 minutes.

4. Turn each shell over, cover, and microwave on medium high for 15 minutes.

5. Remove plastic and let stand 12 to 15 minutes before serving.

Per serving: 17 mg cholesterol, 2.88 gm saturated fat, 5 gm total fat, 2.4 gm fiber, 138 mg sodium, 227 calories, 0 gm trans fat

Obesity contributes to diabetes.

Chilled Mixed
Radicchio, Red Lettuce, and Butter Lettuce
with Low-Calorie Italian Dressing
♦ Pasta Shells with Mushrooms ♦
Steamed Broccoli
Mixed Berries with Light Sour Cream Topping

Pasta Shells with Mushrooms

Serves: 4

Use pasta shells about one inch in size in preparing this recipe, not the ones that are large enough for stuffing.

½ cup minced onion
1 tablespoon extra-virgin olive oil
1 ounce dried porcini mushrooms, soaked in 1 cup dry white wine for 30 minutes (save the strained liquid)
1½ cups thinly sliced fresh mushroom caps
1½ cups cremini mushrooms

½ teaspoon dried Italian herb blend, or 2 teaspoons chopped fresh basil
8 ounces 1-inch whole wheat pasta shells, cooked al dente and drained

1 tablespoon grated Parmesan cheese (optional)

1. Sauté the onion in the oil in a nonstick 1-quart saucepan for several minutes until wilted.

2. Slice the drained porcini mushrooms and add to onions with the sliced fresh mushroom caps and herbs. Sauté 3 minutes.

3. Add the strained soaking liquid and cook 5 minutes.

4. Add the hot cooked pasta shells to the mushroom mixture and mix thoroughly.

To Serve: Mound pasta mixture on a heated serving platter and sprinkle with Parmesan cheese.

Per serving: 0 mg cholesterol, 0.61 gm saturated fat, 4.3 gm total fat, 2.8 gm fiber, 7 mg sodium, 291 calories, 0 gm trans fat

Mixed Grilled Chopped Vegetables with
Low-Calorie Lemon Vinaigrette Dressing
♦ Fresh Tomato, Basil, and Mozzarella Pasta ♦
Crisp Whole Wheat Sourdough Baguette
Cantaloupe Cubes with Fresh Strawberry Sauce (page 319)

Fresh Tomato, Basil, and Mozzarella Pasta Ⓠ

Serves: 2

There is no oil added in this recipe, and the tomatoes in the dish are not cooked—just heated, to give a wonderful, fresh taste.

4 ounces spelt spaghetti, cooked al dente and drained
⅓ cup vegetable broth
2 tablespoon dry white wine
Freshly ground pepper
2 fresh Italian plum tomatoes, diced

2 ounces part-skim mozzarella cheese, diced
1 tablespoon chopped fresh basil leaves

1. While the pasta is cooking, bring the broth, wine, and pepper to a boil. Add the tomatoes and heat *1 minute.* Add the cheese and stir.

2. Immediately pour the tomato mixture and basil over the drained hot pasta and toss to blend.

To Serve: Place on warm plates and serve while hot.

Per serving: 16 mg cholesterol, 2.99 gm saturated fat, 5.4 gm total fat, 2.5 gm fiber, 144 mg sodium, 312 calories, 2 gm trans fat

Vegetarian Dishes

Mixed Green Salad with Garbanzo Beans and
Nancy's Light Russian Dressing
♦ Eggplant Lasagna ♦
Lemony Brussels Sprouts
Baked Sweet Potatoes
Meringues with Fresh Fruit

Eggplant Lasagna Ⓠ Ⓜ

Serves: 6

Many people accustomed to cooking meat-and-potato meals are
stymied by the thought of preparing a vegetarian dinner. The following recipe is simple to make and high in fiber and satisfying flavors.

1 1-pound eggplant, peeled and
cut into 18 slices
1 tablespoon extra-virgin olive oil
8 ounces nonfat ricotta cheese
2 carrots, coarsely shredded
2 green onions, thinly sliced
1 tablespoon chopped fresh
parsley
2 extra-large egg whites, slightly
beaten

1 tablespoon grated Parmesan
cheese
Freshly ground pepper
2–3 cups marinara sauce or tomato
sauce, mixed with 6 sliced fresh
mushrooms and 1 tablespoon
chopped fresh basil
2 Italian plum tomatoes, cut into
12 thin slices

1. Place the eggplant slices on a nonstick cookie sheet and brush one
side lightly with olive oil. Broil until lightly colored on both sides.

2. Combine the ricotta cheese, carrots, onion, parsley, egg whites, 1½
teaspoons of the Parmesan cheese, and the freshly ground pepper.

3. Spoon ⅔ cup of the marinara sauce mixture on the bottom of an
8 × 11 × 3-inch baking pan. Arrange a layer of six slices of eggplant on
the sauce; top each eggplant slice with 1 tablespoon of the ricotta cheese
mixture, 1 tomato slice, and 1 tablespoon of the marinara sauce mixture.

4. Repeat for a second layer, then top with the remaining slices of
eggplant and the remaining marinara sauce. Sprinkle with the Parmesan
cheese and cover with wax paper.

5. Bake on high in a microwave oven for 10 minutes or in a preheated 375° oven for 30 to 35 minutes. Let stand 10 minutes before serving.

Per serving: 12 mg cholesterol, 2.38 gm saturated fat, 5.9 gm total fat, 2.8 gm fiber, 594 mg sodium, 153 calories, 0 gm trans fat

COMPANY DINNER

Wonton Soup with Green Onions
♦ Stir-Fry Vegetables with Tofu ♦
Steamed Bok Choy with Black Mushrooms
Dry String Beans with Garlic
Fried Rice with Egg Whites, Green Onion, and Fresh Pineapple
Pinkberry Green Tea Frozen Yogurt

Stir-Fry Vegetables with Tofu Ⓠ

Serves: 4 (2 cups = 1 serving)

The perfect meal for entertaining vegan friends! Soy protein found in tofu is high in folic acid, calcium, zinc, iron, and genistein, a chemical that is thought to interfere with the reproduction of some cancer cells, particularly prostate cancer cells.*

8 ounces silken low-fat tofu
3 tablespoons low-sodium tamari sauce
¼ cup vegetable broth or water
2 bulbs green garlic or 1 large clove garlic, minced
1½ teaspoons grated fresh ginger root
¼ teaspoon allspice or five-spice seasoning, plus a few grains crushed red pepper flakes (optional)
2 cloves garlic, minced

1 small onion, peeled, quartered, and thinly sliced diagonally
1 cup fresh sliced cremini mushrooms
2 ribs of celery with leaves, sliced
2 large carrots, sliced diagonally
2 cups fresh snow peas
2 cups fresh small broccoli florets
2 cups bean sprouts or soy bean sprouts
¼ cup water or vegetable broth
1 teaspoon cornstarch

1. Dice tofu into 1-inch cubes. Combine tamari sauce, water, garlic, ginger, crushed pepper, and allspice or five-spice in a saucepan. Add tofu and simmer for 5 minutes. Drain tofu and reserve liquid.

2. Coat nonstick wok or skillet with canola-oil cooking spray. Heat and add garlic, onion, mushrooms, celery, and carrots. Stir-fry 4 minutes. Add snow peas and broccoli, and stir-fry 1 minute more.

3. Add reserved tofu and bean sprouts.

4. Blend reserved liquid, water, and cornstarch.

5. Add sauce to vegetables and stir until all the vegetables are coated and sauce coats a spoon.

To Serve: Place stir-fried vegetables and tofu on plates and serve immediately. Follow with other courses one at a time.

Per serving: 0 mg cholesterol, 0.1 gm saturated fat, 1.29 gm total fat, 3.95 gm fiber, 0.0 gm sodium, 19.61 gm carbohydrate, 119.44 calories, 0 gm trans fat

°Dr. James Anderson has found that soy protein lowers LDLs (the bad cholesterol) while not affecting the HDLs (the good cholesterol).

---

*Nutritional yeast (not brewer's or baker's) adds a
cheeselike flavor to sauces and casseroles.*

Steamed Artichokes with Lemon
♦ Tuscan Minestrone ♦
Whole Wheat Sourdough Rolls
Rigatoni with Marinara Sauce
Mixed Fresh Fruit Cup

Tuscan Minestrone

Yield: about 3½ quarts (1½ cups = 1 serving as entrée)

This soup is a hearty meal-in-one, and it's one of my favorites.

1 cup dry kidney beans
1 tablespoon extra-virgin olive oil
3 cloves garlic, minced
1 bay leaf
½ teaspoon crushed red pepper flakes
1 onion, coarsely chopped
2½ quarts water or defatted, sodium-reduced chicken broth
1 leek (white part only), sliced
3 large carrots, sliced
3 stalks celery, with leaves, sliced
2 sweet potatoes (yams), peeled and cubed
1 cup sliced fresh green beans
1½ cups salt-free tomato sauce

1 tablespoon dried Italian herb blend, crushed
Freshly ground pepper
2 zucchini, coarsely chopped
1½ cups canned cannellini or garbanzo beans, drained and rinsed
1 14½-ounce sodium-reduced stewed or peeled tomatoes, chopped
½ cup small macaroni or orzo
1 10-ounce package frozen chopped spinach, defrosted and drained, or 2 cups washed and shredded fresh spinach or Swiss chard

1. Cover the beans with water and soak overnight, or cook in microwave (page 131).

2. Place the oil in a 6-quart saucepan, add the drained beans, garlic, bay leaf, red pepper flakes, and onion. Sauté 5 minutes.

3. Add the water or broth, bring to a boil, and simmer for 1 hour.

4. Add the leek, carrots, celery, potatoes, green beans, tomato sauce, herb blend, and pepper, and cook 30 minutes.

5. Add zucchini, beans, and tomatoes, and cook 15 minutes.

6. Add the macaroni and spinach, and cook 15 minutes. Remove the bay leaf.

Per serving: 0 mg cholesterol, 0.31 gm saturated fat, 2.2 gm total fat, 4.6 gm fiber, 42 mg sodium, 158 calories, 0 gm trans fat

Tomato Bisque
♦ Vegetable Lo Mein ♦
String Beans with Shiitake Mushrooms
Fresh Orange Wedges

Vegetable Lo Mein Ⓠ

Serves: 4

Chinese-style cooking lends itself nicely to meals low in calories, saturated fat, and cholesterol without any animal protein added. Try using a wok to prepare the combination of vegetables, whether alone or with a small amount of chicken, tofu, beef, or pasta.

1 tablespoon canola oil
1 medium onion, thinly sliced and
     separated
1 stalk celery, thinly sliced
2 carrots, thinly sliced with
     vegetable peeler
1 large zucchini, cut into 2-inch
     julienne strips
2 cups chopped broccoli
1 4-ounce can water chestnuts,
     drained and thinly sliced
     (optional)

1 cup fresh snow peas or frozen
     peas or edamame
2 tablespoons sodium-reduced soy
     sauce
6 ounces whole wheat linguine,
     cooked al dente and drained
1 teaspoon sesame oil (optional)
3 green onions, cut into 2-inch
     julienne strips

1. Heat a wok or a nonstick skillet over high heat. Add the oil, swirling it around the pan.

2. Add the onions and stir-fry 2 to 3 minutes.

3. Add the celery and carrots, stir-fry for 2 minutes. Add the zucchini, broccoli, water chestnuts, and pea pods and stir-fry for 2 minutes more.

4. Add the soy sauce; heat 1 minute.

5. Add the hot, well-drained linguine to the vegetable mixture, sprinkle with sesame oil and green onions, and mix until heated through.

Per serving: 0 mg cholesterol, 0.36 gm saturated fat, 4.5 gm total fat, 4.2 gm fiber, 279 mg sodium, 305 calories, 0 gm trans fat

♦ Celery Root, Red Cabbage, and Orange Salad ♦
Breast of Chicken Roasted with
Onions and Leeks
Brown Rice Pilaf
Steamed Brussels Sprouts
Virtual Date Brownies (page 348)

Celery Root, Red Cabbage, and Orange Salad Ⓠ

Serves: 4

Three high-fiber winter vegetables join forces to make a deliciously different salad.

1 cup celery root, peeled and
   shredded
2 cups shredded red cabbage
1 large navel orange, peeled and
   cubed

pomegranate seeds for garnish

Dressing:
¼ cup low-calorie oil-free
   vinaigrette
3 tablespoons fresh orange juice
¼ teaspoon celery seed
2 teaspoons balsamic vinegar

1. Place the celery root, red cabbage, and oranges in a mixing bowl. Toss and chill.
2. Combine the dressing ingredients and blend thoroughly.
3. Just before serving, sprinkle the salad with dressing and toss gently with two forks.

To Serve: Arrange on individual salad plates and sprinkle with pomegranate seeds.

Per serving: 0 mg cholesterol, 0.05 gm saturated fat, 0.3 gm total fat, 1.7 gm fiber, 45 mg sodium, 52 calories, 0 gm trans fat

Hearts of Romaine and Shredded Carrot Salad with
Mustard-Yogurt Dressing
Broiled Orange Roughy
Baked Sweet Potatoes
♦ Angela's Herbed Squash Medley ♦
Red and Green Grapes

Angela's Herbed Squash Medley Ⓠ Ⓜ

Serves: 8 to 10

This vegetable dish makes a large amount (great for guests) and
may be prepared in the morning to be cooked and served for dinner.

4 teaspoons extra-virgin olive oil
6–8 crookneck squash and
zucchinis, cut into ¼-inch slices
4 large cloves garlic, minced, and
1 bunch green onions, thinly
sliced, mixed together
1 pint cherry tomatoes, halved, or
6 plum tomatoes, chopped
¼ cup chopped fresh basil, ¼ cup
chopped fresh Italian parsley,
and 1 tablespoon chopped fresh
thyme, mixed together

Freshly ground pepper
Salt-free vegetable seasoning
1 large beefsteak tomato, thinly
sliced
1 tablespoon grated Parmesan
cheese mixed with 3 tablespoons
dry whole wheat bread crumbs

1. Coat 2-quart shallow oval casserole with butter-flavored nonstick
spray. Sprinkle with 1 teaspoon of the olive oil.
2. Arrange a third of the squash slices in one layer, sprinkle with a third
of the onion and garlic mixture; cover with a third of the tomatoes, sprinkle
with a third of the herb mixture, freshly ground pepper, and vegetable seasoning. Sprinkle 1 teaspoon of the olive oil over the top. Repeat two times.
3. Top with the sliced tomatoes and the cheese mixture.
4. Cover tightly with microwave plastic wrap and microwave on high
for 12 to 15 minutes. (Using a carousel in your microwave oven makes it
unnecessary to rotate the dish a quarter turn after half the cooking time.)

Per serving: 1 mg cholesterol, 0.5 gm saturated fat, 2.9 gm total fat, 1.5 gm fiber,
41 gm sodium, 70 calories

Creamy Cauliflower Soup (page 272)
♦ Lentil Vegetable Salad with
Low-Calorie Tarragon Vinaigrette ♦
Baked Sweet Potato with Nonfat Plain Yogurt
Sliced Fall Fruits with Papaya Puree

Lentil Vegetable Salad with Low-Calorie Tarragon Vinaigrette

Serves: 4

Lentils are a good source of protein and soluble fiber, and this salad makes a nice entrée for a vegetarian meal.

1 cup dried red lentils, washed and drained
2 cups water
2 teaspoons dried thyme, crushed
1 bay leaf
Few grains crushed red pepper
1 large carrot, chopped
2 celery stalks, chopped
½ cup chopped red onion
1 small red or green pepper, seeded and thinly sliced

2 tablespoons chopped fresh Italian parsley
½ cup hearts of palm, sliced
⅓ cup low-calorie oil-free vinaigrette mixed with 1 tablespoon tarragon vinegar and 1 teaspoon extra-virgin olive oil

8 grape tomatoes, for garnish

1. Place the lentils, water, thyme, bay leaf, and crushed pepper in a 2-quart saucepan. Bring to a boil, reduce heat, cover, and simmer 30 to 45 minutes. (*The lentils should be cooked but firm.*)
2. Drain the excess water, remove the bay leaf, and place the lentils in a salad bowl.
3. Add salad dressing and all the vegetables to the lentils; toss lightly and cool to room temperature.

To Serve: Line individual plates with butter lettuce, mound the salad on top of lettuce, and if desired, garnish with tomatoes.

Per serving: 0 mg cholesterol, 0.28 gm saturated fat, 1.9 gm total fat, 6.9 gm fiber, 34 mg sodium, 206 calories, 0 gm trans fat

Endive, Arugula, and Romaine Salad with
Yogurt Dressing (page 92)
♦ Vegetarian Paella ♦
Whole Wheat Rolls
Poached Peaches with Raspberry Sauce

Vegetarian Paella

Serves: 6 to 8

1½ tablespoons extra-virgin olive
oil
2 large onions, thinly sliced
4 garlic cloves, minced
2 cups brown rice, washed
1 small eggplant (about 1 pound),
cubed, or 4 Japanese eggplant,
cut crosswise into ¼-inch slices
1 large red pepper, seeded and
sliced
4½ cups organic vegetable stock
2 celery stalks with leaves, chopped
6 peeled Italian plum tomatoes,
diced, or 2 cups San Marzano
tomatoes

1 can quartered artichoke hearts,
rinsed and drained
Freshly ground pepper
⅛ teaspoon crushed saffron
threads dissolved in 2 teaspoons
hot water
1 cup frozen peas or pea pods
½ cup chopped fresh parsley

2 tablespoons sliced green onions
and 2 tablespoons slivered
toasted almonds, for garnish
(optional)

1. In a 3-quart nonstick saucepan, heat the oil; add the onions and garlic and sauté 5 minutes or until the onions are wilted. Add the rice and stir until opaque.

2. Add the eggplant and red pepper and sauté 3 to 5 minutes.

3. Add the stock, bring to a boil, and reduce the heat to a simmer.

4. Stir in the celery, tomatoes, artichoke hearts, pepper, and saffron.

5. Cover and simmer 35 to 40 minutes or until the rice is tender. Add the peas and parsley and cook 3 to 4 minutes, just until peas are cooked.

To Serve: Turn the paella into a warm serving dish and garnish with sliced green onions and almonds if desired.

Variation: To make paella with animal protein, add 8 skinned chicken thighs (about 1½ pounds), seasoned and broiled, and 1 16-

ounce can sodium-reduced stewed tomatoes in Step 4. If desired, instead of chicken add 18 clams in Step 5 with the peas and parsley.

Per serving: 0 mg cholesterol, 0.65 gm saturated fat, 3.8 gm total fat, 3.5 gm fiber, 51 mg sodium, 255 calories, 0 gm trans fat

Chilled Mixed Green Salad
♦ Stanford Moroccan Vegetable Stew with Couscous and
Spicy Red Pepper Sauce ♦
Seasonal Fresh Fruit
Just a Good Chocolate Cookie (page 342)

Stanford Moroccan Vegetable Stew with Couscous and Spicy Red Pepper Sauce

Yield: 6 servings (2 tablespoons sauce = 1 serving)

This dish is my adaptation of a recipe from the *Sunset International Vegetarian Cookbook.*

1 tablespoon extra-virgin olive oil
1 large onion, finely chopped
1½ teaspoons ground coriander
¾ teaspoon ground cinnamon
2 medium-sized yams, peeled and cut into ½-inch cubes
1 small rutabaga (about 1 cup), peeled and cut into ½-inch cubes
2–3 large tomatoes, peeled and chopped
1¼ cups water or defatted sodium-reduced chicken broth
2 tablespoons lemon juice
½ teaspoon powdered saffron
2 cups cooked, drained chickpeas (garbanzo beans, page 131), or 1

15-ounce can chickpeas, drained and rinsed
Salt (optional)
2 medium-sized zucchini, cut diagonally into ½-inch slices
1 cup chopped broccoli florets
1 large red pepper, seeded and chopped
1 large green pepper, seeded and chopped
4 cups cooked whole wheat couscous, prepared according to package directions (without added fat)

Spicy Red Pepper Sauce (page 235)

1. Heat the oil in a 5-quart kettle over medium heat; add the onion, coriander, and cinnamon, and cook, stirring occasionally, until the onion is soft (about 5 minutes).

2. Stir in the yams and rutabagas and cook, stirring often, for 2 minutes.

3. Add the tomatoes, water or broth, lemon juice, saffron, and chickpeas. Add salt to taste, if desired. Cover, reduce heat, and simmer for 15 minutes, or until the yams are nearly tender.

4. Mix the zucchini, broccoli, and red and green peppers into the potato mixture and cook, covered, until all the vegetables are tender but still crisp (about 7 minutes).

To Serve: Spread the hot couscous around the edges of a deep platter and spoon the vegetable mixture into the center. Pass the Spicy Red Pepper Sauce.

Variation: Hot cooked brown rice, bulgur, buckwheat, quinoa, or millet, prepared according to directions on page 133, can be used instead of couscous.

Per serving: 0 mg cholesterol, 0.77 gm saturated fat, 5.1 gm total fat, 7.8 gm fiber, 25 mg sodium, 345 calories

Spicy Red Pepper Sauce Ⓠ Ⓜ

Yield: about 1½ cups (1 tablespoon = 1 serving)

This sauce will keep for weeks in a tightly closed jar in the refrigerator and may be used as a topping on steamed potatoes, broccoli, or chicken.

3 red peppers, seeded and
  quartered
1½ teaspoons commercial hot red
  pepper sauce, or 1 teaspoon
  cayenne pepper mixed with 1
  teaspoon ground cumin and 3
  cloves garlic

About ½ cup vegetable liquid
  or defatted sodium-reduced
  chicken broth (optional)

1. In a covered dish, microwave the peppers with seasonings for 10 minutes or until soft. Turn dish twice while cooking.

2. Puree the peppers in a food processor or blender. Taste and adjust seasonings.

3. If desired, you may thin the sauce with liquid from vegetables or with chicken broth.

Per serving: 0 mg cholesterol, 0.04 gm saturated fat, 0.3 gm total fat, 0.6 gm fiber, 11 mg sodium, 15 calories

Tofu and Corn Soup (page 277)
♦ Ratatouille ♦
Steamed Carrot Spears
Quinoa with Peas
Baked Apple with Creme Topping (page 316)

Ratatouille Ⓠ Ⓜ

Serves: 8 (1¼ cups = 1 serving)

This menu presents a lovely vegetarian meal for winter. Ratatouille itself, whether served hot as part of a vegetarian meal or as a vegetable side dish with chicken, is a versatile dish that can be made ahead.

1 large onion, coarsely chopped
3 large cloves garlic or green garlic, minced
2 teaspoons extra-virgin olive oil
½ pound fresh mushrooms, sliced
1 green pepper, cut into ½-inch slices
1 red or yellow pepper, cut into ½-inch slices
1 pound eggplant with skin, cut into ¾-inch cubes
1 medium zucchini, cut into ½-inch slices

4 peeled Italian plum tomatoes, cubed, or 8 cherry tomatoes, halved
⅓ cup dry white wine
⅓ cup sodium-reduced V-8 juice
2 tablespoons tomato paste
1 tablespoon Worcestershire sauce
2 tablespoons chopped fresh oregano, thyme, or basil, or 2 teaspoons dried herb
Freshly ground pepper

1. In a large nonstick skillet, sauté the onion and garlic in the oil for several minutes over medium heat.

2. Add the remaining vegetables, stir, and reduce the heat. Combine the remaining ingredients. Add to the vegetables and stir.

3. Cover and simmer the vegetable mixture 35 minutes, stirring occasionally.

To Serve: Serve warm or cold.

To Microwave: Combine the onion, garlic, and oil in a 3-quart oval casserole and cook on high for 3 minutes. Add the remaining ingredients, stir, cover with microwave plastic wrap, and cook on high for about 15 minutes. Mix twice during the cooking time. Let stand, covered, for 10 minutes before serving.

Per serving: 0 mg cholesterol, 0.22 gm saturated fat, 1.6 gm total fat, 2 gm fiber, 29 mg sodium, 62 calories, 0 gm trans fat

Desserts

COMPANY DINNER

Sautéed Mushrooms on Greens with Balsamic Vinaigrette
Broiled Fish with Mustard and Capers
Corn on the Cob
Steamed French-Cut Green Beans
♦ Papaya Ambrosia ♦

Papaya Ambrosia Ⓠ

Serves: 4 (¼ papaya = 1 serving)

This is a busy-day company dinner that allows you to enjoy your guests. Corn is a readily available vegetable, fresh or frozen, that is high in soluble fiber and this refreshing fruit dessert requires little preparation.

2 papayas, quartered and seeded
½ cup small red seedless grapes
½ cup unsweetened pineapple tidbits
½ cup nonfat plain yogurt mixed with 1 teaspoon pure vanilla extract

2 tablespoons toasted slivered almonds, for garnish (optional)

1. Using a grapefruit knife, remove the papaya meat from the shells (reserve the shells) and cube.

2. Combine the papaya, grapes, and pineapple in a bowl and toss lightly to combine.

3. Add the yogurt mixture to the fruit and stir lightly with a fork. Place in the refrigerator to chill.

To Serve: Just before serving, spoon the fruit mixture into the papaya shells and, if desired, sprinkle with toasted almonds.

Per serving: 1 mg cholesterol, 0.12 gm saturated fat, 0.4 gm total fat, 1.6 gm fiber, 26 mg sodium, 92 calories, 0 gm trans fat

Parsley and Tomato Salad
in Basil Vinaigrette (page 96)
Roast Turkey Breast
Stir-Fried Vegetables with Sesame Seeds
Steamed Brown and Wild Rice with Scallions
♦ Fresh White Nectarine Scallop ♦

Fresh White Nectarine Scallop Ⓠ Ⓜ

Serves: 8

Take advantage of fruits that are in season; they are more flavorful and less expensive. Peaches, plums, pears, pineapples, or apples may be substituted for the nectarines in this delicious dessert.

2 pounds fresh white nectarines, cut into ¾-inch slices (about 4 cups sliced)
2 tablespoons minute tapioca
1½ tablespoons lemon juice
2 tablespoons frozen unsweetened apple juice concentrate
1 tablespoon peach brandy or Amaretto

Topping:
3 tablespoons rolled oats, chopped
3 tablespoons sugar-free cold cereal (wheat flakes or oat bran flakes), crushed
2 teaspoons Splenda Brown Sugar blend
½ teaspoon ground cinnamon
2 tablespoons chopped almonds

⅓ cup nonfat plain yogurt mixed with 1 teaspoon peach brandy or Amaretto, for garnish

1. Sprinkle the nectarines with the tapioca, lemon juice, apple juice concentrate, and brandy.

2. Arrange the nectarines in a 10-inch round glass pie plate or quiche pan.°

3. Combine the topping ingredients and blend with your fingers until crumbly.

4. Sprinkle over the nectarines and microwave uncovered on high for 6 minutes or bake in a preheated 350° oven for 25 to 30 minutes.

To Serve: Serve warm with a dollop of flavored yogurt, nonfat milk, or Creme Topping (page 316).

Per serving: 0 mg cholesterol, 0.2 gm saturated fat, 1.9 gm total fat, 2.1 gm fiber, 3 mg sodium, 118 calories, 0 gm trans fat

°Round or oval is the better shape for the microwave because it gives more even cooking.

EASY COMPANY DINNER

Mixed Greens with Shredded Carrots and
Basil Vinaigrette (page 96)
Broiled Salmon with Balsamic Vinegar
Braised Kale
Summer Squash
♦ Baked Alaska Pears ♦

Baked Alaska Pears Ⓠ

Serves: 4

2 large, ripe pears, peeled, halved, and cored, or 4 pear halves canned in juice

2 tablespoons frozen unsweetened apple juice concentrate

3 extra-large egg whites, at room temperature

¼ teaspoon cream of tartar

3 tablespoons Splenda Sugar Blend°

1 teaspoon apricot liqueur

2 tablespoons chopped almonds

4 large unhulled strawberries, for garnish

1. Place the fresh pear halves in a shallow baking dish and sprinkle with the apple juice concentrate. Cover with microwave plastic wrap and mi-

crowave on high for 3 minutes. (This may be prepared in the morning or the day before.) If you are using canned pears, omit this step.

2. Drain the pears on paper towels and place on a baking sheet.

3. Beat the egg whites and cream of tartar with an electric mixer until soft peaks start to form. Add the Splenda, 1 tablespoon at a time, while beating constantly, until stiff peaks form. Add the liqueur and blend.

4. Cover each pear *completely* with the meringue mixture and sprinkle with chopped almonds.

5. Brown quickly in a preheated 400° oven for 5 minutes or until golden brown.

To Serve: Slide a broad spatula under the pears and place on individual dessert plates. Garnish with a fresh unhulled strawberry and serve immediately.

Per serving: 0 mg cholesterol, 0.18 gm saturated fat, 2.6 gm total fat, 2.2 gm fiber, 61 mg sodium, 114 calories, 0 gm trans fat

°You can prepare the meringue without any sugar; however, the texture and taste of the meringue will be affected.

Sliced Beet and Orange Salad with Tarragon Vinaigrette (page 281)
Lump Crabmeat Salad
Asparagus and Roasted Red Peppers
♦ Lemon-Lime Yogurt Pie ♦

Lemon-Lime Yogurt Pie Ⓠ

Serves: 12 (1 slice = 1 serving)

Crust:
1 cup graham cracker crumbs (no animal fat or coconut or palm oils)
4 tablespoons frozen unsweetened apple juice concentrate
1 teaspoon cinnamon
¼ cup chopped almonds

Filling:
2 envelopes unflavored gelatin°

⅓ cup fresh orange juice
8 ounces 2%-fat small-curd cottage cheese
1½ cups fresh raspberries and/or blueberries and 2 limes, thinly sliced, for garnish

4 8-ounce cartons nonfat lemon-lime flavored yogurt
Grated zest and juice of 1½–2 limes

To Make Crust:

1. Combine the graham cracker crumbs, apple juice concentrate, cinnamon, and nuts; mix well with a fork to blend.

2. Sprinkle on the bottom of an 8-inch springform pan coated with butter-flavored nonstick spray. Pat into place.

3. Bake in a preheated 375° oven for 5 to 6 minutes.

To Make Filling:

1. Sprinkle the gelatin over the fresh orange juice in a saucepan. Stir over low heat or hot water until the gelatin is dissolved.

2. Blend the cottage cheese in a food processor or blender *until smooth*.

3. Add the remaining ingredients, including the dissolved gelatin, to the processor and blend until smooth and well combined.

4. Pour the filling into the crust, cover, and chill 1 hour or overnight before serving.

To Serve: Loosen the pie around the edges with a metal spatula and remove the ring from the springform pan. Place the pie on a serving plate and arrange fresh berries and lime slices around the perimeter.

Variation: Save 2 tablespoons graham cracker crumb mixture from the crust to sprinkle on top of the pie.

Per serving: 3 mg cholesterol, 0.45 gm saturated fat, 1.2 gm total fat, 0.8 gm fiber, 171 mg sodium, 84 calories, 0 gm trans fat

°If there is gelatin in your brand of yogurt, use only 1½ tablespoons gelatin instead of two envelopes.

> *3 tablespoons unsweetened cocoa powder + 1 tablespoon canola oil = 1 ounce of chocolate.*

Cauliflower Soup with Whole Wheat Bread Sticks (page 272)
Broiled Chicken Breast
Orzo with Peas and Red Peppers
Steamed Spinach
♦ Chocolate Zucchini Cupcake ♦

Chocolate Zucchini Cupcakes

Yield: 24 cupcakes (1 cupcake = 1 serving)

What a treat to be able to enjoy a no-cholesterol, no-saturated-fat chocolate cupcake!

4 extra-large egg whites
⅓ cup Splenda
¼ cup canola oil
1 12-ounce can nonfat evaporated milk
2 teaspoons pure vanilla extract
2 cups unbleached white flour or whole wheat pastry flour
¼ cup oat bran, processed in blender until fine

1 teaspoon baking soda
2 teaspoons baking powder
1½ teaspoons ground cinnamon
¼ cup unsweetened cocoa
2 cups shredded zucchini
½ cup seeded dark raisins (microwave on high with 2 tablespoons fresh orange juice for about ½ minute)

1. Preheat the oven to 350°. Line two 12-cup muffin tins with paper baking cups.
2. Add the egg whites, sugar, oil, milk, and vanilla to a food processor with a steel blade and process 30 seconds.
3. Combine the flour, oat bran, baking soda, baking powder, cinnamon, and cocoa in a mixing bowl. Blend thoroughly. Add to the food processor and process until smooth.
4. Add the zucchini and raisins and process 5 seconds.
5. Fill the cups with batter and bake at 350° for about 20 minutes or until a toothpick comes out clean.
6. Remove the cupcakes from the tins and cool on a wire rack.

Variation: Mix ¼ cup finely chopped almonds with 1 tablespoon Splenda and ½ teaspoon ground cinnamon and sprinkle ½ teaspoon of the mixture on top of each cupcake *before* baking.

Per serving: 1 mg cholesterol, 0.27 gm saturated fat, 2.7 gm total fat, 0.8 gm fiber, 87 mg sodium, 99 calories, 0 gm trans fat

Bean Curd and Spinach Soup (page 137)
Marinated Cucumbers
Assorted Sashimi and Sushi
with Wasabi and Ginger
♦ Orange Baked Alaska ♦

Orange Baked Alaska ⓠ

Serves: 6 (1 orange = 1 serving)

A quick, attractive dessert that is low in calories. It's also high in vitamin C and potassium.

6 navel oranges
1 small ripe banana, diced
1 tablespoon Grand Marnier or
  orange juice

2 extra-large egg whites
¼ teaspoon cream of tartar
2 tablespoons Splenda sugar blend

1. Cut ⅓-inch off the top of each orange.
2. Cut around flesh close to skin and remove orange meat.
3. Dice fruit into bite-size pieces and mix with banana and brandy.
4. Return fruit mixture to orange cup. Dry outside and rim of orange cup.
5. Beat egg whites until foamy*, add cream of tartar, and continue beating until soft peaks form. Add sugar blend and continue beating until stiff (does not slide in bowl).
6. Spread meringue over each cup and place on baking sheet.
7. Place in preheated 475° oven for 2 to 3 minutes or until meringue is lightly browned.
8. Serve immediately.

Per serving: 0.0 mg cholesterol, .04 gm saturated fat, 0.21 gm total fat, .51 gm fiber, 96.60 calories, 22.35 gm carbohydrate, .51 gm trans fat, 15.85 gm sugar

*Use glass, stainless steel, or copper bowl for better volume in beating egg whites.

Twelve Menus
for Special Occasions

Any meal becomes a special occasion if you give a little extra thought
to your menu planning and food preparation. Healthful foods that are
both delicious and attractively served are not the impossible dream.
To prove it, here are some menus for celebrations and get-togethers
to share with family and friends. With these menus and recipes your
guests will come away feeling satisfied but comfortable, and you can
be sure that the foods you serve are in everyone's best interest.

Enjoying a pleasant meal with family or friends is still one of life's
great pleasures!

MENUS AND RECIPES

AN OUTDOOR BARBECUE   A TRIO OF DIPS

A CHINESE DINNER LION'S HEAD CHINESE MEATBALLS WITH CHINESE CABBAGE

A FRENCH DINNER   CHICKEN BREASTS, MUSHROOMS, AND
                                 WATER CHESTNUTS IN WINE SAUCE

AN ITALIAN DINER   PASTA WITH PESTO

A MEXICAN DINNER   TAMALE PIE

AFTER THE GAME   MANHATTAN CLAM CHOWDER

A COMPANY CASSEROLE DINNER   SHRIMP CASSEROLE

FAMILY FAVORITES FOR OLD FRIENDS   DOWN-HOME MEAT LOAF

IT'S YOUR BIRTHDAY DINNER   MARBLED ANGEL FOOD CAKE

LOTS-OF-COMPANY BUFFET DINNER MUSTARD-BAKED CHICKEN BREASTS

THANKSGIVING DINNER (without the turkey) PUMPKIN PIE CHEESECAKE

LATE FOR DINNER   COLD OR HOT SPICY GAZPACHO

AN OUTDOOR BARBECUE:
A TRIO OF DIPS

Light Style Guacamole

Yield: 3 cups (2 tablespoons = 1 serving)

2 large ripe California avocados
⅔ cup nonfat sour cream or yogurt
2 tablespoons fresh lime juice
¼ cup finely diced red onion
Pinch of kosher salt

Hot pepper sauce to taste
2 ripe Roma tomatoes, seeded and
    cut into ¼-inch dice
¼ cup chopped fresh cilantro
    (optional)

1. Halve, peel, and pit avocados (save pits).
2. Mash avocado in mixing bowl with fork or potato masher.
3. Add sour cream or yogurt, lime juice, red onion, salt, and pepper sauce (blend well).
4. Place in serving bowl over avocado pits (this keeps dip from turning brown).
5. Sprinkle diced tomato over guacamole, cover with plastic, and chill. Serve with baked tortilla chips.

Per serving: 1.44 mg cholesterol, 0.60 gm saturated fat, 4.37 gm total fat, 2.01 gm fiber, 0 mg sodium, 64.22 calories, 0 gm trans fat

Sardine Paté Ⓠ

Yield: 1 tablespoon = 1 serving

3 shallots
2 cans skinless and boneless
    sardines in olive oil, drained
Juice of ½ lemon
4 tablespoons whipped nonfat
    cream cheese

Dash of Tabasco (optional)
Black ground pepper
Capers in vinegar, optional

1. Mince shallots in food processor. Add sardines and lemon juice, process.
2. Add cream cheese and process until smooth. Taste and adjust seasonings.

3. Place in soufflé cups, sprinkle with paprika and capers. Cover with plastic wrap and chill several hours. Serve paté with pita chips or Kashi TLC chips.

Per serving: 9.69 mg cholesterol, 0.1 gm saturated fat, 0.75 gm total fat, 0 gm fiber, 47.5 mg sodium, 16.46 calories, 0 gm trans fat

Asparagus Dip Ⓠ

Yield: About 1¼ cups (2 tablespoons = 1 serving)

It looks like guacamole, but is only about one-fifth the calories!

1 pound green asparagus (tough ends removed), cut into 1-inch pieces
¼ red onion
1 large clove of garlic
1 tablespoon lemon juice

¼ teaspoon Herbes de Provence
2 tablespoons Fage nonfat yogurt
2 teaspoons grated Parmesan cheese
1 tomato, peeled, seeded, and diced

1. Microwave asparagus for about 3 to 4 minutes. Drain well and cool.
2. Place asparagus, onion, garlic, and lemon juice in a food processor and process until finely chopped. Add yogurt and cheese. Blend and chill.
3. To serve, place in hollowed red pepper topped with tomato. Enjoy with blue corn tortilla chips and assorted vegetables.

Per serving: 1.4 mg cholesterol, 0.0 gm saturated fat, 0.8 gm total fat, 8 mg sodium, 14 calories, 0 gm trans fat, 2.5 gm carbohydrate, 0 gm sugar, 0.6 gm fiber

---

2 extra-large egg whites = 1 whole egg =
¼ cup egg substitute

A CHINESE DINNER

Hot and Sour Soup
♦ Lion's Head Chinese Meatballs with Chinese Cabbage ♦
Snow Peas and Red Peppers
Steamed Rice (page 133)
Lychee Nuts and Orange Wedges
Fortune Cookies

This dish originated in Shanghai, but today it is equally at home in Chicago. The oversized meatballs were supposed to be reminiscent of lions' heads. Traditionally, ground pork is used, but I have substituted ground turkey or chicken, which lowers the saturated fat and cholesterol content without sacrificing flavor. Fortune cookies are included in the menu, but enjoy the fortune and forget the cookie.

Lion's Head Chinese Meatballs with Chinese Cabbage

Serves: 6 (about 2 ounces cooked meat = 1 serving)

4 dried shiitake mushrooms (1 ounce), soaked in hot water 20 minutes, drained, and stems removed and discarded

1 pound ground turkey or chicken breast* (see page 144), skin and fat removed

½ cup toasted bread croutons soaked in ½ cup 1% milk

2 extra-large egg whites, slightly beaten

5 finely chopped fresh or canned water chestnuts

2 whole shallots, thinly sliced

1 large clove garlic, minced

2 teaspoons grated fresh ginger root

2 tablespoons dry sherry or dry white wine

1 tablespoon sodium-reduced soy sauce

1 tablespoon cornstarch

1 cup defatted sodium-reduced chicken broth mixed with 1 tablespoon dry sherry

½ fresh Chinese cabbage or bok choy, cut into 6 portions

Freshly ground pepper

6 small green onions, cut into brushes, for garnish

1. Mince the drained mushroom caps.

2. Combine the mushrooms with the turkey, crouton-milk mixture, egg whites, water chestnuts, shallots, garlic, ginger, sherry, soy sauce, and cornstarch, mixing thoroughly. Shape into six equal-sized large meatballs.

3. Brown the meatballs in a hot nonstick skillet coated with nonstick cooking spray.

4. Add the broth and sherry mixture. Bring to a boil, reduce heat, cover, and simmer 20 minutes.

5. Remove the meatballs from the sauce. Layer the Chinese cabbage in the sauce, season with pepper, and then top with the meatballs, basting with sauce.

6. Bring the sauce to a boil, reduce heat, cover, and simmer about another 8 to 10 minutes.

To Serve: Arrange the cooked Chinese cabbage on a warm serving platter, top with the meatballs, and pour sauce over all. Garnish with green onion brushes.

Per serving: 39 mg cholesterol, 0.59 gm saturated fat, 1.9 gm total fat, 1.3 gm fiber, 198 mg sodium, 144 calories, 0 gm trans fat

*Lean pork tenderloin, ground, may be substituted or combined with chicken or turkey.

Use a smaller amount of brown sugar when using in place of white sugar.

♦

If we are what we eat, then we should be concerned about what the animals we eat also eat! (Look for beef that is pastured and 100 percent grass fed.)

A FRENCH DINNER

Red and Green Lettuce Salad with
Dijon Mustard and Shallot Vinaigrette
♦ Chicken Breasts, Mushrooms, and
Water Chestnuts in Wine Sauce ♦
Steamed Wild Rice
Haricot Verte and Baby Carrots
Meringue Shells (page 326) with
Fresh Blueberries and Strawberries with Strawberry Sauce

Chicken Breasts, Mushrooms, and Water Chestnuts in Wine Sauce

Serves: 8 (3½ ounces cooked chicken = 1 serving)

It is always convenient to have a company dish that's not a casserole and yet can be prepared ahead of time or the day before. To complete this meal before your guests arrive, you have only to prepare a salad of mixed greens, generous amounts of rice and vegetables, and raspberries or some other fresh seasonal fruit to serve with meringue shells for dessert. The meringue shells can also be made in advance.

4 whole chicken breasts (about 14–16 ounces each), halved, skinned, boned, and flattened°
2 teaspoons salt-free vegetable seasoning
2 teaspoons Hungarian paprika
Freshly ground pepper
2 teaspoons extra-virgin olive oil
3 large cloves garlic, minced
2 shallots, minced
1 small onion, finely chopped
1 red pepper, seeded and diced
1 cup sliced fresh or drained canned water chestnuts

2½ cups sliced cremini mushrooms
1 10-ounce package frozen small whole onions
1½ tablespoons fresh thyme, chopped, or 1 teaspoon dried thyme, crushed
2 cups canned crushed San Marzano tomatoes in puree
¼ cup white wine
¼ cup dry red wine

Chopped fresh thyme or Italian parsley for garnish

1. Dry the flattened chicken breasts with paper towel and season both sides with vegetable seasoning, paprika, and ground pepper.

2. Coat a 12-inch sauté pan with nonstick spray; add the olive oil and heat the pan.

3. Place chicken breasts in the hot pan and brown lightly on both sides over moderate heat. Remove the chicken to a shallow oven-proof casserole.

4. Add the garlic, shallots, and onion to the sauté pan and sauté, stirring constantly, for 2 to 3 minutes. (If necessary, add a bit of chicken broth.)

5. Add the red pepper, water chestnuts, mushrooms, and whole onions, and sauté 5 minutes.

6. Add the thyme, tomatoes, and wine; stir and bring to a boil. Simmer 5 minutes.

7. Pour the vegetable mixture over the chicken in the shallow baking dish† and cook, uncovered, 25 minutes in a preheated 350° oven.

To Serve: Sprinkle fresh thyme or parsley over the chicken just before serving.

Per serving: 84 mg cholesterol, 1.48 gm saturated fat, 6.1 gm total fat, 1.4 gm fiber, 181 mg sodium, 247 calories, 0 gm trans fat

°To flatten chicken breasts, place a boned breast half between two pieces of waxed paper or plastic wrap and pound with a mallet until it is about ½ inch thick.
†May be prepared a day ahead to this point and refrigerated. If chilled, add 15 minutes to the baking time.

BLTs translates into bites, licks, and tastes, not into bacon, lettuce, and tomato. Mindless eating can cause a weight gain of 1 to 5 pounds per year!

AN ITALIAN DINNER

Panzanella (page 272)
Vegetarian Lentil Soup (page 87)
♦ Pasta with Pesto ♦
Zucchini, Red Peppers, and Mushrooms
Crisp Garlic Toast (page 331)
Compote of Fresh Fruit with Amaretto

Panzanella (a salad using leftover bread and fresh vegetables), a full-bodied vegetarian lentil soup, pasta and pesto, and Amaretto liqueur are all favorites in Italian-style cooking.

Pesto, or basil sauce, is a tradition in Genoa in the northwest part of Italy. If you are fortunate enough to be able to grow your own fresh basil, it should go right from your garden to your food processor. If not, many markets are now selling packaged fresh herbs for your convenience. This flavorful low-fat recipe has much less oil than commercial pesto, and no pine nuts. It is not only wonderful as a sauce with pasta, but a dab enhances the taste of minestrone, steamed or baked potatoes, sliced tomato and onion salad, sandwiches, or warm toast. Fresh pesto will keep for six weeks in the refrigerator in a tightly closed jar, or may be frozen for future use.

Pasta with Pesto ⓠ

Serves: 4 (2 tablespoons pesto = 1 serving)

Pesto:
3 cloves garlic
1 shallot
1 packed cup fresh Italian parsley
  leaves without stems
2½ packed cups fresh basil leaves
  without stems
2 tablespoons extra-virgin olive oil

Few grains crushed red pepper
1–2 tablespoons freshly grated
  Parmesan cheese

8 ounces capellini (angel hair
  pasta), cooked al dente and
  drained, or whole wheat
  linguine

1. Place the garlic, shallot, and parsley in a food processor or blender and chop. Add the basil and process the mixture until chopped.
2. Add the oil, pepper, and cheese, and process until finely blended.

3. Add about half of the sauce to the hot, drained pasta, and stir to blend. (Reserve the rest of the sauce for future use.)

4. Serve immediately while hot, and pass additional Parmesan cheese if desired.

Variations: Two diced peeled Italian plum tomatoes may be added with the pesto sauce before blending with the pasta.

Two and one half cups fresh spinach leaves and 2 tablespoons dried basil may be substituted for the fresh basil in the pesto sauce. However, it won't be nearly as delicious.

Per serving: 1 mg cholesterol, 1.28 gm saturated fat, 8.3 gm total fat, 3 gm fiber, 34 mg sodium, 311 calories

Per 2 tablespoons pesto: 1 mg cholesterol, 1.18 gm saturated fat, 7.5 gm total fat, 1.8 gm fiber, 33 mg sodium, 99 calories, 0 gm trans fat

A MEXICAN DINNER

Sopa de Ajo (Garlic Soup) (page 275)
Quesadilla (page 95)
Sweet Potato Chips (page 270) and Crudités
with Fresh Salsa (page 185)
♦ Tamale Pie ♦
Mixed Green Salad
Mango Fruited Mousse (page 322)

Mexican-style cooking *can* be low fat and low cholesterol, as this tamale pie proves, and still be delicious.

Tamale Pie

Serves: 8

1 recipe Chunky Turkey Chili (page 195); if necessary, add 1 can chili beans with chili gravy to equal 6½ cups total chili mixture
1 cup canned cream-style corn
1 cup fresh corn (about 2 ears) or canned salt-free corn
2 teaspoons dried Italian herb blend, crushed
2 cups cold water

2 cups cold nonfat milk
1¼ cups yellow cornmeal
Freshly ground pepper
1 tablespoon shredded Parmesan cheese

3 tablespoons chopped fresh cilantro or Italian parsley, for garnish

1. Combine the chili, cream-style corn, corn, and 1 teaspoon of the Italian herb blend. Mix thoroughly and pour into a 13 × 9 × 2-inch baking dish coated with nonstick spray.

2. Place the cold water and milk in a 1½-quart saucepan. Add the cornmeal, the remaining teaspoon Italian herb blend, and the pepper. Mix. Cook over medium heat until thick and stiff (about 7 minutes), stirring frequently.

3. Top the chili with eight heaping portions of the cornmeal mixture and flatten with the back of spoon. Sprinkle each portion of cornmeal with a bit of Parmesan cheese.

4. Bake in a preheated 350° oven for 25 to 30 minutes.

To Serve: Sprinkle with cilantro or parsley and serve hot.

Variation: To make a vegetarian meal, use the vegetarian chili recipe on page 196 as a base instead of the Chunky Turkey Chili.

Per serving: 21 mg cholesterol, 0.87 gm saturated fat, 4.8 gm total fat, 6.9 gm fiber, 346 mg sodium, 352 calories, 0 gm trans fat

AFTER THE GAME

♦ Manhattan Clam Chowder ♦
Guacamole and Baked Chips (page 244)
Oven Baked Chinese Chicken Legs (page 299)
Three-Bean Salad • Mixed Fresh Fruit
Today's Coffee Cake (page 340)

This menu will score with family or guests. The tomato-based chowder is filled with vegetables and just enough clams to give a wonderful flavor. It certainly is nutritionally preferable to New England clam chowder!

Manhattan Clam Chowder

Yield: 16 cups (1½ cups = 1 serving as an entrée)

1 large onion, chopped	6 large carrots, coarsely chopped
1 large leek (white part only), washed and chopped	2 large peeled russet potatoes, or yams coarsely chopped
6 stalks celery, chopped	⅓ cup chopped fresh Italian parsley

1 28-ounce can crushed San
  Marzano tomatoes in puree
4 cups water
½ teaspoon crushed red pepper
  flakes
1 bay leaf
2 teaspoons dried oregano, crushed
1 teaspoon dried thyme, crushed
2 cloves garlic, chopped
3 tablespoons unbleached white
  flour

1 cup sodium-reduced canned
  chopped tomatoes
½ cup dry white wine
2 7½ ounce cans chopped
  clams with juice (no MSG or
  preservatives added)
1 8-ounce bottle clam juice
  (optional)

1. Place the onions, leek, celery, carrots, potatoes or yams, parsley, Italian plum tomatoes, water, and seasonings in 4½-quart saucepan. Bring to a boil, reduce to a simmer, cover, and cook 1 hour, stirring occasionally.

2. Lightly brown the flour in a nonstick skillet, stirring constantly. Add the browned flour to the soup and mix thoroughly.

3. Add the chopped tomatoes, wine, and clams and clam juice, and simmer 30 minutes. Remove bay leaf. Freezes well for future use.

Per serving: 18 mg cholesterol, 0.11 gm saturated fat, 0.9 gm total fat, 1.8 gm fiber, 141 mg sodium, 99 calories, 0 gm trans fat

A COMPANY CASSEROLE DINNER

Spicy Cold Tomato Soup (page 88)
Curly Endive, Orange, and Jicama Salad with
Low-Calorie Vinaigrette
♦ Shrimp Casserole with Water Chestnuts and Mushrooms ♦
Assorted Whole Grain Rolls
Steamed Brown Rice
Broccoli Crown (page 305) and Parsleyed Carrot Coins
with Pea Pods
Poached Pear "en Croute" (page 352) with
Blueberry Sauce (page 317)

Whether cooking for four or forty, your preparation for entertaining should allow you time to enjoy your guests. This shrimp casserole may be prepared the day before, and the rest of the menu is simple yet satisfying.

Shrimp Casserole Ⓠ

Serves: 8 (½ cup = 1 serving)

Shrimp is high in cholesterol, but being one of the vegetarians of the sea it is *very* low in saturated fat and contains no trans fat. Besides—it's a snap to make!

2 tablespoons olive or canola oil
½ cup chopped onion
2 shallots, minced
1 cup sliced celery, with leaves
1 small red pepper, seeded and diced
½ teaspoon Herbes de Provence, crushed
1 6½-ounce can sliced water chestnuts, drained
10 ounces sliced cremini mushrooms

2 cans Campbell's Healthy Request mushroom soup
¼ cup dry vermouth or white wine
1½ teaspoons Worcestershire sauce
1 pound large shrimp, raw, peeled and deveined
2 cups toasted herb croutons, optional
4 cups steamed brown rice

1. Preheat oven to 350°.
2. Heat oil in 10-inch nonstick skillet. Add onions, shallots, celery, and red pepper. Sauté about 5 minutes. Add Herbes de Provence, mushrooms, and water chestnuts. Sauté 1 to 2 minutes.
3. Add soup, wine, and Worcestershire sauce to vegetable mixture. Stir to combine. Add shrimp and mix.
4. Pour into 9 × 13-inch glass baking dish.° Top with croutons, and bake about 25 minutes or until mixture bubbles.

To Serve: Top steamed brown rice with a serving of shrimp casserole.

Per serving: 87.71 gm cholesterol, 1.45 gm saturated fat, 6.78 gm total fat, 4.14 gm fiber, 406.41 mg sodium, 279.28 calories, 34.9 gm carbohydrate, 0 gm trans fat

°May be covered with foil and refrigerated, If it is to be baked and served the next day, do not add croutons.

FAMILY FAVORITES FOR OLD FRIENDS

Cole Slaw with Vinaigrette
♦ Down-Home Meat Loaf ♦
Mashed Potatoes with Horseradish and Chives
Braised Kale
Succotash
Bowl of Fresh Seasonal Fruit
Pineapple Cake (page 351)

Considering the resurgence of interest in American cooking, no recipe collection would be complete without a meat loaf recipe. I have added oat bran or rolled oats instead of bread crumbs to provide more soluble fiber and an assortment of vegetables for added flavor. My mother added rolled oats fifty years ago without having any special reason except that it tasted good.

The traditional American recipes in this menu have been adjusted by adding oats to the meat loaf (soluble fiber) and chicken broth, horseradish, and chives to the mashed potatoes. Of course, the cholesterol, saturated fat, and trans-fat content will be lower if you use ground turkey instead of ground round of beef.

Down-Home Meat Loaf ⓠ

Serves: 6 (2 slices = 1 serving)

2 extra-large egg whites
6 ounces sodium-reduced vegetable juice (V-8)
⅔ cup rolled oats
1 tablespoon Worcestershire sauce
Freshly ground pepper
1 small onion, quartered
1 large carrot, quartered
½ red pepper, quartered and diced
1 zucchini, quartered
2 cloves garlic, peeled
½ cup fresh parsley, coarse stems removed, thyme, basil, oregano, chopped

1 pound ground turkey (see page 144) or lean ground round and half-pound ground lean veal
1 teaspoon olive oil

Glaze:
¼ cup salt-free tomato sauce
2 tablespoons frozen unsweetened apple juice concentrate
1 teaspoon Dijon mustard or 3 tablespoons sodium-reduced ketchup mixed with ½ teaspoon dry mustard

1. In a mixing bowl, beat the egg whites slightly with a fork. Add the juice, rolled oats, Worcestershire sauce, and pepper, and let stand 5 to 10 minutes.

2. Place the onion, carrot, zucchini, garlic, and parsley with herbs in a food processor or blender and chop. *Do not puree.* Add diced pepper.

3. Add the vegetable mixture, the ground meat, and olive oil to the egg-white mixture and mix lightly with a fork (or clean hands or plastic gloves) to combine.

4. Mound the meat mixture into a 9-inch square pan coated with non-stick spray and shape into an 8-inch loaf.

5. Bake in a preheated 375° oven for 35 minutes.

6. Mix the glaze ingredients together, brush over the meat loaf, return to the oven, and bake 10 to 12 minutes longer.

7. Remove from the oven and let stand 10 minutes before slicing.

To Serve: Cut the meat loaf into twelve slices and arrange on a heated serving platter. Surround with mashed potatoes sprinkled with chives.

To Microwave:

1. Pack meat mixture into a 9-inch square glass pan and microwave uncovered on high for 8 minutes.

2. Drain juice and cover with glaze. Microwave uncovered on high for 3 to 5 minutes. Let stand 10 minutes before slicing.

Per serving: 40 mg cholesterol, 0.63 gm saturated fat, 3 gm total fat, 3.3 gm fiber, 108 mg sodium, 175 calories, 0 gm trans fat

IT'S YOUR BIRTHDAY DINNER

Herring Antipasto (page 269)
Eggplant Lasagna (page 225)
Vegetable Kabobs with Spicy Red Pepper Sauce (page 235)
Sally's Zucchini (page 313)
♦ Marbled Angel Food Cake (with Three Sauces) ♦

In our family, on your birthday you choose your dinner menu. My daughter Sally selected all of her vegetarian favorites, including Marbled Angel Food Cake.

Marbled Angel Food Cake

Serves: 16 to 20

1 cup cake flour, or 1 cup unbleached white flour, less 2 tablespoons
¼ cup Splenda Sugar Blend
1½ cups liquid egg whites (about 10–12 whites) at room temperature
1 teaspoon cream of tartar

1½ teaspoons pure vanilla extract
¾ cup granulated sugar
3 tablespoons sifted cocoa
Fresh strawberries and Fresh Strawberry Sauce (page 319), fresh blueberries and Blueberry Sauce (page 317), or heated Wax Orchards Fudge Topping

1. Use a 10-inch tube pan, *ungreased*!
2. Sift together the flour and ¼ cup Splenda Sugar Blend.
3. Place the egg whites into the large bowl of an electric mixer, beat until frothy, and add the cream of tartar and extract. Beat until stiff, not dry; gradually add the remaining ¾ cup sugar, 2 tablespoons at a time. Beat well after each addition.
4. Continue beating until the meringue forms stiff peaks and is glossy (*the whites will not slide in the bowl*).
5. Gradually sprinkle the flour-sugar mixture over the meringue, 3 tablespoons at a time, and fold in gently with a rubber spatula to combine.
6. Divide batter in half and fold in 3 tablespoons of sifted cocoa to one half.
7. Put alternate spoonfuls of light and dark batter into 10-inch tube pan. Cut through the batter with a knife to make swirls of light and dark batter.
8. Bake in preheated 375° oven for 30 to 35 minutes or until the cake springs back when touched with finger.
9. Remove cake from oven, invert the pan onto a vinegar or soda bottle, (if angel-food pan does not have legs) and cool upside down for about 1 hour.

To Serve: When cool, loosen the cake from the sides, bottom, and tube with a knife and invert onto a platter. Serve with fruit sauces and/or chocolate sauce.

Hint: Use a serrated knife to cut the cake to prevent squashing.

LOTS-OF-COMPANY BUFFET DINNER

Cold Spicy Gazpacho (page 261)
♦ Mustard-Baked Chicken Breasts ♦
and/or
Oven-Baked Chinese Chicken Legs (page 299)
Salmon Fillets with Dill from Trader Joe's
Fresh Asparagus Salad (page 280)   Assorted Mixed Green Salad
Oven Roasted Vegetables
Fresh White Nectarine Scallop (page 238)
Today's Coffee Cake (page 340)
Chocolate Trifle (page 345)

Somehow when I start inviting guests for dinner, it always ends up a crowd—and I love it. The Mustard-Baked Chicken Breasts, Oven-Baked Chinese Chicken Legs, and easily prepared Dilled Salmon from Trader Joe's give variety without exhausting the hostess. Save room for dessert!

Mustard-Baked Chicken Breasts ⓠ

Serves: 12 (3 ounces cooked chicken = 1 serving)

1 cup buttermilk
2 tablespoons each Dijon mustard
    and coarsely ground mustard
1⅓ cups fine, dry bread crumbs
2 tablespoons grated Parmesan
    cheese

⅓ cup chopped fresh Italian parsley
12 4-ounce halved, boned, skinned,
    and defatted chicken breasts

Watercress and pear tomatoes, for
    garnish

1. Mix the buttermilk and mustard together in a shallow bowl.
2. Mix the bread crumbs, cheese, and parsley together in separate shallow bowl.
3. Coat the chicken with the buttermilk mixture, then dip in the bread crumbs on one side only. Place chicken, *unbreaded*-side-down, on a rack on a nonstick baking sheet. Bake in the upper third of a preheated 475° oven for 25 to 30 minutes or until lightly brown and tender.

To Serve: Place the chicken breasts on a heated platter on a bed of watercress and garnish with tomatoes.

Per serving: 74 mg cholesterol, 1.36 gm saturated fat, 4.8 gm total fat, 0.1 gm fiber, 229 mg sodium, 200 calories, 0 gm trans fat

THANKSGIVING DINNER (*Without the Turkey*)

Mushroom Bisque (page 276)
with Whole Wheat Bread Sticks
Watercress, Radicchio, and Wild Greens Salad
Orange-Glazed Cornish Hens (page 215)
Cranberry-Pineapple Freeze (page 330)
Baked Sweet Potatoes
Stir-Fried Squash and Red Pepper (page 312)
Steamed Tender Whole Green and Yellow Stringbeans
◆ Pumpkin Pie Cheesecake ◆
Persimmon Freeze (page 323)
The Great Pumpkin Muffins (page 334)

For a delicious change at Thanksgiving, I have combined my cheese-cake and pumpkin pie recipes.

Pumpkin Pie Cheesecake

Yield: 1 8-inch cheesecake

Serves: 12 to 14

Graham Cracker Crust:
1¼ cups graham cracker crumbs (with *no* animal or hydrogenated fat, or coconut or palm oil)
½ cup chopped walnuts
1 teaspoon ground cinnamon
Freshly ground nutmeg
3 tablespoons frozen unsweetened apple juice concentrate

Pumpkin-Cheese filling:
16 ounces tofu cream cheese or low-fat Philadelphia cream cheese and 8 ounces low-fat ricotta cheese

2 tablespoons cornstarch
¼ cup Splenda Brown Sugar Blend
2 extra-large egg whites, slightly beaten
½ cup low-fat Silk soy milk
1 1-pound can pumpkin pie filling
1 teaspoon pure vanilla extract

Sour-Cream Topping:
1 cup light-style sour cream
2 teaspoons pure vanilla extract

To Prepare Crust:

1. Combine the crumbs, walnuts, cinnamon, and nutmeg.
2. Moisten the crumb mixture with the apple juice concentrate, mixing with a fork. Reserve 2 to 3 tablespoons of the crumb mixture for garnish.
3. Press the remainder of the crumb mixture firmly into the bottom of an 8-inch springform pan lightly coated with nonstick spray.

To Prepare Filling and Topping:

1. In a food processor or blender blend the cheese, sugar, and cornstarch until smooth.
2. Add the egg whites and blend. Add the soy milk, pumpkin, and vanilla and blend thoroughly.
3. Pour into the prepared crust and bake in a preheated 300° oven for 1 hour or until firm.
4. Cool the pie slightly on a rack for about 10 to 15 minutes. Meanwhile, blend the topping ingredients.
5. Cover the pie with the sour-cream topping and sprinkle with the reserved crumb mixture. Cover and chill until serving time.

To Serve: For an especially festive feeling, place a minipumpkin on the center of the pie before presenting your dessert.

Per serving: 10 mg cholesterol, 1.85 gm saturated fat, 4.5 gm total fat, 1.3 gm fiber, 109 mg sodium, 129 calories, 0 gm trans fat

LATE FOR DINNER

♦ Cold or Hot Spicy Gazpacho ♦
Baked Blue Corn Chips
Broiled Miso-marinated Salmon with Dijon Mustard and Capers
Red Cabbage and Mango Salad
Julienned Green Beans with Toasted Almonds
Virtual Brownies

We have all been in the position of realizing that there's "nothing at home for dinner," or that we'll be getting home too late to prepare it. In Europe, it's not an uncommon practice to stop at the market, see what's available, and use that for the evening meal. With this in mind, if you pick up some fresh salsa for soup, some fresh fish for the entrée, a few fresh vegetables and potatoes for the microwave, and some fresh seasonal fruit—dinner will be ready thirty minutes after you get home!

This spicy gazpacho is fantastic served either cold or hot, and is so easy to make. Make certain that you buy salsa with no preservatives added. It will keep about a week in your refrigerator.

Cold or Hot Spicy Gazpacho Ⓠ

Serves: 5 to 6 (¾ cup = 1 serving)

16 ounces Fresh Salsa (page 185) or canned mild salsa (no preservatives added)
1 large clove garlic
3 6-ounce cans sodium-reduced vegetable juice (V-8)
2–3 tablespoons red wine vinegar

½ teaspoon dried oregano or Italian herb blend
Few drops hot pepper sauce, or to taste

Thinly sliced cucumbers and nonfat plain yogurt, for garnish

1. Place all the ingredients except the garnish in a food processor or blender and process until smooth. Taste and adjust seasonings.

2. Either pour into a storage container, cover, and chill in the freezer for about 20 minutes before serving, or heat and serve either very cold or very hot.

To Serve: Pour into cups or bowls, garnish with cucumber slice, a dollop of nonfat yogurt, and, if desired, 3 shrimp cut into 4 pieces each.

Per serving: 0 mg cholesterol, 0.04 gm saturated fat, 0.2 gm total fat, 1.5 gm fiber, 11 mg sodium, 35 calories, 0 gm trans fat

▼ 6 ▼

Mix and Match:
More Low-Cholesterol
Dishes

The recipes in this chapter may be exchanged for comparable recipes in the menus in the previous chapters and you will still be assured of a cholesterol-controlled diet, low in saturated fat and trans fat. For example, you may decide that you prefer one of the soups or salads in Mix and Match to one of those listed in a menu. Or you may choose one of the fish, poultry, or pasta entrées in this chapter as an exchange for a similar entrée listed in a menu. (All portions of protein are within the guidelines for a healthful lifestyle.) Instead of fruit for dessert, you may have the time or taste for one of the many tempting desserts from this chapter or, occasionally, even a luscious one from Chapter 7.

Whatever you decide, aim for variety to make your mealtimes special. There's no reason that a healthful lifestyle can't be a treat for your palate as well as good for your health.

You can also put together complete menus of your own, based on the patterns of the menus in Chapters 4 and 5. A sample healthful dinner could include:

Soup and/or Salad
4-ounce Cooked Portion of Fish or Poultry
or a Pasta or Casserole Recipe
Rice, Barley, or Corn°
Green or Yellow Vegetables
Dessert (generally fruit or fruit based)

°If the entrée is not a pasta.

Just remember that animal protein should be served at either lunch *or* dinner, *not at both*, and try to have three vegetarian days a week.

REMEMBER THE MEAL PLAN GOAL

Total calories: ♦ about 50 percent from complex carbohydrates
  ♦ no more than 25 percent from protein (animal or vegetable)
  ♦ about 25 percent from vegetables and fruits

Recipes

Appetizers (beginning on page 267):

Spicy Artichoke Hearts
Shrimp or Clam Dip
Russian Dressing Dip
Herring Antipasto
Sweet Potato Chips
Tex-Mex Mini Quiches
Panzanella

Six New Simply Delicious Soups (beginning on page 272):

Creamy Cauliflower Soup
Celery Soup
Sopa de Ajo
Mushroom Bisque
Tofu and Corn Soup
Fresh Vegetable Soup

Salads and Salad Dressings (beginning on page 279):

Cucumber-Buttermilk Dressing
Low-Calorie Salad Dressing
Fresh Asparagus Salad
Sliced Beet and Orange Salad
Black Bean and Corn Salad

Green Bean Salad Piquant with Ginger
Cabbage, Bean Sprout, Tomato, and Carrot Slaw
Cole Slaw Relish Salad
Bristol Farms Fantastic Corn and Eggplant Fiesta
Kasha and Corn Salad
Radish, Celery, and Cucumber Salad
Spinach and Pear Salad
Date Waldorf Salad
Vegetable Antipasto

Entrées (beginning on page 291):

Pasta with Garden Vegetable Marinara Sauce
Turkey Chili and Macaroni
Deviled Turkey Fillets
Grilled Hawaiian Fish with Pineapple Sauce
Red Snapper with Spicy Tomato Sauce
Foil-Baked Fish with Vegetables
Fish Fajitas
Stir-Fried Tuna and Vegetables
Chicken Breasts in Phyllo
Oven-Baked Chinese Chicken Legs
Perfect Chicken Cacciatore
Pasta Pizza Pie
Corn Crêpes with Cheese and Spinach or Vegetable Filling

Vegetarian Dishes (beginning on page 305):

Broccoli Crown
Easy Eggplant Parmesan
Vegetarian Tofu Chili
Gingered Pineapple Carrots
Larry's Scalloped Potatoes and Onions
Sherry's Stuffed Potatoes (with Seven Toppings)
Roast Potatoes with Basil
Different Stuffed Potatoes
Stir-Fried Squash and Red Pepper
Sally's Zucchini

Pasta and Grain Side Dishes (beginning on page 313):

Sweet Pasta Pudding
Cracked Wheat and Tomato Salad
Bulgur Wheat Pilaf
Buckwheat Kernels and Pasta

Desserts (beginning on page 316):

Creme Topping
Blueberry Sauce
Apple Crisp
Poached Pear with Fresh Strawberry Sauce (2 recipes)
Poached Pears and Prunes
Individual Fresh Apple Tart with Apricot Glaze
Fresh Fruit Compote
Fruited Mousse
Persimmon Freeze
Café au Lait Custard
Raisin and Pear Bread Pudding
Bing Cherry Clafouti
Meringue Shells with Fruit
Angel Food Cake

Accompaniments (beginning on page 329):

Mango Salsa
Cranberry-Pineapple Freeze
Cheese Berry Spread
Garlic Toast
High-Fiber Whole Grain Onion Bread
Bran Berry Loaf
The Great Pumpkin Muffins

Snacks (beginning on page 335):

Soy Smoothie Shake
Orange-Yogurt Popsicles

Appetizers

Spicy Artichoke Hearts

Serves: 8

A piquant low-calorie starter.

2 cans quartered artichoke hearts,
   rinsed and squeezed dry, or
   2 9-ounce packages frozen
   artichoke hearts, cooked in
   microwave
2 cups Fresh Salsa (page 185) or
   salt-free canned salsa
1 clove garlic, minced
½ cup crushed San Marzano
   tomatoes

1 teaspoon Italian herb blend,
   crushed, or 1 tablespoon
   chopped fresh oregano
Few drops hot pepper sauce

1 tablespoon chopped fresh
   cilantro or Italian parsley, for
   garnish

1. Combine all the ingredients except the cilantro in a bowl. Stir to blend.
2. Sprinkle with cilantro and chill for at least 1 hour in refrigerator before serving.

Per serving: 0 mg cholesterol, 0.05 gm saturated fat, 0.3 gm total fat, 1.5 gm fiber, 48 mg sodium, 50 calories

Shrimp or Clam Dip

Yield: 1½ cups (2 tablespoons = 1 serving)

A tasty starter to serve with assorted vegetables.

1 cup nonfat Fage plain yogurt or
   1 tablespoon nonfat sour cream
1 tablespoon no-sugar ketchup
1 teaspoon lemon juice
1 tablespoon grated onion
⅛ teaspoon white pepper
½ teaspoon Worcestershire sauce

½ teaspoon dried horseradish
1 tablespoon chopped fresh Italian
   parsley
1 tablespoon capers, rinsed and
   drained (optional)
1 cup cooked bay shrimp, coarsely
   chopped

1. Combine all the ingredients, except shrimp, in a small bowl. Mix well.

2. Add shrimp and chill at least 30 minutes before serving.

To Serve: Serve with raw vegetables for dipping, such as broccoli florets, carrot, zucchini, green and red pepper sticks, jicama, and cherry tomatoes.

Variation: Substitute ½ cup chopped fresh crabmeat or ½ cup scallops poached in 3 tablespoons dry white wine and 1 teaspoon chopped shallot, for the clams.

Per serving: 4 mg cholesterol, 0.03 gm saturated fat, 0.1 gm total fat, 0 gm fiber, 23 mg sodium, 17 calories, 0 gm trans fat

Russian Dressing Dip ⓠ

Yield: 1⅓ cups (1 tablespoon = 1 serving)

This dip may also be used as a salad dressing.

1 cup nonfat sour cream	2 tablespoons red wine vinegar
¼ cup nonfat plain yogurt	1½ tablespoons chili sauce
1 minced shallot	Freshly ground pepper
½ cup minced green pepper and/ or celery	1 tablespoon rinsed capers (optional)

1. Blend first four ingredients until smooth.
2. Add the remaining ingredients and blend just 2 to 3 seconds.
3. Place in a serving bowl, cover, and chill 1 hour or more.

To Serve: Serve cold with assorted raw vegetables.

Per serving: 0 mg cholesterol, 0.07 gm saturated fat, 0.1 gm total fat, 0.1 gm fiber, 22 mg sodium, 12 calories, 0 gm trans fat

Herring Antipasto ⓠ

Serves: 14–16 (2 tablespoons = 1 serving as an appetizer,

½ cup = 1 serving for lunch)

An appetizer that's easy to prepare and high in omega-3 fatty acids. How could anything that tastes so good be so good for you?

1 16-ounce jar of marinated herring, well drained and cut into ¼-inch strips
1 large red bell pepper, seeded and diced
1 small green bell pepper, seeded and diced
1 small red onion, chopped fine
1 16-ounce jar water-packed artichoke hearts, drained and sliced

1 can hearts of palm, drained and sliced
1 cup salt-reduced kidney beans and/or garbanzo beans, drained
2 to 3 caper berries (in vinegar, not brine), drained
¼ cup chopped fresh dill
½ cup chili sauce or no-sugar ketchup
Chopped fresh dill, for garnish

1. Place the herring,* peppers, onions, artichoke hearts, hearts of palm, beans, and capers in a mixing bowl and add dill and chili sauce. Stir to combine. Sprinkle with additional chopped dill.

2. Cover and chill 4 hours or overnight before serving. This will keep up to 2 weeks in the refrigerator—do not freeze.

Per serving: 31.75 mg cholesterol, 0.05 gm saturated fat, 4.71 gm total fat, 4.29 gm fiber, 169.19 calories, 19.32 gm carbohydrate, 5.5 gm sugar, 0 gm trans fat

Note: Drain herring additionally by blotting with paper towel.

Sweet Potato Chips Ⓠ

Serves: 6

Whether served as a snack with Fresh Salsa (page 185), salt-free canned salsa, or store-bought salsa or as an accompaniment in a meal, these sweet potato chips are delicious. They can be frozen for future use and reheated briefly.

2 pounds yams scrubbed, peeled, and sliced ⅛ inch thick
2 tablespoons canola or olive-oil spray

2 tablespoons spicy salt-free vegetable seasoning

1. Place the sliced potatoes in a bowl, sprinkle with oil, and mix thoroughly.
2. Spread the potatoes in a single layer on a nonstick baking sheet and sprinkle with vegetable seasoning.
3. Bake in the upper third of a preheated 450° oven for 12 to 15 minutes, or until nicely browned. Serve immediately.

Variation: Organic russet potatoes can be used instead of sweet potatoes.

Per serving: 0 mg cholesterol, 0.21 gm saturated fat, 3.5 gm total fat, 2.9 gm fiber, 12 mg sodium, 150 calories, 0 gm trans fat

---

> *As the United States population ages and gains weight, the incidence of diabetes increases.*

Tex-Mex Mini Quiches Ⓠ

Yield: 30 mini quiches (1 quiche = 1 serving)

Since you might make this hours ahead of time, to reheat, place on a cookie sheet and bake in a preheated 425° oven for 2 to 3 minutes.

4 extra-large egg whites, slightly beaten
½ cup nonfat evaporated milk or Light Silk Soymilk
½ cup shredded part-skim mozzarella cheese
½ teaspoon chili powder
½ teaspoon ground cumin
2 teaspoons Worcestershire sauce

4 ounces chopped, canned green chilies, drained
2 fresh plum tomatoes, diced
2 whole green onions, sliced
8 6-inch corn tortillas, cut into 30 2½-inch rounds
1 tablespoon grated Parmesan cheese, optional

1. *To make the quiche filling*, place all the ingredients except the tortillas into a mixing bowl and blend thoroughly with a fork.

2. Heat the tortilla circles in a microwave oven for about 1 minute on medium, or until softened, or sprinkle with 1½ tablespoons of water, wrap lightly in foil, and heat in a 375° oven for 5 minutes.

3. Press the tortilla circles into 2½-inch nonstick minimuffin tins.

4. Fill the tortilla-lined cups with quiche filling and bake in a preheated 425° oven for 10 to 12 minutes. Serve warm.

Per serving: 1 mg cholesterol, 0.23 gm saturated fat, 0.6 gm total fat, 0.1 gm fiber, 41 mg sodium, 32 calories, 0 gm trans fat

Panzanella ⓠ

Serves: 8

This delicious no-cholesterol appetizer is often served in Italian restaurants as a first course, and it can easily be prepared at home.

6 Italian plum or heirloom
    tomatoes, cut into chunks
½ red or white onion, diced
½ cucumber, peeled, halved
    lengthwise, seeded, and sliced
½ green pepper, seeded, and sliced
2 tablespoons extra-virgin olive oil
1–2 tablespoons red wine vinegar
    or balsamic vinegar

1 clove garlic, minced
Freshly ground pepper
½ cup chopped fresh Italian
    parsley or chopped fresh basil
1 tablespoon capers, rinsed
4 slices day-old whole wheat
    baguette, cubed

1. Place all the ingredients except the bread in a mixing bowl. Mix lightly but thoroughly with a fork.
2. Chill 30 minutes before serving to marry flavors, but serve at room temperature—it tastes better.

To Serve: Place the bread on a platter, top with the tomato mixture, and serve.

Per serving: 0 mg cholesterol, 0.55 gm saturated fat, 3.8 gm total fat, 1 gm fiber, 147 mg sodium, 81 calories, 0 gm trans fat

Six New Simply Delicious Soups

Creamy Cauliflower Soup

Serves: 8 to 10 (¾ cup = 1 serving)

No butter, no cream, just a smooth, flavorful soup to be served hot or cold on warm summer nights.

2 teaspoons olive oil
½ medium onion, chopped

2 leeks, white part only, washed
    and sliced

2 ounces russet potato, peeled and
  sliced
3 shallots, peeled and sliced
1¾ pounds cauliflower florets
2 sprigs thyme
½ teaspoon Herbes de Provence
1 bay leaf
¼ teaspoon white pepper

¼ teaspoon salt
5 cups Wolfgang Puck's organic
  vegetable soup or low-sodium
  chicken broth
2 cups water

Nonfat sour cream and chopped
  chives, for garnish

1. Coat a 4-quart saucepan with olive-oil spray, add olive oil, and place over medium heat.

2. Add onion, leek, potato, and shallots. "Sweat" the mixture for about 6 minutes or until soft.

3. Add cauliflower and spices. Stir to coat with spices and cook 5 additional minutes.

4. Add soup and water. Bring to boil and then reduce heat to medium-low.

5. Simmer about 25 minutes or until vegetables are soft.

6. Remove from heat, remove the bay leaf, and cool.

7. Insert stick blender, using up and down motion until smooth.

To Serve: Spoon hot soup into bowls or cups and garnish with a dollop of sour cream and chopped chives. Accompany with Stacy's Pita Chips. For cold soup, add 1 cup of 1% milk, blend, and chill overnight until served.

NOTE: To change the consistency of the soup, add water, broth, or 1% milk accordingly.

Variation: For asparagus soup, substitute 1½ pounds of thin asparagus, cut into 1-inch lengths. Proceed as above, simmering for only 15 minutes.

Per serving: 0 mg cholesterol, 0.2 gm saturated fat, 1.61 gm total fat, 3.63 gm fiber, 71.15 calories, 12.51 gm carbohydrate, 5.46 gm sugar, 0 gm trans fat

---

Mark Twain is quoted as saying that "cauliflower is cabbage with a college education."

Celery Soup ⓠ

Serves: 8–10 (Yields 8 cups; 1 cup = 1 serving)

2 teaspoons olive oil
½ onion, sliced
1 leek (white part only) split and cleaned under cold running water, sliced
2 shallots, sliced
4–6 stalks celery with leaves, strings removed and sliced (about 4 cups)

½ knob celery root (celeriac), peeled and sliced
2 sprigs fresh thyme or ½ teaspoon dried
2 bay leaves
3 14-ounce cans of organic, low-sodium vegetable broth
White pepper and salt to taste
1 cup of water as needed

1. Add olive oil, onion, leek, and shallots to 3-quart saucepan. Cook about 5 minutes or until wilted. Stir occasionally to prevent catching.

2. Add celery, celery root, thyme, and bay leaves. Stir. Cook about 5 minutes.

3. Add broth and white pepper. Cover and simmer for 30 minutes or until celery root is fork-tender. Remove bay leaves and thyme.

4. Cool slightly and then puree with stick blender, in food processor, or blender.

5. Garnish with diced red peppers or radishes.

Serve Hot: Heat in a saucepan. It tastes even better the next day!

Per serving: 0 mg cholesterol, 0.19 gm saturated fat, 1.26 gm total fat, 1.31 gm fiber, 44.46 calories, 6.8 gm carbohydrate, 2.0 gm sugar, 0 gm trans fat

Sopa de Ajo Ⓠ
(Garlic soup)

Serves: 8 to 10 (½ cup = 1 serving)

Imagine a flavorful and comforting soup highly seasoned with cloves and cloves of garlic that tastes sweet, yet with a subtle taste of garlic. It may even help lower your blood pressure!

3 tablespoons olive oil
3 teaspoons minced garlic (about 6 large cloves)
2 cups Mrs. Cubbison's or Pepperidge Farms stuffing mix or herbed croutons
3 14-ounce cans of sodium-reduced and fat-free chicken broth

½ teaspoon Hungarian paprika
Few grains of cayenne
2 tablespoons toasted pine nuts (optional)

Chopped Italian parsley, as garnish

1. Heat oil in 3-quart saucepan, add garlic to hot oil and stir over medium heat until lightly colored.
2. Add bread and continue to sauté until lightly colored.
3. Add broth, paprika, and cayenne, and simmer for 25 minutes.
4. Puree with stick blender, food processor, or blender until completely smooth.

To Serve: Serve in small espresso cups as an aperitif and garnish with chopped parsley.

Variation: Place ½ teaspoon toasted pine nuts in cup before adding soup.

Per serving: 3.28 mg cholesterol, 1.64 gm saturated fat, 9.39 gm total fat, 1.18 gm fiber, 154.36 calories, 12.75 gm carbohydrate, 2.77 gm sugar, 0 gm trans fat

Mushroom Bisque

Serves: 8 to 10

This exquisite low-calorie soup will please even the most discerning palate. What a great way to start a Thanksgiving dinner!

2 teaspoons olive oil
½ pound celery root, peeled and thinly sliced
3 large shallots, sliced
1 leek (white part only), washed and sliced
10 ounces sliced cremini mushrooms
10 ounces sliced white button mushrooms
1 ounce dried porcini mushrooms, soaked for 20 minutes in water

3 cups organic vegetable stock
3–4 cups water

Bouquet garni* (2 bay leaves, 1 branch fresh thyme, 4 sprigs Italian parsley, few peppercorns)

½ to 1 teaspoon *freshly ground* nutmeg
Salt and pepper to taste

1. Place oil in saucepan. Add leek, shallots, and celery root. Sauté until wilted (about five minutes).
2. Add fresh mushrooms and drained dry mushrooms. Stir.
3. Add vegetable stock, water, and bouquet garni. Stir.
4. Cook 50 to 60 minutes or until celery root is tender.
5. Remove bouquet garni and puree with stick blender until smooth and satiny.
6. Add salt, pepper, and freshly ground nutmeg to taste.

To Serve: Heat soup and serve in warm white or lightly colored bowls. Then garnish with dollop of sour cream and top with chopped chives.

Per serving: 0 mg cholesterol, 0.25 gm saturated fat, 1.64 gm total fat, 2.66 gm fiber, 71.49 calories, 11.34 gm carbohydrate, 3.47 gm sugar, 0 gm trans fat

*Bouquet garni—a combination of spices placed in a tea caddy or cheesecloth

Tofu and Corn Soup ⓠ

Serves: 8 (1 cup = 1 serving)

This is an easy soup prepared from your pantry, refrigerator, and freezer shelves. The fat in the soup comes from tofu (soybean curd), a product that is relatively low in fat and contains little saturated fat. Tofu is low in sodium, and contains no cholesterol (obviously, since it does not originate from an animal source). However, it is a good source of vegetable protein.

12½ ounces Lite Silken Tofu, drained
1 cup 1% milk or soy milk
½ cup chopped onion
½ red bell pepper, seeded and cut into ¼-inch dice
1 14½-ounce can defatted, sodium-reduced chicken or organic vegetable broth
1 17-ounce can cream-style corn
1 10-ounce package frozen Green Giant white peg corn or 1 12-ounce can sugar-free, salt-free whole-kernel corn

1 teaspoon dried basil, crushed, or 1 tablespoon chopped fresh basil
½ teaspoon ground white pepper

3 tablespoons sliced scallions or chopped Italian flat leaf parsley or fresh cilantro, for garnish

1. Puree the tofu with the milk in a food processor or blender.
2. Sauté the chopped onion in a nonstick saucepan coated with vegetable-oil cooking spray, until wilted (place a lid over the onion to speed sweating process).
3. Add the bell pepper, chicken broth, cream-style corn and corn kernels, basil, white pepper, and pureed tofu mixture. Stir and bring to a simmer; *do not boil.*

To Serve: Serve in warm soup bowls and sprinkle with chopped scallions, chopped parsley, or cilantro. Accompany with fresh vegetable crudités (carrots, broccoli, pepper strips) and crisp whole grain crackers such as Finn Crisp or Rye-Krisp.

Per serving: 1.53 mg cholesterol, 0.24 gm saturated fat, 1.27 gm total fat, 20.33 gm carbohydrate, 1.98 gm fiber, 112.04 calories, 6.81 sugar, 0 gm trans fat

Fresh Vegetable Soup

Serves: 12 to 14 (1 cup = 1 serving)

A vegan delight and favorite of mine made from scratch utilizing all seasonal fresh vegetables and *no meat*.

2 teaspoons olive oil	2 bay leaves
1 onion, chopped	½ teaspoon Herbes de Provence°
4 bulbs fresh green garlic or 2–3 cloves garlic, finely minced	Freshly ground pepper
1 leek, chopped	4–6 cups low-sodium organic fat-free vegetable broth
4 carrots, diced	4–6 cups water
2 cups diced celery, with leaves	¼ cup barley, washed
2 parsnips, diced	¼ cup quick-cooking oats
2 zucchini, quartered lengthwise and diced	6 ounces okra, frozen or fresh, cut into ¾-inch slices

1. Place oil in large stockpot. Add onion, garlic, and leek and sauté for five minutes.

2. Add remaining vegetables, bay leaves, Herbes de Provence, and pepper. Stir.

3. Add broth, water, and barley.

4. Bring to a boil, reduce heat, and simmer for 45 minutes.

5. Add oats and okra, and continue cooking for another 15 to 20 minutes.

6. Taste and adjust seasonings if needed. Remove bay leaves.

Optional: ½ cup chopped Italian parsley, 1 cup shredded cabbage, or spinach may be added at this time.

NOTE: Enjoy the soup for 3 to 4 days, but don't freeze, as this will result in mushy vegetables and affect the flavor. However, soup may be pureed with a stick blender or food processor *and then frozen*.

Per serving: 0 mg cholesterol, 0.18 gm saturated fat, 1.16 gm total fat, 14.46 gm carbohydrate, 3.79 gm fiber, 74.86 calories, 3.85 gm sugar, 0 gm trans fat

°Three cubes Dorot chopped frozen basil may be substituted (available at Trader Joe's).

Salads and Salad Dressings

Cucumber-Buttermilk Dressing Ⓠ

Yield: 1½ cups (1 tablespoon = 1 serving)

This salad dressing provides a welcome change from the usual low-calorie vinaigrette. It keeps for 2 weeks in the refrigerator.

½ cup 1%-fat cottage cheese or
    fat-free sour cream
1 5-inch slice hothouse cucumber,
    cubed, or regular cucumber,
    peeled and seeded
1 slice green onion
1 clove garlic

¾ cup buttermilk (fat removed) or
    nonfat yogurt
¼ teaspoon dried thyme
¼ teaspoon dried basil
1 tablespoon Japanese rice vinegar
⅛ teaspoon white pepper

1. Puree the sour cream, cucumber, onion, and garlic in a blender or stick blender.

2. Add the remaining ingredients and process until well blended and smooth.

3. Taste and adjust seasonings. Store in a tightly closed jar in the refrigerator.

NOTE: Hothouse cucumbers are long thin-skinned cucumbers that are not waxed and need not be peeled before using. They generally come wrapped in plastic.

Per serving: 0 mg cholesterol, 0.07 gm saturated fat, 0.1 gm total fat, 0 gm fiber, 9 mg sodium, 8 calories, 0 gm trans fat

---

HFCS, high-fructose corn syrup, used to sweeten soft drinks and many foods, contributes to increased obesity.

Low-Calorie Salad Dressing Ⓠ

Yield: about 1½ cups (1 tablespoon = 1 serving)

12 ounces sodium-reduced V-8 juice
3 tablespoons fresh lemon juice
2 tablespoons red wine vinegar
1 tablespoon finely chopped onion or shallot
1 tablespoon fresh Italian parsley, minced

1 large clove garlic, minced
½ teaspoon Splenda (optional)
¼ teaspoon celery seed
½ teaspoon dried basil, crushed
Freshly ground pepper
1 teaspoon arrowroot powder
Few drops red pepper sauce (optional)

1. Combine all the ingredients in jar; shake to blend.
2. Pour into a small saucepan and bring to a boil over medium heat, while stirring, until slightly thickened (about 3 minutes).
3. Cool, return to jar, and refrigerate. It keeps for about 3 weeks.

Per serving: 0 mg cholesterol, 0 gm saturated fat, 0 gm total fat, 0.1 gm fiber, 2 mg sodium, 4 calories

Fresh Asparagus Salad Ⓠ Ⓜ

Serves: 4

If you are an asparagus lover, as I am, you'll enjoy this flavorful salad as an accompaniment to either hot or cold chicken breasts.

1 pound fresh asparagus
2 tablespoons water
2 teaspoons extra-virgin olive oil
1 tablespoon dry sherry
2–3 tablespoons brown rice vinegar
1 tablespoon lemon juice
2 teaspoons sodium-reduced soy sauce

1 clove garlic, minced
½ small red onion, minced
½ red pepper, seeded and thinly sliced
½ cup canned water chestnuts, drained and thinly sliced

1. With a vegetable peeler, remove the thin outer skin of the asparagus. Remove the tough ends of the stalks. Cut the stalks into 1½-inch diagonal pieces.

2. Place the asparagus in a microwave dish, add the water, cover, and cook on high for 3 minutes. Drain, rinse under cold water, and drain again.

3. Combine the oil, sherry, vinegar, lemon juice, soy sauce, and garlic in a serving bowl.

4. Add the onion, pepper, water chestnuts, and asparagus. Mix lightly and chill 20 minutes before serving.

Per serving: 0 mg cholesterol, 0.4 gm saturated fat, 2.7 gm total fat, 1.5 gm fiber, 89 mg sodium, 83 calories

Sliced Beet and Orange Salad ⓠ

Serves: 4

2 bunches watercress, washed and
    heavy stems removed
6 cooked beets, peeled and sliced°
2 large navel oranges, peeled and
    sliced

Grated zest of 1 orange, for
    garnish

Dressing:
3 tablespoons low-calorie oil-free
    vinaigrette
1 tablespoon white wine vinegar
1 teaspoon extra-virgin olive oil
1 teaspoon Dijon mustard
½ teaspoon chopped fresh
    tarragon

1. Arrange a bed of watercress on a shallow serving plate.

2. Overlap sliced beets with sliced oranges on the watercress.

3. Combine the dressing ingredients, spoon over the beets and oranges, and garnish with orange zest.

Per serving: 0 mg cholesterol, 0.2 gm saturated fat, 1.5 gm total fat, 2.8 gm fiber, 121 mg sodium, 106 calories, 0 gm trans fat

° Cook beets whole with skin in microwave oven until tender. Cool, peel, and slice.

Black Bean and Corn Salad ⓠ

Serves: 4

In addition to being wonderfully flavorful, beans and corn are both high in complex carbohydrates and soluble fiber.

1 tablespoon canola oil
2 tablespoons sherry or Japanese rice vinegar
2 tablespoons chopped onions or shallots
¼ teaspoon dry ground mustard
¼ teaspoon ground cumin
About ¼ teaspoon hot pepper sauce
2 cups cooked black beans (page 132), or 1 15-ounce can black beans, drained and rinsed

1 12-ounce can sodium-reduced corn, or 1¾ cups fresh corn cooked for 1 minute on high in microwave
½ sweet red pepper, seeded and finely diced
1 tablespoon chopped fresh cilantro
4 cups shredded romaine

1. Place the first six ingredients in a mixing bowl; blend well.
2. Add the beans, corn, red pepper, and cilantro, and toss.
3. Chill 20 minutes in the refrigerator and then bring to room temperature before serving.

To Serve: Place 1 cup shredded romaine on each salad plate and top with a quarter of the salad mixture.

Per serving: 0 mg cholesterol, 0.5 gm saturated fat, 3.8 gm total fat, 9 gm fiber, 16 mg sodium, 282 calories, 0 gm trans fat

Green Bean Salad Piquant with Ginger Ⓠ

Serves: 4

3 cloves garlic, minced
2 green onions, finely chopped
1–2 tablespoons grated fresh
  ginger root
2 teaspoons canola oil
½ teaspoon crushed red pepper
  flakes
2 tablespoons Japanese rice
  vinegar

2 teaspoons hoisin sauce
1 pound Chinese long beans or
  young, tender green beans, cut
  into 3-inch lengths

2 peeled toasted red peppers, for
  garnish

1. Place the garlic, onion, ginger, oil, and pepper flakes in small glass bowl. Microwave uncovered on high for 1 minute.

2. Add the vinegar and hoisin sauce. Place beans in large bowl and stir to combine. Cover tightly with microwave plastic wrap and microwave on high for 4 to 5 minutes. Mix and cook 4 to 5 minutes more.

3. Remove from oven, stir, cover, and chill at least 30 minutes before serving.

To Serve: Place on a serving platter and garnish generously with roasted red pepper strips. Or, to serve as individual salads, arrange green bean bundles in roasted red pepper halves.

Per serving: 0 mg cholesterol, 0.21 gm saturated fat, 2.7 gm total fat, 2.2 gm fiber, 125 mg sodium, 69 calories, 0 gm trans fat

Cabbage, Bean Sprout, Tomato, and Carrot Slaw Ⓠ

Serves: 4

Winter vegetables can also make interesting salad combinations varied to suit your palate.

1½ cups shredded red cabbage
1½ cups shredded green cabbage
4 ounces fresh bean sprouts,
   washed and drained
4 plum tomatoes, diced
3 carrots, shredded

Salad Dressing:
½ cup low-calorie vinaigrette
2 teaspoons Hungarian paprika
1 teaspoon Splenda
2 teaspoons Japanese rice vinegar

4 thin slices avocado, for garnish
   (optional)

1. Combine the cabbages, bean sprouts, tomatoes, and carrots and toss lightly in a bowl.

2. Mix the dressing ingredients together, pour over the salad, and toss lightly.

To Serve: Mound the salad on chilled plates and garnish each with a thin slice of avocado.

Per serving: 0 mg cholesterol, 0.09 gm saturated fat, 0.7 gm total fat, 3.4 gm fiber, 42 mg sodium, 91 calories, 0 gm trans fat

Cole Slaw Relish Salad ⓠ

Serves: 16 (½ cup = 1 serving)

This salad goes particularly well with chicken, turkey, or meat loaf. Using your food processor for chopping will really speed up the preparation time.

1 small head (about 1 pound) green cabbage, finely chopped
½ small head red cabbage, finely chopped
½ cup chopped seeded green pepper
½ cup chopped seeded red pepper
1 cup chopped carrots
½ small onion, finely chopped

1½ teaspoons celery seed
Freshly ground pepper
3 tablespoons light-style mayonnaise mixed with ¾ cup nonfat plain yogurt and 2 tablespoons lemon juice
1 tablespoon Splenda
3 tablespoons chopped fresh dill (optional)

1. Combine the vegetables. Add the celery seed and freshly ground pepper to taste.
2. Add the yogurt mixture and stir well.
3. Cover and refrigerate at least 2 hours before serving.

Per serving: 1 mg cholesterol, 0.05 gm saturated fat, 1.2 gm total fat, 1.5 gm fiber, 47 mg sodium, 45 calories, 0 gm trans fat

---

Broccoli florets are more nutritious than the stalks.

Bristol Farms Fantastic Corn and Eggplant Fiesta

Serves: about 10 (⅔ cup = 1 serving)

Bristol Farms Market sells this delicious, habit-forming salad in their takeout section. This is my adaptation to make it a more viable recipe for home use.

10 ears fresh corn° (about 5 cups), or 5 cups canned (if fresh is unavailable)
⅔ pound eggplant, diced into about ½-inch cubes
1 tablespoon extra-virgin olive oil
1 red pepper, seeded and diced
1 green pepper, seeded and diced
1 small red onion, finely chopped
1 2-ounce can chopped green chilies, drained, or 2 Anaheim chilies, roasted, peeled, and diced

¼ cup chopped fresh Italian parsley
½ bunch fresh cilantro, chopped

Dressing:
¼ cup fresh lemon juice
1 tablespoon extra-virgin olive oil
1 tablespoon cold-pressed safflower oil
Freshly ground pepper

1. Remove the kernels from the cob with a sharp knife and place in a bowl and microwave on high for 2 minutes.
2. Place the eggplant on a nonstick baking sheet and brush lightly with the 1 tablespoon olive oil. Place under the broiler and brown lightly.
3. Add the diced eggplant and all the remaining salad ingredients to the corn. Mix to combine.
4. Combine the dressing ingredients and sprinkle over the corn mixture. Blend thoroughly. Taste and adjust seasonings.
5. Cover and refrigerate for at least 1 hour before serving.

Per serving: 0 mg cholesterol, 0.6 gm saturated fat, 5.1 gm total fat, 2.1 gm fiber, 16 mg sodium, 124 calories, 0 gm trans fat

°If you can, use fresh white corn; it's divine.

Kasha and Corn Salad Ⓠ

Serves: 6 (½ cup = 1 serving)

This hearty dish—high in complex carbohydrates, B-complex vitamins, and iron—may be served as a side dish or a salad.

½ cup cooked buckwheat (kasha), quinoa, or millet (page 133)
1 cup (about 2 ears) cooked fresh corn (save cooking liquid) or sodium-reduced canned corn
⅓ cup sliced green onion
⅓ cup minced fresh Italian parsley
½ cup chopped carrots
⅓ cup chopped celery
1 tablespoon extra-virgin olive oil
2 tablespoons lemon juice
3 tablespoons juice from corn or Low-Calorie Salad Dressing (page 280)

1½ teaspoons chopped fresh basil, or ½ teaspoon dried basil
1 teaspoon chopped fresh oregano or ½ teaspoon dried oregano

Thinly sliced hothouse cucumber, for garnish
2 Italian plum tomatoes, chopped, for garnish

1. Place the first six ingredients in a mixing bowl and toss lightly.
2. Combine the oil, lemon juice, vegetable juice, basil, and oregano in a small jar and shake to combine.
3. Pour over the corn mixture and toss to blend. Marinate at least 15 minutes.

To Serve: Arrange on a platter and garnish with cucumber slices and chopped tomato.

Per serving: 0 mg cholesterol, 0.38 gm saturated fat, 2.7 gm total fat, 1.2 gm fiber, 53 mg sodium, 70 calories, 0 gm trans fat

Radish, Celery, and Cucumber Salad Ⓠ

Serves: 4

2 cups red radishes, trimmed and
 halved
3 celery stalks, cut into ¼-inch
 slices
1 cup diced hothouse cucumber or
 regular cucumber, peeled and
 seeded
1 teaspoon chopped fresh chervil
1 teaspoon chopped fresh tarragon
 or ⅓ teaspoon dried tarragon

Freshly ground pepper
Butter lettuce, for lining plates
2 tablespoons chopped almonds,
 for garnish (optional)

Dressing:
½ cup nonfat plain yogurt
1 tablespoon light-style
 mayonnaise
1 tablespoon apple cider vinegar

1. Combine the radishes, celery, and cucumbers in a bowl. Sprinkle with the chervil, tarragon, and pepper; toss lightly.
2. Blend the dressing ingredients, add to the radish mixture, and combine.

To Serve: Line a platter with butter lettuce and mound the salad mixture on top. Sprinkle with chopped almonds if desired.

Per serving: 2 mg cholesterol, 0.07 gm saturated fat, 1.6 gm total fat, 0.8 gm fiber, 86 mg sodium, 47 calories, 0 gm trans fat

Spinach and Pear Salad Ⓠ

Serves: 4

Pears are high in soluble fiber; however, since fruits always have better flavor when in season, you may substitute nectarines or peaches in their season.

4 cups spinach leaves, washed
 thoroughly, dried, and torn
2 cups red leaf lettuce, washed
 thoroughly, dried, and torn

3 tablespoons low-calorie
 vinaigrette
1 tablespoon lemon juice
2 tablespoons orange juice

½ teaspoon Dijon mustard
Freshly ground pepper
2 small ripe pears or papaya,
  halved, cored, and sliced

2 tablespoons coarsely chopped
  walnuts

1. Toss the spinach and lettuce together in a bowl. Divide evenly among four plates.
2. Combine the dressing, lemon and orange juices, mustard, and pepper. Beat with a fork to blend.
3. Arrange a quarter of the pear slices in a fan shape on the greens on each plate.
4. Sprinkle with dressing and chopped toasted walnuts, and serve.

Optional: Top each plate with 1 teaspoon low-fat goat cheese.

NOTE: The salad may be prepared ahead (sprinkle the fruit *lightly* with lemon juice to prevent discoloring). Cover with plastic wrap and refrigerate. Drizzle with dressing just before serving.

Per serving: 0 mg cholesterol, 0.06 gm saturated fat, 0.6 gm total fat, 4.6 gm fiber, 56 mg sodium, 73 calories

Date Waldorf Salad ⓠ

Serves: 4

This combination of ingredients is a pleasant change from the traditional Waldorf salad.

2 large red apples, cored and
  diced
2 teaspoons lemon juice
1 raw turnip, peeled and shredded
8 dates, pitted and chopped

¼ cup soy Silk nondairy vanilla
  yogurt

2 carrots, shredded, for garnish

1. Combine the apples, lemon juice, turnips, and dates in a bowl; toss lightly.
2. Add the yogurt and blend with a fork.

To Serve: Place on a platter and surround with shredded carrot.

Per serving: 0 mg cholesterol, 0.09 gm saturated fat, 0.3 gm total fat, 3.7 gm fiber, 21 mg sodium, 96 calories, 0 gm trans fat

Vegetable Antipasto Ⓜ

Serves: 8

An easy and attractive salad, first course, or buffet dish for entertaining.

¼ cup white wine vinegar
3 tablespoons water
½ tablespoon extra-virgin olive oil
½ teaspoon Dijon mustard
Freshly ground pepper
1 tablespoon chopped fresh thyme, or 1 teaspoon crushed dried thyme
3 cups combined fresh broccoli and cauliflower florets and sliced carrots
1 cup cut green beans

½ green pepper, seeded and cut into thin strips
½ red pepper, seeded and cut into thin strips
½ cup kalamata olives
½ mild white onion, thinly sliced

Butter lettuce, for lining platter
2 plum tomatoes, diced, and 1 tablespoon chopped fresh thyme or parsley, for garnish

1. Place the first six ingredients in a microwave casserole and combine.
2. Add all the vegetables except the peppers. Stir, cover tightly with plastic wrap, and microwave on high for 3 to 5 minutes.
3. Stir. Add the peppers, olives, and onion slices.
4. Toss, cover, or place in a plastic bag, seal, and chill 2 hours or overnight.

To Serve: Remove the vegetable mixture with a slotted spoon to a platter lined with butter lettuce and sprinkle with chopped tomato and chopped fresh thyme.

Variations: A 16-ounce package of any frozen vegetable mixture of your choice may be substituted for the broccoli mixture.

Instead of the first six ingredients, use ½ cup oil-free low-calorie Italian dressing plus 1 teaspoon olive oil and ½ teaspoon Dijon mustard.

Per serving: 0 mg cholesterol, 0.23 gm saturated fat, 1.5 gm total fat, 1.5 gm fiber, 57 mg sodium, 38 calories, 0 gm trans fat

Entrées

Pasta with Garden Vegetable Marinara Sauce

Serves: about 10

Yield: 5 to 6 cups sauce (⅔ cup = 1 serving)

This meatless sauce for pasta helps make a vegetarian dinner special. It may be prepared ahead of time and frozen for future use. Any egg-free pasta may be used (or spelt, soba, or brown rice pasta).

Sauce:

1 medium onion, finely chopped
3 cloves garlic, minced
1 tablespoon extra-virgin olive oil
2 carrots, finely chopped
1 stalk celery with leaves, finely chopped
1 medium zucchini, coarsely chopped
1 crookneck squash, coarsely chopped
½ green pepper, seeded and finely chopped
1 28-ounce can San Marzano chopped plum tomatoes in puree
3 tablespoons tomato paste

1 teaspoon dried Italian herb blend, crushed
½ teaspoon crushed dried basil, or 1½ teaspoons chopped fresh basil
½ teaspoon crushed dried red pepper flakes
Optional: 1 cup sliced cremini mushrooms

1¼ pounds angel hair pasta or whole wheat linguine, cooked al dente and drained
Freshly grated Parmesan cheese (optional)

1. Sauté the onions and garlic in the oil in a 3-quart saucepan for 3 to 5 minutes, stirring constantly.
2. Add the carrots, celery, zucchini, squash, and pepper. Stir and sauté 5 minutes.
3. Add the tomatoes, tomato paste, herbs, and pepper flakes.
4. Bring to a boil, reduce to a simmer, and cook for 30 minutes. Place hot pasta in large pasta bowl. Spoon one-half of the sauce over hot pasta

and blend. Serve remaining sauce at the table and allow each person to use with cheese as desired.

Per serving: 0 mg cholesterol, 0.29 gm saturated fat, 2 gm total fat, 2.5 gm fiber, 119 mg sodium, 217 calories, 0 gm trans fat

Turkey Chili and Macaroni

Serves: 6 (1½ ounces cooked turkey = 1 serving)

A meal in one.

10 ounces ground turkey breast (see page 144)

1 14½-ounce can San Marzano chopped tomatoes

2 6-ounce cans sodium-reduced V-8 juice

1 cup chopped onion

2 cloves garlic, minced

1 tablespoon chili powder

½ teaspoon ground cumin

1 teaspoon dried oregano, crushed

Freshly ground pepper

1 bay leaf

1½ cups cooked kidney beans (page 132) or canned beans, drained and rinsed

2 cups fresh or frozen mixed vegetables

6 ounces elbow macaroni, cooked al dente and drained

1. Put the turkey into a 4-quart nonstick saucepan and cook until the meat is no longer pink, stirring frequently.
2. Add the tomatoes, juice, onion, garlic, and seasonings. Simmer, covered, for 20 minutes. Remove the bay leaf.
3. Add the beans and vegetables and simmer, covered, for 12 minutes.
4. Add the cooked macaroni and heat 5 minutes.

To Serve: Serve with mixed green salad and crisp sourdough rolls, with fruit for dessert.

Per serving: 28 mg cholesterol, 0.44 gm saturated fat, 2 gm total fat, 5.7 gm fiber, 90 mg sodium, 307 calories, 0 gm trans fat

Deviled Turkey Fillets Ⓠ

Serves: 4 (3 ounces cooked turkey = 1 serving)

2 8-ounce turkey breast fillets
Juice of ½ lemon
2 teaspoons onion powder
2 teaspoons salt-free vegetable
   seasoning
2 tablespoons Dijon mustard
2 tablespoons dry white wine

½ teaspoon red pepper sauce
2 teaspoons Worcestershire sauce
1 cup dry whole wheat or rye
   bread crumbs

Watercress and cherry tomatoes,
   for garnish

1. Sprinkle the fillets with the lemon juice and seasonings, cover, and let stand in the refrigerator for 30 minutes or overnight.

2. Combine the mustard, wine, red pepper sauce, and Worcestershire sauce.

3. Brush the fillets with the mustard sauce and coat one side with bread crumbs.

4. Place on a nonstick baking sheet, crumbed-side-up, and bake in the upper third of a preheated 375° oven for about 20 minutes or until lightly browned.

To Serve: Cut the turkey into sixteen diagonal slices and arrange on a platter with watercress and tomatoes.

Per serving: 60 mg cholesterol, 0.9 gm saturated fat, 4.1 gm total fat, 0.2 gm fiber, 322 mg sodium, 222 calories, 0 gm trans fat

---

Splenda is a calorie-free sweetener made from cane syrup to which chlorine has been added—which increases the sweetening power of the final product.

Grilled Hawaiian Fish with Pineapple Sauce Ⓠ

Serves: 4 (4 ounces cooked fish = 1 serving)

The fish of Hawaii is combined tastefully with its native fruit.

1 cup fresh or canned crushed
  pineapple with its juice
2 teaspoons cornstarch
½ teaspoon crushed red pepper
  flakes
1 tablespoon chopped fresh cilantro

1 tablespoon chopped fresh
  parsley
4 5-ounce fillets of ahi, mahimahi,
  or hebi (halibut or tuna may be
  substituted for Hawaiian fish)

1. Combine the first three ingredients in a saucepan and bring to a boil. Add the cilantro and parsley.
2. Grill or broil the fish about 3 minutes on each side.

To Serve: Place fish on a heated serving platter and top with warmed sauce. Accompany with fresh broccoli and wild rice.

Per serving: 62 mg cholesterol, 0.2 gm saturated fat, 1.1 gm total fat, 0.5 gm fiber, 90 mg sodium, 163 calories, 0 gm trans fat

Red Snapper with Spicy Tomato Sauce Ⓠ

Serves: 4 (3½ ounces cooked fish = 1 serving)

4 5-ounce red snapper, tilapia, or
  ocean perch fillets
2 teaspoons extra-virgin olive oil
¼ cup dry bread crumbs mixed
  with 2 teaspoons salt-free
  vegetable seasoning and ⅛
  teaspoon white pepper

1 tablespoon chopped fresh
  cilantro or parsley, for garnish

Spicy Tomato Sauce:
2 cups crushed San Marzano plum
  tomatoes, in puree
1 large shallot, finely minced
2 cloves garlic, finely minced
2 tablespoons chopped fresh
  cilantro
Few grains crushed red pepper
  flakes
Few drops red pepper sauce

1. Combine the sauce ingredients in a saucepan and bring to a boil. Set aside.

2. Coat a baking dish with nonstick butter-flavored cooking spray, arrange the fish fillets in the pan, and brush lightly with the olive oil. Bake in a preheated 375° oven for 5 minutes.

3. Sprinkle the fish with the seasoned bread crumbs, return to the oven, and bake 10 minutes or until lightly browned.

To Serve: Spoon ½ cup hot tomato sauce onto each dinner plate. Top with a fish fillet and sprinkle with chopped cilantro.

Per serving: 40 mg cholesterol, 0.73 gm saturated fat, 4.3 gm total fat, 1 gm fiber, 294 mg sodium, 189 calories, 0 gm trans fat

Foil-Baked Fish with Vegetables ⓠ

Serves: 2 (3 ounces cooked fish = 1 serving)

This dish may be prepared *en papillote* (in parchment paper) but it works quite well with foil. It can be prepared and refrigerated hours ahead.

Sauce:

1 shallot, minced
2 teaspoons extra-virgin olive oil
2 green onions, cut into matchstick slices 2 inches long
1 leek (white part only), well washed, cut into matchstick slices 2 inches long
1 teaspoon peeled grated fresh ginger root
1 carrot, cut into matchstick slices 2 inches long
1 small zucchini, cut into matchstick slices 2 inches long

4 fresh mushroom caps, thinly sliced
4 canned water chestnuts, thinly sliced
1 tablespoon fresh lime or lemon juice
2 teaspoons sodium-reduced soy sauce
Freshly ground white pepper
2 4-ounce halibut, salmon, or monkfish fillets
Parsleyed lemon wedges, for garnish

1. Sauté shallot in the oil for ½ minute. Add the green onions, leek, and ginger root and cook 1 minute.

2. Add the carrot, zucchini, mushrooms, and water chestnuts, stirring over heat for about 2 minutes.

3. Add the lime or lemon juice, soy sauce, and pepper.

4. Place the fish fillets on a 20 × 12-inch piece of lightweight foil and top each fillet with half of the vegetable mixture. Fold the foil over the fish-vegetable mixture and crimp the edges to seal the packet.

5. Place on a baking sheet and bake in a preheated 450° oven for 8 to 10 minutes per inch of thickness of the fish.

To Serve: Place the packet on a heated plate, slit open, slide the fish and vegetables onto the plate, remove from the foil, and serve immediately with parsleyed lemon wedges.

Per serving: 35 mg cholesterol, 1.32 gm saturated fat, 9.6 gm total fat, 1.7 gm fiber, 242 mg sodium, 239 calories, 0 gm trans fat

Fish Fajitas Ⓠ

Serves: 4 (1 fajita = 1 serving)

A meal-in-one suitable for lunch or supper.

2 tablespoons rice vinegar
Juice of 2 limes
1 tablespoon cumin
2 dashes of pepper sauce (optional)
3 cloves of garlic, crushed
1 tablespoon canola oil
1 medium red onion, halved and thinly sliced

1 each green, yellow, and red pepper, halved and sliced
12 ounces red snapper, halibut, or haddock°
4 whole wheat or corn tortillas, and fresh salsa (optional)

1. Mix vinegar, lime juice, cumin, garlic, and ½ tablespoon canola oil in 1-gallon plastic bag.

2. Add vegetables and marinate 3 to 4 hours

3. Heat 1 teaspoon oil in 10- to 12-inch nonstick skillet. Add vegetables and sauté over medium heat until peppers are tender. Remove vegetables from pan.

4. Heat remaining oil, add sliced fish or shrimp, and sauté 3 to 4 minutes or until lightly browned.

5. Return veggies to skillet and mix with fish over low heat.

6. Remove from heat. Spoon over warm tortillas and add salsa. Roll up and serve immediately.

To Serve: Serve with black beans and rice.

Per serving: 28.25 mg cholesterol, 0.53 gm saturated fat, 8.33 gm total fat, 4.57 gm fiber, 323.41 calories, 32.67 gm carbohydrate, 4.91 gm sugar, 0.01 gm trans fat

°Halibut or haddock cut into ½-inch strips, or shrimp, may be added to marinated veggies just before sautéing. (Do not marinate fish, as it gets mushy.)

Stir-Fried Tuna and Vegetables ⓠ

Serves: 4

This tuna dish is a convenient fish meal that can be prepared in minutes. Remember to always use tuna packed in water because it has only a trace of fat, whereas there are about 18 grams of fat in a 3½-ounce can of tuna packed in oil.

2 teaspoons canola oil
3 cloves garlic, minced
1 teaspoon grated fresh ginger root
3 cups chopped fresh broccoli florets, or 1 16-ounce package frozen broccoli, red peppers, and corn, defrosted and drained
1 small red onion, thinly sliced into rings

3 tablespoons organic vegetable broth
1 cup fresh snow peas
2 cups sliced fresh mushrooms
1 6½-ounce can albacore tuna in water, drained and flaked
1–2 tablespoons sodium-reduced soy sauce
3 cups hot steamed brown rice (page 133)

1. Heat the oil in a nonstick skillet. Add the garlic and ginger and stir-fry briefly.

2. Add the broccoli and onion rings and stir-fry 3 minutes.

3. Add the chicken broth, snow peas, and mushrooms and stir-fry 3 minutes more.

4. Add the tuna and soy sauce, and stir-fry just to heat.

To Serve: Mound the hot rice on a warm serving platter, spoon the hot tuna and vegetables over the top, and serve immediately.

Per serving: 19 mg cholesterol, 0.51 gm saturated fat, 3.9 gm total fat, 2.1 gm fiber, 323 mg sodium, 143 calories, 0 gm trans fat

Chicken Breasts in Phyllo

Serves: 4 (3 ounces cooked chicken = 1 serving)

I used to teach a version of this elegant and delicious dish years ago in my French cooking classes. Of course, then each leaf of phyllo was drenched with melted butter.

4 4-ounce boned, skinned, and defatted chicken breasts, flattened
Juice of ½ lemon
Freshly ground pepper
1 tablespoon chopped fresh thyme, or 1 teaspoon dried thyme
1 shallot, minced
1 large clove garlic, minced
¾ cup each chopped onion, chopped celery, and chopped fresh mushrooms, mixed together (reserve ½ cup mixture for sauce)
2 teaspoons extra-virgin olive oil

2 tablespoons defatted sodium-reduced chicken broth mixed with 1 tablespoon dry white wine and ½ teaspoon fines herbes or Herbes de Provence
8 sheets phyllo, defrosted if frozen
Butter-flavored nonstick cooking spray
Extra-virgin olive oil (optional)

Sauce:
½ cup reserved vegetable mixture
½ cup defatted sodium-reduced chicken broth
1 tablespoon dry white wine
Pinch dried Herbes de Provence

1. Season the chicken with the lemon juice, pepper, and thyme.
2. Sear the chicken in a heated nonstick skillet coated with nonstick spray, cooking about 2 minutes on each side. Cool.
3. Sauté the shallot, garlic, and mixed vegetables in the oil in a separate skillet for about 2 minutes. Add the broth mixture and cook 3 minutes or until excess moisture evaporates. Save ½ cup for sauce.
4. Coat a nonstick baking sheet with nonstick spray. Place a sheet of phyllo on the counter and coat with butter-flavored nonstick spray. Fold in half; coat with a light layer of spray. Place 1 chicken breast on the folded phyllo, 4 inches from the bottom. Spread a quarter of the vegetable mixture on the chicken. Fold the sides of the phyllo over the chicken and roll up, enclosing chicken entirely in phyllo.° Place the phyllo packet on the baking sheet seam-side-down. Repeat for the remaining chicken and phyllo.
5. Coat the phyllo packets with a light layer of cooking spray or brush them lightly with olive oil and bake in a preheated 425° oven for 12 to 15 minutes until golden brown.

To Make Sauce:

1. Puree the vegetables with the broth in a food processor or blender until smooth.

2. Place in a saucepan, add the wine and herbs. Bring to a simmer, taste, and adjust seasonings.

To Serve: Serve immediately with a selection of crisp cooked fresh vegetables such as snow peas, carrots, and zucchini and stir-fried cherry tomatoes with chives. Serve sauce on side.

Per serving: 72 mg cholesterol, 1.42 gm saturated fat, 6.3 gm total fat, 0.7 gm fiber, 88 mg sodium, 206 calories, 0 gm trans fat

*Phyllo packets may be prepared several hours ahead of time to this point and refrigerated or frozen for future use. Defrost in the refrigerator for several hours before baking.

Oven-Baked Chinese Chicken Legs

Serves: 6 (2 legs = 1 serving)

These chicken legs are a favorite of mine. They are delicious served hot or cold at a picnic with potato or rice salad.

12 chicken drumsticks, skin and fat removed (cut tendon at tip of leg to prevent splitting)
Juice of 1 large lemon (about 3 tablespoons)
2 tablespoons sodium-reduced soy sauce
1 clove garlic, minced
2 tablespoons dry sherry or rice wine
2 tablespoons hoisin sauce

1. Place the drumsticks in a plastic bag. Combine the remaining ingredients and add to the chicken. Coat the chicken thoroughly and marinate overnight in the refrigerator, turning the bag from time to time to distribute the marinade.

2. Drain the drumsticks, place on a nonstick baking sheet, and bake in the upper third of a preheated 425° oven, turning and basting occasionally with marinade, about 25 to 30 minutes, or until golden brown.

Per serving: 80 mg cholesterol, 1.27 gm saturated fat, 4.9 gm total fat, 0 gm fiber, 243 mg sodium, 154 calories, 0 gm trans fat

Perfect Chicken Cacciatore Ⓠ

Serves: 4 (1 serving = 181 calories)

1 16-ounce can San Marzano
   tomatoes, crushed
⅓ cup dry white wine
1 small onion, chopped
1 small green pepper, chopped
1 red pepper, chopped
2 cloves garlic, minced
1 bay leaf
½ teaspoon fennel seeds, crushed
½ teaspoon basil

½ teaspoonn coriander
¼ teaspoon cinnamon
¼ teaspoon crushed red pepper
Juice of ½ lemon
1 broiler chicken, cut into serving
   pieces, skinned, and all visible
   fat and wing tips removed or 2
   whole chicken breasts, halved
½ lemon

1. Place tomatoes in a small saucepan.

2. Add all remaining ingredients, except lemon juice, cover, and simmer 5 minutes.

3. Season chicken with lemon juice and broil on both sides until lightly browned.

4. Arrange chicken pieces in a baking dish sprayed with nonstick spray. Pour sauce over chicken, covering pieces with sauce. Remove bay leaf.

5. Cover and bake in a preheated 350° oven for 1 hour or until tender.

To Serve: Serve with steamed brown rice and steamed vegetables, such as zucchini, green beans, or peas and carrots.

NOTE: May be fully prepared the day before. To reheat, place in a 350° oven for 20 minutes or microwave for 7 to 10 minutes. It may also be frozen for future use.

Variation: Four slices of firm tofu, cut into ½-inch-thick slices, may be seasoned with soy sauce and garlic, then browned in a nonstick skillet. Use instead of chicken.

Per serving: 115.15 mg cholesterol, 1.35 gm saturated fat, 5.53 gm total fat, 3.2 gm fiber, 268.42 calories, 14.22 gm carbohydrate, 8.07 gm sugar, 0 gm trans fat

Pasta Pizza Pie

Serves: 10 to 12

Instead of taking the time to make a pizza crust, I use pasta as the crust and fill it with a generous tomato-vegetable filling. Add an easy salad and fresh fruit for dessert and it fills the bill for lunch or dinner.

Filling:
1 small onion, finely chopped
2 cloves garlic, minced
2 teaspoons extra-virgin olive oil
½ red pepper, seeded and thinly sliced
½ green pepper, seeded and thinly sliced
1 small zucchini, diced
1 crookneck squash, diced
1 Japanese eggplant, diced
1 cup thinly sliced fresh mushrooms
1 28-ounce can crushed San Marzano plum tomatoes in puree
2 tablespoons dry red wine
2 tablespoons chopped fresh basil, or 1 teaspoon dried Italian herb blend

Crust:
½ cup dry bread crumbs
1 green onion, thinly sliced
2 extra-large egg whites, slightly beaten
Few drops red pepper sauce
Freshly ground pepper
¼ cup shredded part-skim mozzarella cheese mixed with 2 tablespoons shredded Parmesan cheese
⅓ cup filling
About 2 cups (4 ounces dry) cooked capellini (angel hair pasta), drained

2 plum tomatoes, cut crosswise into 10 to 12 slices, for top
Fresh basil leaves, for garnish

To Make the Filling:

1. Sauté the onion and garlic in the oil in a nonstick saucepan for 2 to 3 minutes.

2. Add the peppers, squashes, eggplant, and mushrooms and sauté 3 minutes.

3. Add the remaining ingredients except the garnishes, bring to a boil, reduce to a simmer, and cook 15 minutes, stirring occasionally.

To Make the Crust:

1. Combine all the ingredients except the sauce and the pasta in a large mixing bowl. Add ⅓ cup sauce and blend with a fork; add the pasta and blend.

2. Coat a 10-inch glass pie plate with nonstick spray. Spread the pasta mixture around the bottom and sides of the plate.

3. Pour the vegetable filling into the crust and arrange the tomato slices on top.

4. Bake in the upper third of a preheated 425° oven for about 20 minutes.

To Serve: Let stand 20 minutes; garnish with basil leaves and cut into 10 or 12 pie-shaped pieces and serve with crushed red pepper, if desired.

Per serving: 2 mg cholesterol, 0.61 gm saturated fat, 1.9 gm total fat, 1.3 gm fiber, 177 mg sodium, 89 calories, 0 gm trans fat

Corn Crêpes with Cheese and Spinach or Vegetable Filling

Yield: about 15 crêpes

(2 filled crêpes = 1 serving as entrée; 1 crêpe = 1 serving as appetizer)

These crêpes are easy to make and extremely versatile. With a filling they make a wonderful entrée to serve with soup, salad, and dessert. Or they may be used in any recipe instead of tortillas. They may also be sprinkled lightly with Parmesan cheese, folded into quarters, heated in a microwave, and served as an accompaniment to chicken or turkey.

4 extra-large egg whites
1½ cups 1% milk or soy milk
1 tablespoon canola oil
½ cup whole wheat flour or cornmeal
1 cup unbleached white flour
⅛ teaspoon white pepper
1 teaspoon dried thyme
Pinch of salt (optional)
1 tablespoon grated onion
2 tablespoons canned chopped green chilies

1 cup fresh corn kernels (about 2 ears corn) or sodium-reduced canned corn
4 tablespoons chopped fresh cilantro or Italian parsley (optional)

Cheese and Spinach Filling (page 304) or Vegetable Filling (page 303)

To Make the Batter:

1. Place the egg whites, milk, oil, flours, pepper, thyme, and salt in a blender or the food processor. Blend until smooth.

2. Add the onion, green chilies, corn, and cilantro. *Blend just to combine*, not until smooth.

3. Place in a bowl, cover, and chill at least 1 hour before preparing crêpes.

To Prepare the Crêpes:

1. Heat a 6-inch nonstick skillet coated with nonstick spray until hot. (A few drops of water will dance on the skillet.)

2. Stir the batter and pour ¼ scant cup (about 3 tablespoons) on the hot skillet, tilting to cover the bottom.

3. Brown the bottom of the crêpe; turn and just dry the second side.

4. Flip the hot crêpe onto a flat clean dish towel before cooking the next one. Do not stack the warm crêpes.

5. If you plan to use the crêpes right away, cover them loosely with dish towels to keep them warm and pliable. Fill and bake as directed in the filling recipes below.

6. If you plan to use the crêpes later, let them cool. As the crêpes are cooled, stack them in layers using wax paper or plastic bags between them to prevent sticking. Then wrap the stacked crêpes in foil. They will keep in the refrigerator for 2 to 3 days or the freezer for 6 to 8 weeks.

To Freeze for Future Use:

Seal the foil-wrapped crêpes in a freezer bag. *To defrost*, heat the foil packet of crêpes in a 350° oven for 5 to 7 minutes or remove the foil and defrost in the microwave on medium for 2 minutes.

Per crêpe: 0 mg cholesterol, 0.16 gm saturated fat, 1.2 gm total fat, 0.7 gm fiber, 31 mg sodium, 73 calories, 0 gm trans fat

Vegetable Filling for 8 Corn Crêpes:

1 tablespoon canola oil	Freshly ground pepper
1 small onion, chopped	1 teaspoon dried marjoram
1 clove garlic, minced	2 tablespoons grated Parmesan
4 carrots, cut into julienne strips	cheese
2 zucchini, cut into julienne strips	
1 red pepper, seeded and cut into julienne strips	

1. Place the oil, onion, and garlic in a 9-inch glass pie plate. Microwave on high for 2 minutes, or sauté in a nonstick skillet for 5 minutes.

2. Add the remaining vegetables, stir, cover with plastic, and microwave on high for 3 minutes, or stir-fry for about 2 minutes and cook covered for 6 minutes.

3. Season with pepper and marjoram. Place ⅛ of the mixture on each of 8 crêpes, roll, and place seam-side-down in the pie plate.

4. Top each crêpe with 1 scant teaspoon of cheese and microwave on high for 1 minute.

To Serve: Place 2 crêpes on a warm plate and accompany with broccoli spears and broiled tomato half.

Per crêpe: 0 mg cholesterol, 0.08 gm saturated fat, 0.7 gm total fat, 1.3 gm fiber, 14 mg sodium, 32 calories, 0 gm trans fat

Cheese and Spinach Filling for 8 Crêpes:

1½ cups part-skim ricotta cheese	3 green onions, finely chopped
¼ cup nonfat whipped cream cheese or tofu cheese	2 tablespoons chopped fresh cilantro (optional)
½ 10-ounce package frozen chopped spinach, defrosted and squeezed dry	About 1½ cups Fresh Salsa (page 185) or canned salsa

1. Place all the ingredients except the salsa in a bowl and stir to blend.

2. Spread about 3 tablespoons onto each crêpe and fold the crêpe into thirds.

3. Arrange in a shallow baking pan, spoon 2 tablespoons fresh salsa over each crêpe, and bake in a preheated 375° oven for 5 to 7 minutes to heat before serving.

To Serve: Place 2 hot crêpes on a serving dish, top with salsa and/or light sour cream and accompany with steamed broccoli.

Per crêpe: 15 mg cholesterol, 2.28 gm saturated fat, 3.8 gm total fat, 1 gm fiber, 75 mg sodium, 76 calories, 0 gm trans fat

Broccoli Crown Ⓠ Ⓜ

Serves: 4 to 6

This colorful dish may be served hot or cold, as part of a vegetable plate or as a salad. Broccoli is high in insoluble fiber, and also a great source of calcium and vitamin A.

1½ pounds fresh broccoli, or
   ¾ pound fresh broccoli and
   ¾ pound fresh cauliflower
½ red pepper, seeded and cut into
   1-inch squares
1 tablespoon water

2 tablespoons Low-Calorie Salad
   Dressing (page 280—optional)

Sliced tomatoes or broiled halved
   tomatoes, for garnish

1. Peel the broccoli stems and remove the florets. Cut the stems into 1-inch pieces.
2. Sprinkle the red pepper pieces into the bottom and sides of a 2-quart glass mixing bowl.
3. Arrange the broccoli florets, stem-side-up, around the bowl. Sprinkle with the water and fill the center with the remaining broccoli stems.
4. Cover tightly with microwave plastic wrap and microwave on high for 6 minutes. Puncture holes in the plastic with a fork to allow steam to escape.
5. Place a 2-pound can on top of the plastic to mold the broccoli and let stand 10 minutes before serving or chilling for future use.

To Serve: Remove the plastic and drain the bowl of any liquid. Unmold on a serving plate and drizzle with salad dressing if desired. Surround with sliced tomatoes or broiled halved tomatoes.

Per serving: 0 mg cholesterol, 0.1 gm saturated fat, 0.6 gm total fat, 2.3 gm fiber, 46 mg sodium, 50 calories, 0 gm trans fat

Easy Eggplant Parmesan Ⓠ Ⓜ

Serves: 4 as an entrée, 8 as a vegetable

1 1½-pound eggplant, cut into 16 ½-inch slices with the skin
3 tablespoons part-skim ricotta cheese
4 plum tomatoes, cut into 16 lengthwise slices

1 cup marinara sauce mixed with ½ teaspoon dried Italian herb blend
1 tablespoon grated Parmesan cheese

1. Place the sliced eggplant in an 11 × 14 × 2-inch microwave baking dish and cover tightly with microwave plastic wrap.

2. Microwave on high for about 2 minutes, or broil in the broiler until lightly browned on both sides.

3. Remove the plastic wrap and spread 8 slices of the eggplant lightly with about 1 teaspoon ricotta cheese each, then top with 2 tomato slices each and the remaining slices of eggplant.

4. Spoon the sauce over the eggplant and sprinkle with the Parmesan cheese.

5. Bake on high in the microwave oven for 5 minutes, or uncovered in a preheated 375° oven for 15 to 20 minutes.

Per serving as an entrée: 5 mg cholesterol, 1.31 gm saturated fat, 5.1 gm total fat, 3.8 gm fiber, 61 mg sodium, 134 calories, 0 gm trans fat

Per serving as a vegetable: 2 mg cholesterol, 0.66 gm saturated fat, 0.86 gm total fat, 1.9 gm fiber, 2 mg sodium, 52 calories, 0 gm trans fat

Vegetarian Tofu Chili Ⓠ

Yield: 9–10 cups (1 cup = 1 serving)

This chili is a welcome addition to any barbecue or informal menu. It offers a healthy choice to vegetarians as well as meat eaters.

2 cups firm tofu, drained and crumbled
3 cloves garlic, minced
2 tablespoons chili powder

1–2 tablespoons ground cumin
1–2 tablespoons Worcestershire sauce
1 onion, chopped

1 red or green bell pepper,
  stemmed, cored, seeded, and
  chopped
2 ribs of celery, chopped
1 4-ounce can mild green chilies
1 14-ounce can diced San Marzano
  tomatoes
1 15-ounce salt-reduced, drained
  kidney beans or black beans

1 15-ounce can chili beans with
  sauce
1 teaspoon dried basil
½ teaspoon dried oregano

½ cup chopped onion, light sour
  cream, or veggie cheese for
  garnish (optional)

1. In a mixing bowl, combine the tofu, garlic, chili powder, cumin, and Worcestershire sauce. Set aside for at least 30 minutes to absorb flavors.

2. Coat a large nonstick skillet with cooking spray. Heat and add onion, pepper, and celery; sauté until onion is transparent.

3. Add marinated tofu mixture, sauté, and stir 3 additional minutes.

4. Add tomatoes, beans, basil, and oregano.

5. Stir well to combine; bring to a simmer over low heat.

6. Simmer for 30 minutes. Taste and adjust seasoning to suit your palate.

To Serve: Serve in an individual casserole and garnish with shredded tofu cheddar cheese, chopped red and/or green onion, and light sour cream. When served as an entrée, accompany with large mixed green salad, a crisp whole wheat baguette, and fresh berries with low- or nonfat sour cream. This chili may be frozen for future use.

Per serving: 8.03 mg cholesterol, 1.46 gm saturated fat, 5.42 gm total fat, 7.02 gm fiber, 171.25 calories, 21.15 gm carbohydrate, 5.05 gm sugar, 0 gm trans fat

Gingered Pineapple Carrots Ⓠ Ⓜ

Serves: 6

6 medium carrots, cut into 3 × ½-
  inch spears
2 tablespoons water
1 8-ounce can sugar-free crushed
  pineapple with juice

2 teaspoons cornstarch
¼ teaspoon ground ginger
¼ teaspoon freshly grated nutmeg

1. Microwave the carrots in the water in a tightly covered casserole on high for 3 minutes or until barely tender.

2. Mix the remaining ingredients, add to the carrots, stir, and microwave on high for 2 to 3 minutes or until the juice is slightly thickened.

To Serve: Place on a warm platter and serve immediately.

Per serving: 0 mg cholesterol, 0.04 gm saturated fat, 0.2 gm total fat, 2 gm fiber, 25 mg sodium, 57 calories, 0 gm trans fat

Larry's Scalloped Potatoes and Onions

Serves: 6 to 8

When our family decided to follow a healthier lifestyle, I thought my son would never get over the trauma of my not preparing his favorite scalloped potatoes. He did, and indeed, now even prefers these to my archaic fat- and calorie-laden old recipe!

1 onion, halved and thinly sliced
1 large clove garlic, minced
1 tablespoon extra-virgin olive oil
    or canola oil
3 unpeeled russet potatoes,
    scrubbed and cut into ¼-inch
    slices
Freshly ground pepper

1 teaspoon dried thyme, or 1
    tablespoon chopped fresh
    thyme
1½ cups defatted sodium-reduced
    chicken broth or ½% milk
1 tablespoon shredded Parmesan
    cheese

1. Sauté the onions and garlic in the oil in a nonstick skillet briefly, for about 4 to 5 minutes.
2. Place a layer of potatoes in a 9-inch square baking dish. Add a layer of the onions and garlic, and sprinkle with thyme, pepper, and half of the cheese. Repeat.
3. Pour broth or milk over potato mixture, sprinkle with cheese, and cover with foil.
4. Bake in a preheated 425° oven for 40 minutes.
5. Uncover and bake about 15 more minutes, or until browned.

Per serving: 0 mg cholesterol, 0.3 gm saturated fat, 1.4 gm total fat, 0.4 gm fiber, 17 mg sodium, 73 calories, 0 gm trans fat

Sherry's Stuffed Potatoes Ⓠ Ⓜ

Serves: 4 (2 halves = 1 serving)

4 6-ounce russet baking potatoes
  or sweet potatoes, scrubbed
1 cup diced cooked turkey breast
1 4-ounce can chopped green
  chilies, drained
1 cup coarsely chopped steamed
  broccoli
2 whole green onions, sliced

About 1½ cups Fresh Salsa (page
  185) or canned salt-free salsa
3 slices shredded Galaxy
  mozzarella cheese
2 Italian plum tomatoes, sliced
1 tablespoon grated Parmesan
  cheese

1. Pierce the potatoes with a fork and microwave on high for about 12 to 15 minutes or until soft to the touch, or bake in a preheated 425° oven for about 45 minutes.

2. Slice the potatoes lengthwise; scoop out the pulp into a mixing bowl and mash.

3. Add the turkey, chilies, broccoli, green onions, salsa, and mozzarella cheese. Mix well.

4. Fill the potato skins with the mixture; top each half with 2 slices of tomato and sprinkle with Parmesan cheese.

5. Place in a shallow microwave-safe round dish and bake on high for 10 minutes or in a 350° oven for 25 to 30 minutes.

Variations: Instead of stuffing your potatoes, try serving split baked potatoes with one or several of the following toppings:

Per serving: 31 mg cholesterol, 1.46 gm saturated fat, 3.6 gm total fat, 3.7 gm fiber, 107 mg sodium, 347 calories

---

Seven Toppings for Split Baked Potatoes
(Measurements Are for 1 Potato)

START WITH	ADD	SEASON WITH
½ cup 1%-fat cottage cheese, blended until smooth	3 tbsp. chopped fresh broccoli or spinach 1 tbsp. chopped red pepper	Freshly ground pepper 1 tsp chopped fresh dill

START WITH	ADD	SEASON WITH
⅓ cup nonfat plain yogurt	3 tbsp. shredded carrots 1 tbsp. chopped chives	Freshly ground pepper 1 tsp. Parmesan cheese
⅓ cup nonfat plain yogurt	1 tbsp. chopped green onion ½ clove garlic, chopped 3 tbsp. frozen peas, defrosted	Freshly ground pepper About 1 tsp. curry powder ½ tsp. Worcestershire sauce
½ cup chopped fresh tomato	1 tbsp. chopped onion 1 tbsp. chopped green chilies ½ tbsp. lime juice	¼ tsp. dried oregano Freshly ground pepper Top with nonfat plain yogurt and chopped fresh cilantro
½ small red onion, sliced, with 1 tsp. olive oil. Microwave covered in a 1-cup measure on high for 1 min.	3 fresh mushrooms, sliced 2 tbsp. chopped green pepper 1 tbsp. defatted sodium-reduced chicken broth or 1 chopped Italian plum tomato Microwave all together on high for ½ min. in 1-cup glass measure	Salt-free vegetable seasoning Freshly ground pepper Few drops red pepper sauce
1 tbsp. each: chopped green & red peppers, zucchini, & 1 small clove garlic in 1 tbsp. defatted sodium-reduced chicken broth Microwave on high for 1 min. and place on split potato	1 slice mozzarella cheese or cheddar Galaxy Veggie slice over potato Microwave on high for 30 seconds	Spicy vegetable seasoning Chopped chives
¼ cup salt-free canned salsa or Fresh Salsa (page 185)	2 tbsp. nonfat plain yogurt (Fage) Greek	Chopped fresh cilantro

Roast Potatoes with Basil

Serves: 6

1 recipe Basil Vinaigrette (page 96)
1 tablespoon extra-virgin olive oil
½ small onion, finely chopped

3 pounds small new potatoes, scrubbed and quartered
Freshly ground pepper
Hungarian paprika

1. Combine the vinaigrette, olive oil, and onions and place in a shallow nonstick roasting pan.
2. Add the potatoes and stir to coat potatoes. Sprinkle with pepper and paprika.
3. Roast the potatoes in a preheated 425° oven for 35 to 40 minutes, stirring occasionally, until browned and tender.

Per serving: 0 mg cholesterol, 0.25 gm saturated fat, 1.5 gm total fat, 0.6 gm fiber, 12 mg sodium, 136 calories, 0 gm trans fat

Different Stuffed Potatoes Ⓜ

Serves: 8 (½ potato = 1 serving)

By combining sweet and white potatoes, this recipe takes on an interesting new taste. For special occasions, use a pastry tube to fill the potato shells.

4 6-ounce russet potatoes, scrubbed
8 ounces sweet potatoes, scrubbed
About ⅔ cup Light Silk Soymilk
1 teaspoon ground cinnamon

¼ teaspoon freshly grated nutmeg
¼ teaspoon white pepper
2 whole green onions, thinly sliced
1 cup frozen peas

1. Pierce the russet potatoes with a fork and microwave with the sweet potatoes on high for about 15 minutes, or bake in a preheated 425° oven for about 1 hour.
2. Halve and scoop out the centers of the russet potatoes, leaving ¼-inch shells. Scoop out the pulp of the sweet potatoes and discard the skins.
3. Mash the white potato and sweet potato pulp together.
4. Add the remaining ingredients and combine well.

5. Mound the mixture into the russet potato shells° and heat in a 450° oven for 10 to 15 minutes or until warm and lightly browned or heat on high in microwave for 5 minutes.

Per serving: 1 mg cholesterol, 0.09 gm saturated fat, 0.3 gm total fat, 2.3 gm fiber, 43 mg sodium, 150 calories, 0 gm trans fat

°May be prepared ahead of time to this point, or frozen for future use.

Stir-Fried Squash and Red Pepper Ⓠ Ⓜ

Serves: 6

I particularly enjoy this recipe because squash is so delicious, and it cooks so quickly! You may, of course, use other combinations of vegetables in stir-frying.

2 teaspoons canola oil or 3 tablespoons organic vegetable broth

2 summer squash, sliced ¼ inch thick

2 crookneck squash, sliced ¼ inch thick

2 zucchini, cut into 3-inch spears

¼ red pepper, seeded and sliced ¼ inch thick

1 teaspoon onion powder

Freshly ground pepper

1 tablespoon low-sodium soy sauce (optional)

1. Heat the oil or broth in a 12-inch nonstick skillet over medium-high heat.

2. Add the squashes and stir-fry 2 to 3 minutes. Add the pepper and seasonings and stir.

3. Cover and cook 3 to 5 minutes.

To Microwave:

Place all the ingredients in a microwave dish, cover, and cook on high for 3 minutes. Mix and cook 1 additional minute.

NOTE: If you have any vegetables left over, add to a mixed green salad the next day, or serve by themselves with a bit of oil-free vinaigrette.

Per serving: 0 mg cholesterol, 0.14 gm saturated fat, 1.8 gm total fat, 1.5 gm fiber, 2 mg sodium, 36 calories, 0 gm trans fat

Sally's Zucchini Ⓠ Ⓜ

Serves: 4 (2 halves = 1 serving)

4 whole zucchini (about 1 pound),
  steamed or microwaved until
  barely tender and halved
  lengthwise
2 teaspoons salt-free vegetable
  seasoning
Freshly ground pepper

¼ cup nonfat sour cream
3 tablespoons shredded tofu
  cheddar cheese

Fresh thyme sprigs or watercress,
  for garnish

1. Remove a ½-inch strip from the center of each zucchini with a grapefruit spoon or knife.
2. Sprinkle with vegetable seasoning and pepper.
3. Spoon 2 teaspoons of the sour cream down the center of each zucchini half; sprinkle with cheese.
4. Place on a microwave-safe dish and microwave on medium for 1 minute or until the cheese is melted. Top with fresh thyme.

Per serving: 2 mg cholesterol, 0.41 gm saturated fat, 0.8 gm total fat, 0.6 gm fiber, 33 mg sodium, 36.5 calories, 0 gm trans fat

Pasta and Grain Side Dishes

Sweet Pasta Pudding

Serves: 8 (1 wedge = 1 serving)

A pleasant change from rice or potatoes with roast turkey or chicken.

8 ounces whole wheat linguini
  or capellini (angel hair pasta),
  cooked al dente and drained
4 extra-large egg whites, beaten
  until slightly thickened
3 tablespoons Splenda Brown
  Sugar Blend

1 teaspoon ground cinnamon
½ cup dark seeded raisins
1½ tablespoons canola oil

Fresh pineapple spears and red
  grapes, as garnish

1. Combine all the ingredients except the oil in a mixing bowl and blend well.

2. Heat the oil in a 10-inch glass pie plate in a preheated oven. Add the hot oil to the pasta mixture and blend well.

3. Pour the mixture into the hot pie plate that has been coated with oil from heating. Bake in a preheated 375° oven for 30 to 40 minutes or until the bottom is golden brown.

To Serve: Invert the pudding on a serving dish, unmold, and cut into eight wedges. Surround with pineapple spears and sprigs of red grapes.

Per serving: 0 mg cholesterol, 0.34 gm saturated fat, 4 gm total fat, 3.1 gm fiber, 37 mg sodium, 189 calories, 0 gm trans fat

Cracked Wheat and Tomato Salad Ⓠ

Serves: 6

Grain dishes like this one offer an inexpensive source of complex carbohydrates, B-complex vitamins, and iron.

1⅓ cups cracked wheat, soaked in cold water 20 minutes and drained

4 tablespoons chopped fresh Italian parsley

2 tablespoons chopped fresh mint

4 green onions, sliced

4 plum tomatoes, diced

3 tablespoons lemon juice

1½ tablespoons extra-virgin olive oil

1 teaspoon freshly ground pepper

Romaine leaves, for lining salad bowl

12 cucumber slices and 1 quartered tomato, for garnish

1. Place the cracked wheat, parsley, mint, green onions, and tomatoes in a bowl and mix with a fork.

2. Combine the lemon juice, olive oil, and pepper. Blend with a fork and sprinkle over the wheat mixture.

To Serve: Line a salad bowl with romaine, add the cracked wheat mixture, and garnish with sliced cucumbers and tomato wedges.

Per serving: 0 mg cholesterol, 0.56 gm saturated fat, 4.1 gm total fat, 3.1 gm fiber, 8 mg sodium, 136 calories, 0 gm trans fat

Bulgur Wheat Pilaf

Serves: 4

There are some packaged wheat pilaf mixes that may be prepared without added fat. But in case you can't find one at your market, here's a recipe that can be made from scratch.

1 small onion, finely chopped
2 teaspoons extra-virgin olive oil
¾ cup bulgur wheat (cracked
    wheat), washed
1 stalk celery, thinly sliced
1 carrot, thinly sliced
½ green pepper, seeded and thinly
    sliced

1 teaspoon salt-free vegetable
    seasoning
⅛ teaspoon white pepper
2 cups organic vegetable broth
¼ cup orzo

¼ cup slivered almonds, lightly
    toasted, for garnish (optional)

1. In a 2-quart saucepan, sauté the onion in the olive oil for 3 to 5 minutes or until wilted. Add the bulgur and cook, stirring constantly, for 2 to 3 minutes.
2. Stir in the celery, carrot, green peppers, seasoning, and pepper. Add the vegetable broth and bring to a boil. Add orzo.
3. Reduce to a simmer, cover, and cook over low heat 20 minutes.
4. Remove from heat and let stand until all the liquid is absorbed.
5. Fluff with a fork and serve, sprinkling with almonds if desired.

Variation: After removing from heat, add ½ cup muscat raisins, chopped dates, or frozen peas.

Per serving: 0 mg cholesterol, 0.39 gm saturated fat, 2.9 gm total fat, 3.7 gm fiber, 18 mg sodium, 157 calories, 0 gm trans fat

---

To control hunger, eat a healthy breakfast and don't skip meals.

Buckwheat Kernels and Pasta Ⓠ Ⓜ

Serves: 4

1 large clove garlic, chopped
1 small onion, finely chopped
½ red pepper, seeded and diced
2 teaspoons canola oil
½ 10-ounce package frozen peas

1 cup cooked buckwheat (prepared according to package directions)
4 ounces farfalle (macaroni bows), cooked al dente and drained
Freshly ground pepper, to taste

1. Microwave the garlic, onions, peppers, and oil on high until soft (about 2 minutes). Add the frozen peas.
2. Combine with the hot cooked buckwheat, toss with the cooked pasta, season with pepper, and serve.

Variation: For Black-Eyed Peas and Tomatoes with Pasta, add ⅔ cup cooked black-eyed peas and 1 cup chopped tomatoes to the frozen peas and buckwheat.

Per serving: 0 mg cholesterol, 0.82 gm saturated fat, 3 gm total fat, 2.0 gm fiber, 150 mg sodium, 155 calories, 0 gm trans fat

Desserts

Creme Topping Ⓠ

Yield: 1 cup (1 tablespoon = 1 serving)

This low-calorie sauce makes a delicious no-fat, no-cholesterol topping for fruit or pudding to use instead of whipped cream or heavy cream (remember them?).

½ cup nonfat powdered skim milk
¼ cup frozen unsweetened apple
   juice concentrate

¼ cup *very* cold water
½ teaspoon vanilla extract

1. Place all the ingredients into a chilled 2-cup measure.
2. Beat with a stick blender until thick.
3. Store in the refrigerator until serving time—up to 1½ hours.

Variation: Your favorite chilled fruit juice may be substituted for the apple juice concentrate.

Per serving: 1 mg cholesterol, 0.02 gm saturated fat, 0 gm total fat, 0 gm fiber, 21 mg sodium, 21 calories, 0 gm trans fat

Blueberry Sauce Ⓜ

Yield: 1½ cups (3 tablespoons = 1 serving)

This may be used as a topping for frozen nonfat vanilla yogurt, sliced pears, or angel food cake as dessert, or without the liqueur, on pancakes, French toast, or waffles.

1 pint fresh blueberries, washed, or 2 cups frozen unsweetened blueberries

1 teaspoon Splenda
2 tablespoons pear brandy or Grand Marnier

1. Combine the blueberries with the apple juice concentrate in a 4-cup glass measure.
2. Cover tightly with microwave plastic wrap and microwave on high for 3 minutes.
3. Add the brandy and stir to blend. Store in tightly covered container in refrigerator until serving time.

Per serving: 0 mg cholesterol, 0.01 gm saturated fat, 0.2 gm total fat, 1.1 gm fiber, 3 mg sodium, 36 calories, 0 gm trans fat

---

Melted frozen nonfat vanilla yogurt makes a tasty topping for fruit and fruit desserts.

Apple Crisp Ⓠ Ⓜ

Serves: 8

4 medium apples (McIntosh or
Golden Delicious) or pears,
peeled, cored, and cut into ½-
inch slices
3 tablespoons unsweetened papaya
juice or frozen unsweetened
apple juice concentrate mixed
with ½ teaspoon ground
cinnamon and ½ teaspoon
freshly ground nutmeg

Topping:
⅓ cup rolled oats, chopped
3 tablespoons whole wheat flour
1 tablespoon Splenda Brown
Sugar Blend
½ teaspoon cinnamon
1 teaspoon canola oil
2 tablespoons chopped almonds or
walnuts (optional)

1. In a mixing bowl, toss the apples and juice mixture together.
2. Place in 8-inch round° or square microwave baking dish.
3. Combine the topping ingredients and blend with your fingers until crumbly. Sprinkle over the apples.
4. Bake on high in a microwave oven for 12 to 15 minutes, or in a preheated 350° oven for 35 to 40 minutes.

To Serve: Serve warm with a pitcher of nonfat cold milk or Creme Topping (page 316).

Per serving: 0 mg cholesterol, 0.17 gm saturated fat, 1.1 gm total fat, 2.2 gm fiber, 2 mg sodium, 81 calories, 0 gm trans fat

°Use of a round baking dish on a turntable in the microwave gives more even cooking.

Poached Pears with Fresh Strawberry Sauce Ⓠ Ⓜ

Serves: 4 (1 pear = 1 serving)

This is a repeat performance of the popular Perfect Pear recipe found in my first book *Deliciously Low*. It makes such a special dessert that it bears repeating, and this time around it sits on a bed of pureed fresh strawberries. Of course, you may just serve it with some of its cooking liquid if you wish. A microwave is the only way to cook these pears (and apples, too, for that matter).

4 ripe Bosc, Bartlett, or d'Anjou pears, peeled
3 tablespoons fresh orange juice or papaya nectar
½ teaspoon ground cinnamon

½ teaspoon freshly ground nutmeg
1 cup Fresh Strawberry Sauce (page 319)
Lemon or camellia leaves, for garnish

1. Core each pear starting at the bottom, leaving the stem intact, and peel.

2. Place the pears upright in a microwave dish; sprinkle with the juice, cinnamon, and nutmeg.

3. Cover the dish with microwave plastic wrap (airtight but not stretched) and microwave on high for about 5 to 6 minutes or until barely fork-tender. *Do not overcook.*

To Serve: Spoon ¼ cup strawberry sauce on each of four flat dessert plates. Place a warm or chilled pear in the center of each plate and garnish with a green lemon or camellia leaf or fresh mint leaves.

Variation: Pears may also be served with the Blueberry Sauce on page 317 or nonfat vanilla yogurt and Wax Orchards Fudge Topping (see footnote page 328).

Per serving: 0 mg cholesterol, 0.10 gm saturated fat, 0.6 gm total fat, 3.1 gm fiber, 0 mg sodium, 82 calories

Fresh Strawberry Sauce ⓠ

Yield: 1 cup (¼ cup = 1 serving)

This sauce may be used with fresh cantaloupe cubes or peaches, as a sauce over nonfat frozen yogurt, or as a topping on angel food cake.

1¼ cups fresh strawberries, washed and hulled

Frozen unsweetened apple juice concentrate or Grand Marnier

1. Place the strawberries in a food processor or blender and puree until smooth.

2. Taste and adjust the flavor with apple juice concentrate or Grand Marnier. Store in a covered container in the refrigerator until ready to use, or freeze for future use.

Per serving: 0 mg cholesterol, 0.12 gm saturated fat, 1 gm total fat, 5.2 gm fiber, 1 mg sodium, 121 calories

Poached Pears and Prunes ⓆⓂ

Serves: 4

2 Bartlett pears, peeled, cored, and cut into a total of 12 slices in all

12 pitted prunes

3 tablespoons frozen unsweetened apple juice concentrate

½ teaspoon ground cinnamon

1 lemon or lime, quartered, for garnish

1. Place the pears and prunes in a 1½-quart microwave casserole.
2. Sprinkle with the apple juice concentrate and cinnamon. Cover and microwave on high for about 4 minutes.
3. Serve warm or at room temperature.

Per serving: 0 mg cholesterol, 0.04 gm saturated fat, 0.5 gm total fat, 6.2 gm fiber, 4 mg sodium, 132 calories, 0 gm trans fat

Individual Fresh Apple Tart with Apricot Glaze ⓆⓂ

Yield: 6 tarts (1 tart = 1 serving)

6 Granny Smith or Golden Delicious apples, peeled, cored, and sliced ½ inch thick

1 cup papaya nectar or fresh orange juice

1 tablespoon Grand Marnier

2 teaspoons honey

1 teaspoon orange zest

½ teaspoon ground cinnamon

Freshly ground nutmeg

9 sheets frozen phyllo, thawed

Butter-flavored nonstick cooking spray

Glaze:

6 pitted fresh or dried apricots

¼ cup apple juice

½ split vanilla bean

1. Place the apples in a microwave dish. Mix the juice, Grand Marnier, honey, zest, and spices together and pour over the apples. Microwave on high for 3 minutes, drain the juice, return the juice to the microwave, and reduce to ¼ cup.

2. Fold the phyllo leaves in half and cut out two 6-inch circles from each.

3. Place six circles of phyllo on a nonstick baking sheet, coat with butter-flavored nonstick spray. Place another phyllo circle on each of the six circles and spray. Repeat with the last six circles.

4. Arrange the drained apple pieces on each of the six phyllo stacks. Pour 2 tablespoons reduced sauce over each apple tart.

5. Bake in a preheated 425° oven for 5 to 7 minutes or until lightly browned.

6. *To make the glaze*, cook the apricots with the apple juice and vanilla bean in a saucepan for about 15 minutes until tender. Remove the vanilla bean and puree in the food processor. If necessary, use apple juice to thin the glaze.

To Serve: Drizzle the warm apricot glaze over the apple tarts and serve immediately.

Variations: Use fresh peaches or nectarines instead of apples and Amaretto instead of Grand Marnier.

For a quick glaze, use sugar-free apricot preserves thinned with apple juice.

To Microwave:

Cook all the ingredients in a 3-cup glass measure covered with microwave plastic wrap for 5 minutes on high. Then proceed as above.

Per serving: 0 mg cholesterol, 0.12 gm saturated fat, 0.7 gm total fat, 4.3 gm fiber, 3 mg sodium, 147 calories, 0 gm trans fat

Fresh Fruit Compote Ⓠ

Serves: 8

1 cup diced fresh pineapple
1 orange, peeled and cubed
1 peach or nectarine, cubed
1 banana, sliced

1 apple, cored and cubed
1 cup red or green seedless grapes
½ cup unsweetened papaya nectar
    or fresh orange juice

1. Place all the fruits in a bowl and toss lightly.
2. Sprinkle with papaya nectar, cover, and chill at least 20 minutes before serving.

Per serving: 0 mg cholesterol, 0.09 gm saturated fat, 0.4 gm total fat, 2.2 gm fiber, 2 mg sodium, 71 calories, 0 gm trans fat

Fruited Mousse Ⓠ

Serves: 8

This fresh fruit dessert is a wonderful light ending to a meal. It is best if served within 1 hour of preparation. You may use frozen mangos, papayas, strawberries, or nectarines instead of peaches.

12 ounces frozen unsweetened
    peaches (packaged, or flash-
    freeze your own in season)
2 extra-large egg whites
1 tablespoon fresh lemon juice

2–3 tablespoons frozen
    unsweetened apple juice
    concentrate
1 teaspoon almond extract, or 1
    tablespoon Amaretto

1. Chop the frozen fruit with the metal blade of a food processor or with a stick blender.
2. Add the remaining ingredients and process until thick and fluffy, about 3 to 4 minutes.

To Serve: Spoon into 8 wine glasses or glass fruit coupes and serve or chill up to 1 hour before serving.

Per serving: 0 mg cholesterol, 0 gm saturated fat, 0.1 gm total fat, 0.6 gm fiber, 16 mg sodium, 32 calories, 0 gm trans fat

Persimmon Freeze Ⓠ

Serves: 4

This wonderful fresh fruit sorbet is made by simply freezing ripe persimmons when they're in season. The taste is incredibly delicious!

4 ripe persimmons, unwashed and frozen solid

4 teaspoons frozen unsweetened apple juice concentrate, defrosted, Cointreau, or Creme Topping (page 316)

1. Defrost the frozen persimmons at room temperature for about 1 hour (depending on the size of the persimmon) until slightly soft.
2. Peel the defrosted persimmons in petal-like fashion and place in a fruit dish or on dessert plates.
3. Drizzle each persimmon with 1 teaspoon apple juice concentrate and serve with a grapefruit spoon.

Per serving: 0 mg cholesterol, 0 gm saturated fat, 0.1 gm total fat, 0.4 gm fiber, 2 mg sodium, 41 calories, 0 gm trans fat

Café au Lait Custard

Serves: 10 (⅓ cup = 1 serving)

Baked custard has always been one of my husband's favorite desserts, and since it is easy to prepare, it appeared frequently as a family dessert in our "prior life." However, when we converted to a healthier lifestyle, I thought "Never again."

A traditional custard conjures up visions of lots of egg yolks and cream but not so with my Café au Lait Custard, which uses egg whites and nonfat evaporated milk. It sets up beautifully and has a delectable velvety texture and delicious flavor.

6 extra-large egg whites, or 3 extra-large egg whites and 1 Eggland's Best egg
⅓ cup Splenda
1½ cups instant decaffeinated coffee

2 teaspoons pure vanilla extract
1½ cups nonfat evaporated milk, scalded
2 teaspoons cocoa mixed with a dash of ground cinnamon (optional)

1. Beat the egg whites lightly; add sugar, coffee, and vanilla.
2. Slowly add the scalded milk, stirring constantly.
3. Pour into 10 custard cups or 5-ounce soufflé dishes or espresso cups and if desired, sprinkle with the cocoa mixture. Place the cups in a rectangular pan containing very hot water to just below the level of the custard.
4. Bake in a preheated 375° oven for 20 minutes or until a knife comes out clean when inserted in the custard. Cool slightly, cover, and refrigerate at least 1 hour before serving.

Per serving: 2 mg cholesterol, 0.05 gm saturated fat, 0.1 gm total fat, 0 gm fiber, 81 mg sodium, 71 calories, 0 gm trans fat

Raisin and Pear Bread Pudding

Serves: 12 (½ cup = 1 serving)

1 pear with skin, cored and sliced
5 cups day-old whole wheat raisin bread, cubed
3 cups Light Silk Soymilk
1 12-ounce can nonfat evaporated milk
2 tablespoons Splenda Brown Sugar Blend

2 teaspoons pure vanilla extract
2 teaspoons ground cinnamon
4 extra-large egg whites, slightly beaten with a fork
½ teaspoon freshly grated nutmeg
2 tablespoons chopped walnuts (optional)

1. Coat an 8-inch-square glass baking dish with butter-flavored cooking spray.
2. Mix the apple with the bread cubes and spread in the baking dish.
3. Combine the milks, Splenda, vanilla, and half of the cinnamon with the egg whites. Beat with a fork to blend.
4. Pour the milk mixture over the bread and let soak 10 minutes.
5. Sprinkle with the remaining cinnamon, nutmeg, and nuts if desired and bake in a preheated 350° oven for 40 to 45 minutes.

To Serve: While warm or at room temperature, spoon into serving dishes. Accompany with Creme Topping (page 316) or Fresh Strawberry or Blueberry Sauce (pages 319 and 317).

Per serving: 2 mg cholesterol, 0.14 gm saturated fat, 0.5 gm total fat, 1.3 gm fiber, 114 mg sodium, 74 calories

Bing Cherry Clafouti

Serves: 12

1½ pounds (about 4 cups) fresh
    pitted black bing or Royal Anne
    cherries or frozen unsweetened
    cherries, thawed and drained
Zest of 1 orange
1 tablespoon Grand Marnier
1⅓ cups Light Silk Soymilk or
    nonfat milk

2 teaspoons pure vanilla extract
4 extra-large egg whites
1 cup unbleached white flour
¼ cup sugar or 2 tablespoons
    Splenda

Confectioner's sugar (optional)

1. Preheat the oven to 400°.
2. Macerate the cherries with the zest and Grand Marnier in a bowl for about 5 to 10 minutes.
3. Place the milk, vanilla, egg whites, flour, and sugar in a blender or food processor and blend until smooth, or mix by hand.
4. Pour a third of the mixture into a 9-inch round nonstick baking pan or springform pan.
5. Spread the cherries over the batter; pour the remaining batter over the cherries.
6. Bake at 400° for 5 minutes; lower the temperature to 375° and bake for about 40 minutes or until a knife comes out clean.

To Serve: Cool about 30 minutes. Sprinkle with confectioner's sugar if desired, and serve while still warm.

Per serving: 2 mg cholesterol, 0.38 gm saturated fat, 0.8 gm total fat, 0.9 gm fiber, 36 mg sodium, 107 calories

---

Old-fashioned oatmeal—not the instant or one-minute variety—helps to control blood sugar.

Meringue Shells with Fruit

Yield: 12 shells (1 shell = 1 serving)

Although this dessert has more sugar than I normally use or recommend, it is fat- and cholesterol-free and makes a lovely occasional dessert treat. When watching your cholesterol, you sometimes need something a little sweet so that you don't feel completely deprived.

5 extra-large egg whites, *at room temperature*
¼ teaspoon cream of tartar
2 teaspoons pure vanilla extract
⅓ cup extra fine granulated sugar
⅓ cup Splenda Sugar Blend

6 cups fresh blueberries or sliced strawberries, peaches, pears, or nectarines

Blueberry Sauce (page 317) or Fresh Strawberry sauce (page 319), optional

1. Preheat the oven to 200°. Lightly coat a nonstick cookie sheet with nonstick cooking spray; then coat it lightly with flour, shaking off any excess.

2. Combine the egg whites, cream of tartar, and vanilla in the large bowl of an electric mixer and beat until the egg whites form soft peaks.

3. Gradually add the sugar, a tablespoon at a time, while beating continually.

4. Beat until the meringue is shiny and forms very stiff (not dry) peaks.

5. Using a tablespoon, shape the meringue into twelve individual shells on the prepared baking sheet, pressing the centers with the back of a spoon to form nests.

6. Bake at 200° for 30 minutes. For optimum texture and taste, the meringues should be totally dry and not change color. (Technically, meringues are dried, not baked.)

7. Turn off the heat, leave the oven door partially ajar, and leave the meringues in the oven until cool. Remove carefully with a spatula.

To Serve: Fill the meringue shells with fruit and serve with Blueberry Sauce or Strawberry Sauce if you like.

NOTE: These meringue shells may be made in advance, placed in a container or plastic bag (not airtight), and stored for up to a week at room temperature or for several months in the freezer.

Per serving: 0 mg cholesterol, 0.01 gm saturated fat, 0.3 gm total fat, 1.7 gm fiber, 30 mg sodium, 62 calories, 0 gm trans fat

Angel Food Cake

Serves: 16 to 20

No collection of recipes for a healthful lifestyle would be complete without a recipe for angel food cake. In my prior life, angel food cake was not one of my favorites. I used to lust for a piece of rich home-made pound cake. I'd settle for chiffon cake made with oil or sponge cake made with lots of egg yolks! Today, it's old faithful angel food cake that I can have in the freezer and serve with fresh fruit or fresh-fruit sauce for dessert. You can vary the recipe by adding cocoa or spices, or you can top the cake with Wax Orchards Fudge Topping—a wonderful, virtually fat-free chocolate sauce (only 16 calories in a teaspoon). If you'd rather use a commercial cake mix, the result will be the same nutritionally, but the taste will not be nearly as good.

1 cup cake flour or 1 cup unbleached white flour less 2 tablespoons
½ cup granulated sugar
1½ cups egg whites° (about 10–12), at room temperature
1 teaspoon cream of tartar
1½ teaspoons pure vanilla extract

½ teaspoon pure almond extract ·
¾ cup Splenda Sugar Blend

Fresh Strawberry sauce (page 319), Blueberry Sauce (page 317), or heated Wax Orchards Fudge Topping† (optional)

1. Sift the flour and ½ cup sugar together.
2. Place the egg whites into the large bowl of an electric mixer, beat until frothy, and add the cream of tartar and extracts. Beat until stiff, not dry, then gradually add the remaining ¾ cup sugar, 2 tablespoons at a time. Beat well after each addition.
3. Continue beating until the meringue forms stiff peaks and is glossy (the whites will not slide in the bowl).
4. Gradually sprinkle the flour-sugar mixture over the meringue, 3 table-spoons at a time, and fold in gently with a rubber spatula to combine.
5. Quickly but gently push the batter into an *ungreased* 10-inch tube pan.
6. Bake in a preheated 375° oven for 30 to 35 minutes or until the cake springs back when touched with fingers.
7. Remove from the oven, invert the pan onto a vinegar or soda bottle, and cool upside-down for about 1 hour.

To Serve: When cool, loosen the cake from the sides, bottom, and tube of the pan with a long knife and invert onto a platter. Pass fruit sauce or chocolate sauce if desired.

Hint:

Use a serrated knife to cut the cake so that the slices are not squashed.

Variations:

Marbled Angel Food Cake:
Follow the basic recipe, omitting the almond extract. Divide the batter in half and fold in 3 tablespoons sifted cocoa to one half. Put alternate spoonfuls of white and dark batter into the pan. Cut through the batter with a knife to make swirls of dark and light batter, and bake as directed in the basic recipe.

Spicy Angel Food Cake:
Add 2½ teaspoons pumpkin pie spice to the sifted flour mixture and stir lightly to blend. Proceed as in the basic recipe.

Per serving: 0 mg cholesterol, 0.01 gm saturated fat, 0 gm total fat, 0.1 gm fiber, 38 mg sodium, 76 calories

*Separate the eggs when cold (it's easier), then let the whites stand to reach room temperature. *Caution:* When separating the eggs, do not get a speck of egg yolk into the whites or they will not beat stiff. Be certain to use a stainless steel or glass bowl for beating whites. Plastic bowls frequently retain grease from previous use.
†This delicious sauce is made from fruits only. Use it hot on frozen nonfat yogurt with a few almonds, and would you believe—a hot fudge sundae! I almost feel guilty eating it, and my guests still don't believe it when I say it has no cholesterol or saturated fat. The sauce may be available at specialty food stores in your area, or contact the manufacturer: Wax Orchards, Route 4-320, Vashon Island, WA 98070.

Mango Salsa

Yield: 1½ cups (2 tablespoons = 1 serving)

A lovely fruited salsa to serve with grilled chicken, turkey breast slices, or broiled fish. It tastes better if it marinates for 30 minutes before being served.

1 large mango, halved and seeded
½ small red onion, diced
1 tablespoon finely diced jalapeño
  pepper, seeds removed, or 2
  plum tomatoes, seeded and
  chopped

Juice of 1 lime (2 tablespoons)
2 tablespoons chopped cilantro or
  mint or 3 sliced caper berries

1. Remove the mango pulp with a grapefruit knife and dice.
2. Add all the remaining ingredients to the diced mango and combine thoroughly. Taste and adjust seasoning. Chill in a covered container in the refrigerator for 30 minutes before serving. Bring to room temperature before serving.

Variation: A fresh papaya and 1 small ripe pear may be substituted for the mango.

Per serving: 0 mg cholesterol, 0.01 gm saturated fat, 0 gm total fat, 0.2 gm fiber, 0 mg sodium, 9 calories, 0 gm trans fat

Cranberry-Pineapple Freeze

Yield: 24 foil cups (1 foil cup = 1 serving)

Freezes are delicious served either as an accompaniment to roast chicken or turkey or as a dessert. In my book *Deliciously Low*, I prepared this recipe with fresh cranberries; however, there are now available delicious sugar-free cranberry or cranberry-orange marmalades that make it even easier to prepare. This revised recipe can be made in minutes.

2 8-ounce jars sugar-free cranberry or cranberry-orange marmalade
1 20-ounce can crushed unsweetened pineapple, drained

1 pint nonfat plain vanilla or lemon yogurt
¼ cup chopped walnuts (optional)

1. Combine all the ingredients in a mixing bowl and stir with a fork.
2. Line muffin tins with foil cupcake liners and fill each cup two-thirds full with the yogurt mixture.
3. Freeze for several hours or until firm.

To Serve: Remove from freezer 15 minutes before serving.

To Freeze for Future Use:

When firmly frozen, remove the foil cups from the muffin tins and store in an airtight container in the freezer.

Per serving: 0 mg cholesterol, 0.03 gm saturated fat, 0.1 gm total fat, 0.4 gm fiber, 17 mg sodium, 73 calories, 0 gm trans fat

Cheese Berry Spread

Yield: about 1¼ cups (1 tablespoon = 1 serving)

A delicious low-fat, low-cholesterol spread to use on your daily Oat Bran Muffins or on whole wheat toast or English muffins. This is also excellent as a sandwich spread instead of the usual peanut butter (which may contain hydrogenated oil) and jelly.

8 ounces part-skim ricotta cheese
or nonfat whipped cream
cheese

3 tablespoons sugar-free
strawberry or raspberry
preserves

1. Process the ricotta cheese in a food processor or blender until smooth.
2. Add the preserves and process until smooth.
3. Place in a covered container and chill at least 1 hour before serving. This keeps up to a week in the refrigerator.

Per serving: 4 mg cholesterol, 0.56 gm saturated fat, 0.9 gm total fat, 0 gm fiber, 14 mg sodium, 18 calories, 0 gm trans fat

Garlic Toast ⓠ

Yield: 8 slices (1 slice = 1 serving)

8 slices whole wheat,
pumpernickel, or rye bread,
thinly sliced
2 tablespoons extra-virgin olive
oil mixed with 3 cloves garlic,
minced, and 1 teaspoon Herbes
de Provence

3 tablespoons shredded Parmesan
cheese (optional)
Crushed red pepper flakes,
optional

1. Arrange the bread slices on a baking sheet and brush one side lightly with the olive-oil mixture.
2. Sprinkle each slice with 1 teaspoon of the Parmesan cheese.°
3. Place under a preheated boiler until lightly browned. Serve immediately.

Variation: For an oil-free toast, toast the bread lightly in the toaster and rub with cut garlic cloves while the toast is still hot, so that the garlic melts into the bread.

Per serving: 1 mg cholesterol, 0.58 gm saturated fat, 3.8 gm total fat, 0.3 gm fiber, 109 mg sodium, 86 calories, 0 gm trans fat

° Bread may be prepared ahead of time through Step 2 and just broiled at serving time.

High-Fiber Whole Grain
Onion Bread

Yield: 1 loaf cut into 20 slices

This bread freezes well and is terrific toasted. It is great for sandwiches or just spread with nonfat cream cheese.

4 tablespoons dehydrated onion
    flakes or rolled oats, or a
    combination of the two
1 cup 7-grain cereal
2 cups whole wheat flour
1 cup rolled oats
½ cup oat bran

2 tablespoons brown sugar
½ cup lightly toasted onion flakes
1 envelope quick-rising yeast
1 teaspoon salt
2 cups *hot* water or nonfat milk
    (130°)

1. Preheat the oven to 425°. Coat a 9 × 5 × 4-inch loaf pan with butter-flavored nonstick spray and sprinkle with 2 tablespoons of the onion flakes. Reserve the remaining 2 tablespoons onion flakes for topping.

2. Place the remaining dry ingredients in a mixing bowl and combine with a fork or your fingers.

3. Add the liquid ingredients to the dry and stir with a wooden spoon until all the flour is completely moistened.

4. Put the batter into the prepared pan and sprinkle with the remaining onion flakes. Cover with a towel and allow to rise in a warm place for 20 minutes or until the dough reaches the top of the pan.

5. Lower the oven temperature to 400° and bake for 45 minutes.

6. Remove the bread from the pan and cool on a rack before slicing.

To Freeze for Future Use:

Slice and wrap the cool bread in an airtight plastic bag.

Per serving: 0 mg cholesterol, 0.09 gm saturated fat, 0.7 gm total fat, 2.1 gm fiber, 134 mg sodium, 83 calories, 0 gm trans fat

Bran Berry Loaf

Yield: 1 loaf cut into 18 slices (1 slice = 1 serving)

This lovely loaf provides a pleasant change from Oat Bran Muffins; however, it does not contain quite as much soluble fiber per serving.

¾ cup Kamut flour
½ cup unbleached white flour
1 cup oat bran
1 tablespoon baking powder
½ teaspoon baking soda
3 tablespoons Splenda Brown
   Sugar Blend
1½ teaspoons cinnamon

2 extra-large egg whites, slightly
   beaten
1 tablespoon canola or walnut oil
¾ cup fresh orange juice
1 teaspoon grated orange zest
¼ cup nonfat evaporated milk
1 cup fresh or frozen blueberries
   (do not defrost before using)

1. Preheat the oven to 350° and coat a 9 × 5 × 4-inch loaf pan with nonstick spray.
2. Combine the first seven ingredients in a mixing bowl and blend thoroughly.
3. In a separate bowl, mix together the egg whites, oil, orange juice, zest, and milk.
4. Add the liquid ingredients to the dry and stir until the dry ingredients are complete moistened.
5. Add the blueberries and blend gently.
6. Pour into the prepared loaf pan and bake at 350° for 50 minutes, or until loaf is lightly browned and starts to pull from sides of pan. Cool before slicing. This freezes nicely for future use.

Per serving: 0 mg cholesterol, 0.10 gm saturated fat, 1.4 gm total fat, 1.8 gm fiber, 84 mg sodium, 70 calories, 0 gm trans fat

The Great Pumpkin Muffins

Yield: 12-14 muffins (1 muffin = 1 serving)

There is no need to wait for Thanksgiving to savor the special flavor of pumpkin. These muffins are delicious for breakfast or with meals. In fact, they are so delicious you can even serve them as dessert. The pumpkin muffins you prepare from this recipe are different from the ones you buy commercially, since they contain *no* cholesterol, no saturated fat, no trans fat, and are *low* in all fat and *high* in good soluble fiber.

1 cup whole wheat flour
1½ cups oat bran
½ cup barley flour
1½ tablespoons baking powder
½ cup Splenda Brown Sugar Blend
2 teaspoons ground cinnamon
½ teaspoon ground nutmeg
½ cup dark raisins or dried cranberries

3 extra-large egg whites, slightly beaten
1¼ cups canned pumpkin
1 cup nonfat evaporated milk or Light Silk Soymilk
2 tablespoons canola oil
2 teaspoons pure vanilla extract
¼ cup chopped walnuts

1. Preheat the oven to 425° and coat muffin tins with nonstick spray or line with paper cupcake liners.

2. Mix the first eight ingredients together in a bowl; blend thoroughly with a fork or slotted spoon.

3. Combine the liquid ingredients in another bowl and blend thoroughly.

4. Add the pumpkin mixture to the dry ingredients and stir with a fork until all the flour disappears and is moistened.

5. Fill the prepared muffin tins, place in oven, and lower temperature to 400°. Bake for 20 to 25 minutes or until lightly browned.

6. Cool slightly on a rack before serving.

Per serving: 1 mg cholesterol, 0.22 gm saturated fat, 3.5 gm total fat, 4.7 gm fiber, 137 mg sodium, 164 calories, 0 gm trans fat

Snacks

Soy Smoothie Shake Ⓠ

A quick breakfast alternative!

Serves: 1

½ cup fresh orange juice, soy milk, or low-fat Lactaid

½ cup green tea (steeped for 3 minutes)

½ cup soy protein isolate powder (Genisoy), in any flavor°

3 frozen unsweetened strawberries, or ¼ cup of frozen unsweetened peaches or blueberries

½ banana, sliced

1 teaspoon vanilla extract or grated orange zest (optional)

1. In a blender, or using a stick blender, combine all of the ingredients until smooth; serve immediately.

Per serving: 0 mg cholesterol, 0.1 gm saturated fat, 4.49 gm total fat, 2.56 gm fiber, 415.87 calories, 30.13 gm carbohydrate, 19.33 gm sugar, 0 gm trans fat

°Refer to nutrients panel on the back of the package of the powdered soy protein powder for nutritional analysis.

Orange-Yogurt Popsicles

Yield: 8 popsicles (1 popsicle = 1 serving)

A wonderful snack—and not just for children!

16 ounces nonfat plain yogurt

1 ripe banana, sliced

6 ounces frozen unsweetened orange juice, pear-grape juice, or pineapple-orange juice concentrate

2–3 teaspoons pure vanilla extract

8 4-ounce paper cups

8 wooden popsicle sticks or tongue depressors°

1. Place the yogurt, banana, orange juice, and vanilla in a food processor or blender and blend thoroughly until smooth.

2. Pour into the paper cups, place in the freezer, and chill.

3. When half-frozen, add the popsicle sticks or tongue depressors and freeze until solid.

To Serve: Place the cup in hot water *briefly* to just loosen the paper.

Variation: Instead of using paper cups, for smaller popsicles you can use plastic ice cube trays, pouring the yogurt mixture into each ice cube cup and using plastic stirrers for sticks.

Per serving: 1 mg cholesterol, 0.1 gm saturated fat, 0.2 gm total fat, 0.5 gm fiber, 44 mg sodium, 74 calories

°Ask your doctor or pharmacist.

▼ 7 ▼

Family Favorites
Made Healthful

When it comes to dessert, fruit° is obviously the most nutritionally sound selection, but realistically, everyone wants an occasional indulgence. The day I decided it was past time for my family to change to a low-fat, low-cholesterol lifestyle, I started to look at some of our favorite recipes—ones that I made "by popular request." I had thought I had been cooking in a healthful manner until I really examined some of these recipes more closely, particularly the desserts. What I found were high-fat, high-cholesterol killers. I soon discovered that all the fat, both saturated and trans fats, egg yolks, chocolate, and sugar I had previously added were unnecessary to produce a delicious product. By making substitutions, I proved that we could enjoy delicious desserts without feeling guilty *or* clogging our arteries.

In the following pages I have included some of our favorite desserts, changed to satisfy our revised style of eating as well as our palates. And to help you begin converting your own recipes, I am sharing a few tricks of the trade in the chart on page 338—substitutions that will cut the cholesterol and saturated fat content of baked goods dramatically.

Recipes

(beginning on page 340)

Today's Coffee Cake
Almost Edie's Coffee Cake
Just a Good Chocolate Cookie

°Remember to buy fruit in season and wash before eating not storing.

Spiced Honey Tea Loaf
Chocoholic's Chocolate Cake
Chocolate Trifle
Blueberry Meringue Cobbler
Virtual Date Brownies
Cranberry Oatmeal Cookies
Oat Nut Slices with Jam
Pineapple Cake
Poached Pear "en Croute"
Apple Streudel

Simple Tricks of the Trade for Baking and Dessert Making

INSTEAD OF:	TRY:
Butter, margarine, or vegetable shortening (for conversion, see page 356)	Canola, sunflower, cold-pressed safflower oil, or walnut oil
Sugar	Frozen unsweetened apple juice concentrate, date sugar, or cut amount of sugar in recipe by ⅓ to ½ of the amount listed. You can use smaller amounts of brown sugar when used instead of white sugar or substitute Splenda Brown Sugar Blend or Splenda Sugar Blend.
Sour cream	Nonfat plain yogurt and/or strained buttermilk, or at most, plain low-fat yogurt or nonfat or light sour cream
Whole milk	Nonfat milk or nonfat evaporated milk (also called skim), 1% milk, or Light Silk Soymilk

INSTEAD OF:	TRY:
Egg yolks or whole eggs	Egg whites (2 extra-large egg whites equal 1 whole egg), or low-cholesterol egg substitute, liquid egg whites, Eggland eggs, or egg replacement powder
Chocolate	Sugar-free cocoa (3 tablespoons cocoa plus 1 tablespoon canola oil equal 1 ounce chocolate)
All white flour	Whole wheat or sometimes a combination of whole wheat or Kamut and unbleached white flour. Substitute some oat bran for some of the flour when possible in cookies, cakes, sweet breads, and plain breads.
Melted butter or margarine (for conversion, see page 356)	Butter-flavored nonstick spray for coating pans. Use slightly beaten egg white as glaze or a base for spreading filling on coffee cakes.
Nuts in cake or cookies	Crushed cereals, dried fruits (e.g., raisins and dates), or reduce the amount of nuts

For many years, I prepared a quick and easy coffee cake for my family and unexpected guests. It, like most of the baking in my "previous life," started with butter, eggs, sour cream or whole milk, and lots of sugar! But that was long ago. Today, I am much wiser, and healthier alternatives are available. This recipe uses egg whites—no yolks; canola oil—no butter or margarine, 1% fat milk or Light Silk Soymilk instead of whole milk, and less sugar courtesy of Splenda! The result is a low–saturated fat, trans fat–free delicious coffee cake. By the way, *don't forget your portion control!*

Today's Coffee Cake

Yield: 1 cake cut into 30 squares (1 square = 1 serving)

1⅓ cups unbleached white flour
1⅓ cups whole wheat pastry flour
½ cup oat bran
½ cup Splenda Sugar Blend
½ cup Splenda Brown Sugar Blend
½ cup canola oil
1 teaspoon freshly ground nutmeg
½ cup rolled oats, chopped

⅓ cup chopped walnuts
2 teaspoons ground cinnamon
1½ teaspoons baking powder
1 12-ounce can nonfat evaporated milk or Light Silk Soymilk
4 extra-large egg whites, slightly beaten

1. Preheat the oven to 350°. Coat a 9 × 13-inch metal* baking pan with butter-flavored nonstick spray.

2. Combine the first seven ingredients in the large mixing bowl of an electric mixer. Blend well.

3. Remove ⅔ cup of the mixture and combine with the oats, nuts, and cinnamon to be used as topping. Set aside.

4. Combine the baking powder, milk, and eggs, and beat slightly with a fork. Add to the remaining flour mixture and beat thoroughly with electric beater on medium speed.

5. Pour half of the batter into the prepared baking pan and sprinkle half of the oat mixture evenly over the batter. Add the remaining batter and sprinkle with the remaining oat mixture.

6. Bake about 30 minutes or until cake springs back when lightly touched or a toothpick comes out clean.

7. Cool slightly in pan on a rack before cutting and serving.

NOTE: This cake freezes quite well. Sometimes I bake the recipes in two 9-inch loaf pans (baking time reduced to about 25 minutes) and freeze one for future use.

Per serving: 0 mg cholesterol, 0.34 gm saturated fat, 4.8 gm total fat, 0.8 gm fiber, 73 mg sodium, 121 calories, 0 gm trans fat

°If you use a glass baking dish, lower the oven temperature to 325°.

The tricks in this delicious and healthful coffee cake? I've cut the sugar in the original recipe by half, added whole wheat pastry flour, and substituted yogurt for whole sour cream, egg whites for whole eggs, and oil for stick margarine, and it still tastes delicious!

Almost Edie's Coffee Cake

Yield: 1 cake cut into 40 slices (1 slice = 1 serving)

⅓ cup canola oil or walnut oil
1⅔ cups Splenda Sugar Blend
3 teaspoons pure vanilla
1 whole Eggland egg
4 extra-large egg whites, slightly beaten
1¾ cups whole wheat pastry flour
1¾ cups unbleached white flour
1 tablespoon baking powder
2 teaspoons baking soda
1 pint nonfat plain or vanilla yogurt or nonfat or low-fat sour cream

1 cup seeded manuka raisins and/ or sun-dried apricots, plumped in 2 tablespoons apricot brandy or fresh orange juice°

Streusel:
½ cup finely chopped toasted walnuts
⅓ cup finely chopped rolled oats
2 tablespoons Splenda Brown Sugar Blend
2 teaspoons cinnamon

1. Preheat the oven to 375°. Coat a 10-inch tube pan (angel-food cake pan) with butter-flavored nonstick spray.
2. Pour the oil in the bowl of an electric mixer. Add the sugar and beat until smooth. Add the vanilla and blend.
3. Add the egg and egg whites gradually and beat for 3 minutes.

4. In a separate bowl, combine the flours, baking powder, and baking soda and mix thoroughly.

5. Alternately place a third of the flour mixture, then half of yogurt, into the batter, starting and ending with flour. Beat until smooth after each addition.

6. Mix together the streusel ingredients.

7. Place a third of the batter in the bottom of the prepared tube pan. Sprinkle with a third of the streusel and half of the raisins. Repeat; then top with the remaining third of batter and streusel.

8. Bake at 375° for 25 minutes. Lower the temperature to 325° and bake for about 30 minutes more or until the cake starts to pull away from sides of pan.

9. Cool in the pan on a rack and then loosen with a metal spatula and remove from pan. May be frozen for future use.

Per serving: 0 mg cholesterol, 0.33 gm saturated fat, 2.2 gm total fat, 0.9 gm fiber, 110 mg sodium, 102 calories, 0 gm trans fat

*Put in microwave for 1 minute on high, covered tightly with microwave plastic wrap. If your raisins are really fresh, just combine with hot brandy or juice.

Everybody is always asking for "just a good chocolate cookie." Well, here's one for your files—and it's trans fat– and saturated fat–free!

Just a Good Chocolate Cookie

Yield: 45 cookies (2 cookies = 1 serving)

1½ cups Splenda Sugar Blend
⅓ cup confectioners' sugar
2 cups walnuts, lightly toasted and chopped in food processor

½ cup unsweetened cocoa powder
2 extra-large egg whites, slightly beaten with a fork
½ teaspoon pure vanilla extract

1. Preheat 350° oven and line baking sheets with parchment paper.

2. In a large mixing bowl whisk together Splenda Sugar Blend, confectioners' sugar, ground walnuts, and cocoa powder.

3. Add slightly beaten egg whites and vanilla. Stir until mixture is well combined and moistened.

4. Form rounded teaspoons of mixture into balls; place on baking sheet lined with parchment paper.

5. Using a small glass, press balls with bottom of glass until flattened.

6. Bake in preheated oven for 15 minutes or until tops of cookies appear dry.

7. Remove cookies and cool on rack. Yields about 45 cookies.

Per serving: 0 mg cholesterol, 0.69 gm saturated fat, 7.38 gm total fat, 1.88 gm fiber, 87.68 calories, 5.49 gm carbohydrate, 1.79 gm sugar, 0 gm trans fat

I have changed my traditional recipe by cutting the amount of sugar in half, the amount of oil in half, using egg whites only, and substituting part whole wheat flour and part oat bran for all white flour. This no-cholesterol, low-fat loaf is lovely to serve with tea or as a light dessert with fresh fruit.

Spiced Honey Tea Loaf

Yield: 2 loaves cut into 36 slices and halved (½ slice = 1 serving)

1 cup honey
1⅓ cups hot decaffeinated coffee
2 cups unbleached white flour
1 cup whole wheat pastry flour
1 tablespoon baking powder
1 teaspoon baking soda
2 teaspoons cinnamon
½ teaspoon allspice
¼ cup canola or walnut oil

2 extra-large egg whites
⅓ cup Splenda Sugar Blend
4 extra-large egg whites, at room temperature
¼ teaspoon cream of tartar

¼ cup sliced almonds, or chopped walnuts for garnish

1. Preheat the oven to 350°. Lightly coat the bottoms of two 9 × 5 × 4-inch loaf pans with nonstick spray and line with wax paper.

2. Dissolve the honey in the hot coffee and cool.

3. Combine the flours, baking powder, baking soda, cinnamon, and allspice and mix together with a spoon.

4. Beat the coffee mixture, oil, 2 egg whites, and 3 tablespoons of Splenda in the bowl of an electric mixer. Add the dry ingredients and mix until smooth.

5. In a separate bowl, beat the 4 egg whites with the cream of tartar until slightly thick. Add the remaining 3 tablespoons Splenda, a tablespoon at a time, and beat until stiff (the whites will not slide in the bowl).

6. Fold the beaten egg whites into the cake mixture gently, just until blended.

7. Pour into the prepared loaf pans, sprinkle the tops of the loaves with the nuts, and bake at 350° for about 1 hour or until the cake starts to pull away from the sides of the pans.

8. Invert the pans onto a cake rack to cool completely.

9. Loosen the sides of the loaves with a spatula and remove from the pans. Remove the wax paper and slice.

To Freeze for Future Use:

Wrap the sliced loaf in plastic wrap, then foil.

Per serving: 0 mg cholesterol, 0.05 gm saturated fat, 0.9 gm total fat, 0.4 gm fiber, 30 mg sodium, 47 calories, 0 gm trans fat

Devil's food cake has always been a favorite in our house. In fact, I made it as a standard birthday cake. How could I sacrifice this tradition? Happily I don't have to since I concocted this delicious, moist cake which we all just love. I fight being a chocoholic; however, when I do use chocolate, it's in the form of cocoa powder, not chocolate squares that are high in saturated fat (which raises cholesterol). This cake has no cholesterol and virtually no saturated fat so that you can enjoy each mouthful. It also freezes beautifully.

Chocoholic's Chocolate Cake

Yield: 1 cake cut into 20 pieces (1 piece = 1 serving)

1½ cups cake flour
½ cup unsweetened cocoa
½ cup Splenda Brown Sugar Blend
2 teaspoons baking powder
1 teaspoon baking soda
⅓ cup canola oil
1 cup cold water or fresh orange
    juice

2 teaspoons pure vanilla extract
2 tablespoons white vinegar
2 tablespoons Kahlua (optional)

Cocoa and confectioners' sugar,
    for sifting over cooled cake
    (optional)

1. Preheat the oven to 375° and spray the bottom of an 8 × 8 × 2-inch baking pan or an 8-inch round springform pan (for a fudgier cake) with butter-flavored nonstick cooking spray.

2. Combine the flour, cocoa, sugar, baking powder, and baking soda in a mixing bowl and blend thoroughly with a slotted spoon.

3. Combine the oil, water, vanilla, and Kahlua (if desired) in a separate bowl, and beat thoroughly with a fork.

4. Add the liquid ingredients to the dry and mix quickly with a slotted spoon until all the flour is moistened and the batter is smooth. Add vinegar to batter and stir quickly to blend.

5. Pour the batter into the prepared baking pan *immediately* and bake at 375° for 20 to 25 minutes, or until the cake starts to shrink from the sides of the pan.

6. Cool on a rack. Sift the cocoa powder on the top of half of the cake and confectioners' sugar onto the remaining half if you like.

Variation: Drizzle 2 tablespoons of Wax Orchards Fudge Topping (see page 328) over hot cake before cooling.

Per serving: 0 mg cholesterol, 0.38 gm saturated fat, 4.1 gm total fat, 0.5 gm fiber, 78 mg sodium, 94 calories, 0 gm trans fat

Personally, I really never cared much for trifle as a dessert, but I did prepare it as a tradition for holiday dinners. When I look back on the ingredients, I cringe: eggs in the cake, eggs in the custard, and heavy cream on top of all that! How could anybody who cooked like that change her culinary habits enough to make something that looked good, tasted delicious, and didn't perpetuate atherosclerosis? Well, I did—and so can you, while you enjoy your family's enjoyment!

Chocolate Trifle ⓠ

Serves: about 16

⅓ Chocoholic's Chocolate Cake (page 344), cut into ½-inch slices
3 tablespoons sugar-free raspberry preserves mixed with 1 tablespoon Framboise liqueur
1 pint frozen nonfat vanilla yogurt

1 pint frozen Soy Delicious chocolate yogurt
2 tablespoons chopped toasted almonds (optional)
½ cup fresh raspberries

1. Place a layer of chocolate cake slices on the bottom of a glass soufflé dish or a crystal bowl.

2. Spread the cake with half of the raspberry preserve mixture.

3. Cover the preserves with half of the vanilla and chocolate yogurt, giving a marbled or checkerboard effect.

4. Repeat the procedure and sprinkle the top with chopped almonds, if desired.

5. Cover with plastic wrap and place in the freezer until serving time, or until solid.

To Serve: Remove from freezer 20 to 30 minutes before serving.

Variation: This may be served with a fresh raspberry sauce and/or fresh raspberries.

Per serving: 1 mg cholesterol, 0.2 gm saturated fat, 1.5 gm total fat, 0.3 gm fiber, 70 mg sodium, 69 calories, 0 gm trans fat

An all-time family favorite for dessert in our home for many years was the traditional blueberry cobbler. Since cobblers have only a top crust, I thought that by not making my usual pie (with 387 calories and 17 grams of fat per serving), I was really cutting calories and fat. However, I now realize that was not nearly enough. The cobbler was made with three cans of blueberry pie filling and a topping of a very short and flaky (albeit delicious) pastry crust. Per serving, it was "reduced" to a whopping 320 calories and 12.8 grams of fat. As if this weren't bad enough, we frequently added a blob of French vanilla ice cream! I can hardly believe I made this, let alone ate it and fed it to my family.

Since we now realize that this calorically dense dessert is nutritionally unacceptable, I have come up with a delicious version of a cobbler that can be served and savored without qualms. It does have some sugar, but as a healthy dessert trade-off, with literally no saturated fat and no trans fat, it wins hands-down.

Blueberry Meringue Cobbler ⓠ

Serves: 8

1 can blueberry pie filling
3 cups fresh or frozen blueberries, unsweetened
½ teaspoon ground cinnamon
4 extra-large egg whites, at room temperature

¼ teaspoon cream of tartar
⅓ cup sifted confectioners' sugar
1 teaspoon pure vanilla extract

1. Combine the blueberry filling with the fresh blueberries in a bowl. Pour into an 8-inch-square glass baking dish and sprinkle lightly with cinnamon.

2. Place the egg whites and cream of tartar in the bowl of an electric mixer and beat until frothy.

3. Gradually beat in the sugar, a tablespoon at a time. Continue beating until stiff and glossy (not dry).

4. Pile the meringue by spoonfuls onto the blueberries and *seal the meringue to the edges of the dish all around to prevent shrinking.* Swirl with back of a spoon or spatula for a decorative top.

5. Bake in a preheated 425° oven for 5 to 7 minutes or until delicately browned. Cool gradually, away from drafts, before serving.

To Serve: Take the dessert to the table (it looks so pretty) and spoon onto dessert plates, with a portion of meringue on top of each serving.

Variation: Use Comstock cherry pie filling and 3 cups frozen or pitted fresh cherries.

Per serving: 0 mg cholesterol, 0.02 gm saturated fat, 0.3 gm total fat, 1.7 gm fiber, 41 mg sodium, 127 calories, 0 gm trans fat

As in many American families, brownies are a favorite in our home. My old recipe contained 12 ounces of chocolate and 1⅓ sticks of butter—both ingredients high in saturated fat—whole eggs (a total of 550 milligrams of cholesterol), and lots of sugar! Since we all do love an occasional chocolate treat, I came up with this healthier recipe for brownies, using

cocoa instead of chocolate and canola oil instead of butter, virtually eliminating saturated fat. I use only 1 egg and egg white, so the cholesterol is
minimal, and I use Splenda Sugar Blend and dates instead of sugar. Let's
face it, these are not the same as those decadent morsels, but it satisfies
your sweet tooth without endangering your health.

Virtual Date Brownies Ⓠ

Yield: 20 bars (1 bar = 1 serving)

⅓ cup unbleached white flour
1 cup whole wheat pastry flour
¾ cup unsweetened cocoa
2 teaspoons baking powder
¼ teaspoon baking soda
½ cup chopped dates
1 extra-large egg white
1 Eggland egg

⅔ cup Splenda Sugar Blend
2 tablespoons Kahlua (coffee
   liqueur) or coffee
⅓ cup canola oil
2 teaspoons vanilla extract
½ cup chopped walnuts (optional)
2 tablespoons fudge topping,
   optional

1. Preheat the oven to 375°. Coat an 8 × 8 × 2-inch baking dish with
butter-flavored nonstick spray.
2. Place the first five ingredients in a mixing bowl and blend thoroughly
with a spoon. Add the dates and mix.
3. In a separate bowl, beat the egg white and egg with a fork until foamy.
Add the Splenda Sugar Blend, Kahlua, oil, and vanilla. Mix thoroughly.
4. Add the liquid ingredients to the dry and stir until the flour is completely absorbed.
5. Spread in the prepared baking dish, sprinkle with nuts, and bake at
375° for 20 minutes.
6. Cool and cut into twenty bars. Drizzle with fudge topping if
desired.

Per serving: 10 mg cholesterol, 0.40 gm saturated fat, 4.3 gm total fat, 1 gm fiber,
51 mg sodium, 92 calories, 0 gm trans fat

Whether you are six or sixty, everybody likes to eat a cookie occasionally. This is an adaptation of a cookie that I made years ago. Then,
I thought it was especially healthy, because I used rolled oats. I didn't

count the half pound of butter, the egg yolks, and the huge amount of sugar I used! This revised recipe *is* healthy, *and* high in soluble fiber. It is cholesterol free and *low* in fat, though not fat free; however, the fat I do use is polyunsaturated canola oil, and the amount is *greatly* reduced (about 1 gram in each cookie!).

Cranberry Oatmeal Cookies

Yield: about 60-65 cookies (1 cookie = 1 serving)

3 extra-large egg whites, slightly beaten
½ cup Splenda Brown Sugar Blend
3 tablespoons canola oil
2 teaspoons pure vanilla extract
½ cup whole wheat flour

2 teaspoons ground cinnamon
1 teaspoon freshly ground nutmeg
4 teaspoons baking powder
3 cups quick-cooking rolled oats
½ cup dried cranberries
½ cup finely chopped walnuts

1. Preheat the oven to 375°. Coat a nonstick cookie sheet with butter-flavored nonstick spray.
2. Combine the egg whites, Splenda Brown Sugar Blend, oil, and vanilla in a bowl. Beat in electric mixer for 2 minutes or until thick.
3. In a separate bowl, combine the flour, cinnamon, nutmeg, baking powder, oats, cranberries, and nuts and mix thoroughly with a spoon.
4. Add the dry ingredients to the egg whites and blend until the flour disappears.
5. Drop rounded teaspoonfuls of cookie mixture onto cookie sheet.
6. Bake at 375° for 10 to 12 minutes or until lightly browned.
7. Loosen the cookies from the cookie sheet and cool. Store in a container that is *not* airtight, so that the cookies remain crisp.

Per serving: 0 mg cholesterol, 0.1 gm saturated fat, 1 gm total fat, 0.4 gm fiber, 23 mg sodium, 37 calories, 0 gm trans fat

There was a marvelous cookie I made years ago called the "thumbprint cookie." It contained butter, eggs, nuts, and all those terrible things. I have adjusted the recipe to eliminate *any* added fat or shortening and egg yolks. The result is a superdelicious, cholesterol-free sliced bar with jam that brings rave reviews. Caution: These cookies may be habit-forming. Remember, they still have calories.

Oat Nut Slices with Jam

Yield: 32 ½-inch slices (1 slice = 1 serving)

¾ cup ground nuts (walnuts and/or almonds)
¾ cup rolled oats, chopped
¼ cup oat bran
¼ cup Splenda Brown Sugar Blend
2 extra-large egg whites and 1 teaspoon pure vanilla extract, slightly beaten with a fork

About 2 tablespoons sugar-free preserves (apricot, strawberry, or raspberry)

1. Preheat the oven to 350° and coat a nonstick baking sheet with butter-flavored nonstick spray.
2. Mix the nuts, oats, and oat bran with the Splenda Brown Sugar Blend.
3. Add enough of the egg white and vanilla mixture to just make a mixture firm enough so that the nuts, oats, and Splenda Brown Sugar Blend all adhere.
4. Shape two rolls 1½ inches in diameter and about 12 inches long and place on the prepared baking sheet.
5. Dip your finger in cold water and make a deep ridge down the center of each roll.
6. Bake for 15 to 20 minutes or until lightly browned.
7. Remove from the oven, spoon jam into each ridge, and cool.
8. When cool, cut into ½-inch slices.

Variation: Use Wax Orchards Fudge Topping (page 328) instead of jam.

Per serving: 0 mg cholesterol, 0.14 gm saturated fat, 1.9 gm total fat, 0.4 gm fiber, 4 mg sodium, 35 calories, 0 gm trans fat

We have a family friend whose nemesis was pineapple upside-down cake. One slice was always just a beginning to his eating orgy. With all the butter and eggs in the recipe, I had to make a change before I could serve this to him without regret. This no-cholesterol cake tastes rather like the traditional pineapple upside-down cake but has a delicious flavor of its own. Although there is no added fat or cholesterol, the fat in the nuts still makes it necessary to limit the portion size (even though it is principally a polyunsaturated fat).

Pineapple Cake

Yield: 28 pieces (1 piece = 1 serving)

2 cups unbleached white flour mixed with ⅔ cup finely chopped walnuts
1 cup whole wheat pastry flour
1 teaspoon cinnamon
¾ teaspoon allspice
¼ teaspoon freshly ground nutmeg
½ cup dark Mannouka raisins
4 extra-large egg whites, at room temperature
¼ teaspoon cream of tartar

¾ cup Splenda Sugar Blend
2 teaspoons pure vanilla extract
2 teaspoons each lemon and orange zest
1 20-ounce can crushed pineapple in natural juice
2 teaspoons baking soda mixed with ¼ cup pineapple juice drained from crushed pineapple
¼ cup chopped walnuts for topping

1. Lightly coat the bottom only of a 13 × 9 × 2-inch glass baking pan with butter-flavored nonstick cooking spray, and preheat the oven to 325°

2. Combine the flours, nuts, spices, and raisins and mix until well combined.

3. Beat the egg whites with the cream of tartar until frothy. Gradually add the sugar, a tablespoon at a time, beating until the mixture forms soft peaks.

4. Add the vanilla, zests, baking soda mixture, and crushed pineapple with its remaining juice and blend.

5. Add the flour mixture to the pineapple mixture, and stir gently until the flour disappears.

6. Pour the batter into the prepared baking pan and bake 35 to 40 minutes or until the cake starts to pull from the sides of the pan.

7. Cool in the pan on a rack. Cut into 28 serving pieces.

Variations: This cake may be served with Creme Topping (page 316) that is made with chilled pineapple juice instead of apple juice concentrate, and topped with sliced strawberries

Per serving: 0 mg cholesterol, 0.16 gm saturated fat, 1.8 gm total fat, 1 gm fiber, 70 mg sodium, 113 calories, 0 gm trans fat

My daughter always loved fruit, especially when it was combined with a rich pastry. My new Pear "en Croute" recipe is her favorite now that she too has changed to a healthier lifestyle. She doesn't mind the reduction in calories that goes with it either. I've taken "culinary license" by referring to this recipe as "en croute." Obviously, we can't use flaky puff pastry with all its fat and cholesterol. I have substituted phyllo dough, which is nothing more than flour and water but results in a delicate, crisp packet in which to enclose the fruit. When a peeled, poached apple is substituted for the pear, it resembles a fancy apple turnover.

Poached Pear "en Croute" Ⓠ

Serves: 4 (1 pear = 1 serving)

4 phyllo leaves
4 small poached Comice pears,
  drained
Butter-flavored nonstick cooking
  spray
1 cup papaya, mango, strawberry,
  or blueberry puree mixed with
  1 tablespoon Grand Marnier or
  pear poaching liquid

Lemon leaf or fresh mint, as
  garnish

1. Lightly coat the phyllo with butter-flavored nonstick cooking spray and fold in half. Coat again. Place a poached pear in the center of the folded leaf.

2. Wrap the pear tightly, twisting at the stem. Lightly coat the outside of the phyllo with butter-flavored cooking spray.

3. Repeat for the other three pears.

4. Place on a nonstick baking sheet and bake in a preheated 350° oven about 7 to 10 minutes, until the phyllo is crisped and lightly colored.

5. Spoon ¼ cup puree onto each of four dessert plates, place a hot pear in the center of the sauce, and garnish with a lemon leaf or fresh mint.

Variation: Strawberry Sauce (page 319) or Blueberry Sauce (page 317) may be used instead of the puree.

Per serving: 0 mg cholesterol, 0.12 gm saturated fat, 0.7 gm total fat, 3.4 gm fiber, 1 mg sodium, 106 calories, 0 gm trans fat

It's not exactly like Mama used to make, but I think your heart will like it better without all the melted butter.

Apple Streudel ⓠ

Serves: 8

½ cup frozen unsweetened apple juice concentrate
3 cups thinly sliced McIntosh, Golden Delicious, or Granny Smith apples
½ cup seeded dark raisins
1 tablespoon Splenda Brown Sugar Blend
½ teaspoon grated lemon zest
1 teaspoon ground cinnamon
¼ teaspoon freshly ground nutmeg
3 sheets phyllo pastry

Butter-flavored nonstick cooking spray or 2 tablespoons canola oil
2 tablespoons dry bread-crumbs

Apricot topping:
⅓ cup sugar-free apricot jam mixed with 2 teaspoons Splenda Brown Sugar Blend, 1 teaspoon lemon juice, and mix until syrupy

1. Heat the apple juice concentrate, add the apples, and sauté until tender, about 10 minutes.

2. Add the raisins, Splenda Brown Sugar Blend, lemon zest, cinnamon, and nutmeg and mix well. Cool.

3. Coat each phyllo sheet lightly with cooking spray and lay phyllo sheets on top of one another on plastic wrap. Sprinkle lightly with bread-crumbs.

4. Spoon the apple mixture along the short edge of the phyllo and roll up into a long roll.

5. Place the roll on a nonstick baking sheet. Coat lightly with cooking spray. Score the top diagonally into eight equal sections with a knife.

6. Bake in a preheated 400° oven for 15 to 20 minutes. Remove from oven and cut into eight diagonal serving portions.

To Serve: Serve warm on individual dessert plates with apricot topping.

Per serving: 0 mg cholesterol, 0.08 gm saturated fat, 0.3 gm total fat, 1.8 gm fiber, 17 mg sodium, 93 calories

Appendix

In 1988, C. Everett Koop, M.D., former U.S. Surgeon General, issued the first report on nutrition and disease. He urged the public to increase its consumption of fresh fruit, vegetables, and whole grain products and to decrease the consumption of dietary fat. He observed that "your diet can influence your long-term health prospects more than any other action you may take."

As of 2004, U.S. Surgeon General Richard H. Carmona, M.D., M.P.H., F.A.C.S., has followed in his predecessor's footsteps by urging the public to focus on good nutrition and emphasizing the prevention of childhood obesity.

Besides limiting the intake of cholesterol, the most important change the average person can make in his diet is to reduce the amount of total fat he eats, *especially the bad fats—saturated fat and trans fat.* Ideally, only 15 to 20 percent of the total calories in your diet should come from fat. If you know your total daily intake of calories, you can determine the total amount of fat and the total calories from fat you should eat daily from the table on page 357. For example, if you consume 1,200 calories a day, only 240 of those calories should be from fat (using the more comfortable 20 percent figure). That means that you are allowed 27 grams of fat per day (there are about 9 calories in each gram of fat). Remember that of this amount, *no more than 10 percent of your daily calories* should come from both saturated fat and trans fat.

The recipes in this book, which focus on helping you lower your total fat intake as well as your cholesterol intake, give you the number of grams of fat they contain per serving. The table beginning on page

358 will help you determine how many grams of fat and what types of fat a given food or commercial product contains per serving as well as the sodium and cholesterol content and calorie count. Current food labels can also help you find out how many grams of saturated and trans fat are contained in packaged foods.

Finally, you can increase the amount of fiber you eat daily by being aware of the fiber content of the foods you eat. The table starting on page 396 will help you.

KITCHEN CONVERSIONS
Metric Equivalents by Volume

1 teaspoon = ⅓ tablespoon = 5 mL
1½ teaspoons = ½ tablespoon
3 teaspoons = 1 tablespoon = 15 mL
4 tablespoons = ¼ cup = 59 mL
5⅓ tablespoons = ⅓ cup = 79 mL
8 tablespoons = ½ cup = 118.4 mL
16 tablespoons = 1 cup = 236 mL
1 cup = 8 fluid ounces = .237 liters (approx. ¼ liter) = 237 mL
2 cups = 1 pint = .473 liters (approx. ½ liter) = 473 mL
4 cups or 2 pints = 1 quart = .9463 liters (approx. 1 liter) = 946 mL
4 quarts = 1 gallon = 3785 mL

Measurements by Weight

1 ounce = approx. 28 grams
3½ ounces = 100 grams
16 ounces = 1 pound
1 pound = 454 grams
2.2 pounds = 1 kilogram

Do You Need an Oil Change?

Substitute vegetable oil for solid fats in a recipe and you'll cut the total fat called for by about 10 percent. Not only have you switched to a healthier alternative but you have reduced the total fat in your baked goods! Use the following chart to experiment with your recipes that ask for solid fat.

Oil Baking Substitution Chart

SOLID FAT TO OIL IMPERIAL CONVERSION°	SOLID FAT TO OIL METRIC CONVERSION
1 cup → ¾ cup	250 mL → 175mL
¾ cup → ⅔ cup	175 mL → 150mL
½ cup → ⅓ cup	125 mL → 75 mL
¼ cup → 3 tablespoons	50 mL → 45 mL
1 tablespoon → 2 teaspoons	15 mL → 10 mL
1 teaspoon → ¾ teaspoon	5 mL → 4 mL

°As used in the United States

Note: No more than 7 percent of your daily calories should come from saturated fat. Trans fat should be as low as possible and *no more* than 2 grams per day.

How much fat should I eat daily to achieve a diet that provides 20 percent of energy from fat?

IF YOU CONSUME THIS MANY CALORIES (ENERGY) DAILY . . .	EAT THIS NUMBER OF GRAMS OF FAT DAILY TO ACHIEVE A DIET PROVIDING 20% OF ENERGY FROM FAT.
1,200 kcal	27 grams
1,500 kcal	33 grams
2,000 kcal	44 grams
2,500 kcal	56 grams
3,000 kcal	67 grams

Temperatures

To convert degrees Fahrenheit to Celsius, subtract 32 then multiply by .56.

To convert degrees Celsius to Fahrenheit, multiply by 1.8 then add 32.

The Calorie, Fat, Sodium, and Cholesterol Content
of Commonly Used Foods*

	PORTION	K CAL (CALORIES)	FAT (GM.)	SATU-RATED FAT (GM.)	SODIUM (MG.)	CHOLES-TEROL (MG.)	TRANS FAT (MG.)
Beverages							
Alcoholic:							
Beer:							
regular	12 fl. oz.	146	0	0	18	0	0
light	12 fl. oz.	99	0	0	11	0	0
Gin, Rum, Vodka, & Whiskey:							
80 proof	1½ fl. oz.	95	0	0	0	0	0
86 proof	1½ fl. oz.	105	0	0	0	0	0
90 proof	1½ fl. oz.	110	0	0	0	0	0
Wines:							
Champagne	6 fl. oz.	128	0	0	18	0	0
red	6 fl. oz.	127	0	0	18	0	0
white, dry	6 fl. oz.	122	0	0	7	0	0
sweet dessert wine	6 fl. oz.	283	0	0	16	0	0
dry dessert wine	6 fl. oz.	269	0	0	16	0	0
sherry, dry	6 fl. oz.	205	0	0	11	0	0
Carbonated:							
club soda	12 fl. oz.	0	0	0	75	0	0
Perrier or comparable mineral water	8 fl. oz.	0	0	0	5	0	0
Colas:							
regular	12 fl. oz.	154	0	0	28	0	0
diet (artificially sweetened)	12 fl. oz.	2	0	0	6	0	0
Ginger ale	12 fl. oz.	124	0	0	29	0	0

TR = nutrient present in trace amount
N/A = not available

*For carbohydrate and sugar content in over 3,000 foods, refer to *Harrriet Roth's Fat Counter*, 3rd edition (2007).

	PORTION	K CAL (CALORIES)	FAT (GM.)	SATU- RATED FAT (GM.)	SODIUM (MG.)	CHOLES- TEROL (MG.)	TRANS FAT (MG.)
Grape soda	12 fl. oz.	160	0	0	53	0	0
Lemon-lime soda	12 fl. oz.	150	0	0	82	0	0
Orange soda	12 fl. oz.	179	0	0	43	0	0
Root beer	12 fl. oz.	152	0	0	46	0	0
Cocoa & chocolate-flavored beverages (see Dairy Products)							
Coffee:							
brewed	6 fl. oz.	4	0.0	0.0	4	0	0
instant	6 fl. oz.	4	0.0	0.0	TR	0	0
Tea:							
brewed	6 fl. oz.	0.0	0.0	0.0	5	0	0.0
instant, unsweetened	8 fl. oz.	0.0	0.0	0.0	1	0	0.0
instant, sweetened	8 fl. oz.	70	0.0	0.0	TR	0	0.0
Breads & Grain Products							
Breads:							
Bagels, Bruegger's plain°	1	300	2.0	0.0	440	0	0.0
Biscuits, Gold Medal (from mix)	1	170	8.0	3.0	620	0	N/A
Boston brown bread, canned	1 slice	95	1	0.3	113	3	N/A
Bread crumbs, plain	1 oz.	111	1.5	0.0	244	0	0.0
Bread stuffing, seasoned	¾ cup	220	16.0	3.0	326	71	N/A
Ezekiel bread	1 slice	80	0.5	0.0	80	0	0.0
French or Vienna bread	1 oz.	78	0.9	0.2	145	1	0.0

° Egg bagels have 45 mg cholesterol per bagel.

	PORTION	K CAL (CALORIES)	FAT (GM.)	SATU-RATED FAT (GM.)	SODIUM (MG.)	CHOLES-TEROL (MG.)	TRANS FAT (MG.)
Breads (cont.)							
Italian bread	2 oz.	154	2.0	0.5	140	0	0.0
Oatmeal bread, enriched	1 slice	73	1.2	0.2	72	0	0.0
Pita, whole wheat	1 6" ½ pita	154	0.0	0.0	330	0	0.0
Pumpernickel, dark	1 slice	80	1.0	0.5	176	0	0.0
Raisin bread, enriched	1 slice	80	0.5	0.0	91	0	0.0
Rye	1 slice	80	1.0	0.0	139	0	0.0
Sourdough bread	1 slice	150	0.0	0.0	260	0	0.0
Wheat, Oroweat	1 slice	120	2.0	1.0	190	0	0.0
White, Oroweat	1 slice	70	1.0	0.0	163	0	0.0
Whole grain bread, enriched	1 slice	65	1	0.2	106	0	0.0
Whole wheat	1 slice	69	1.2	0.3	120	0	0.0
Breakfast Cereals, Hot, Cooked:							
Corn (hominy grits): regular & quick	1 cup	143	0.5	0.1	0	0	0.0
instant, plain, dry	1 oz.	97	0.3	0.0	440	0	0.0
Country Choice organic steel cut oats, dry	¼ cup	150	3	0	0	0	0.0
Cream of Wheat: regular, quick, instant	1 cup	140	0.0	0.0	46	0	0.0
mix & eat	1 packet	100	0.0	0.0	241	0	0.0
Malt-o-Meal	1 cup	120	0.0	0.0	2	0	0.0
Oat Bran O's	½ cups	67	0.0	0.0	90	0	0.0
Oatmeal or Rolled Oats: regular, quick, instant	1 cup	145	2	0.4	2	0	0.0

TR = nutrient present in trace amount
N/A = not available

	PORTION	K CAL (CALORIES)	FAT (GM.)	SATU-RATED FAT (GM.)	SODIUM (MG.)	CHOLES-TEROL (MG.)	TRANS FAT (MG.)
instant, fortified, organic apple	1 packet	150	1.5	0.0	90	0	0.0

Breakfast Cereals, Cold (all 1-ounce equivalents):

	PORTION	K CAL (CALORIES)	FAT (GM.)	SATU-RATED FAT (GM.)	SODIUM (MG.)	CHOLES-TEROL (MG.)	TRANS FAT (MG.)
All-Bran, Kellogg's	½ cup	80	1	0.0	80	0	0.0
Cheerios	1 cup	100	2	0.0	190	0	0.0
Corn Flakes, Kellogg's	1 cup	101	0.2	0.1	300	0	0.0
40% Bran Flakes, Kellogg's	1 cup	127	0.7	0.12	363	0	0.0
Crispy Brown Rice	1 cup	110	0.0	0.0	240	0	0.0
Fruit Loops	1 cup	118	0.9	0.5	150	0	0.0
Golden Grahams	¾ cup	112	1.1	0.2	280	0	0.0
Go Lean, Kashi	1 cup	140	1	0.0	85	0	0.0
Grape-nuts	⅓ cup	137	0.7	0.2	263	0	0.0
Health Valley Granola	⅔ cup	190	2.0	0.0	90	0	0.0
Honey Nut Cheerios	1 cup	112	1.2	0.2	299	0	0.0
Oat Bran O's	½ cup	67	0.0	0.0	90	0	0.0
100% Natural Cereal	¼ cup	135	6	4.1	12	TR	0.0
Product 19	1 cup	100	0.4	0.1	371	0	0.0
Raisin Bran, Kellogg's	1 cup	195	1.5	0.3	390	0	0.0
Rice Krispies	1 cup	95	0.3	0.1	340	0	0.0
Shredded Wheat, Barbara's	2 biscuits	140	1.0	0.0	0	0	0.0
Special K, Kellogg's	1 cup	117	0.5	0.1	199	0	0.0
Super Bran Flakes, Arrowhead	1 cup	110	1.0	0.0	230	0	0.0
Total Whole Grain	1 cup	130	1.0	0.2	189	0	0.0
Trix	1 cup	117	1.1	0.2	181	0	0.0
Wheaties	1 cup	107	1.0	0.2	354	0	0.0

	PORTION	K CAL (CALORIES)	FAT (GM.)	SATU-RATED FAT (GM.)	SODIUM (MG.)	CHOLES-TEROL (MG.)	TRANS FAT (MG.)
Breads & Grain Products, Miscellaneous:							
Barley, pearled & cooked	1 cup	193	0.7	0.1	2	0	0.0
Bulgur, cooked	1 cup	151	0.4	0.1	5	0	0.0
Corn chips, unsalted	1 oz.	111	6.0	1.0	26	0	0.0
Cornmeal, degermed,	1 cup	489	2.4	0.6	4	0	0.0
Crackers:							
Cheez-It plain	27-1" squares	156	8.4	1.7	224	2	0.0
sandwich-type, peanut butter	1	181	8.7	1.7	90	1	1.0
Graham, plain	4	80	2.0	0.0	86	0	0.0
Melba toast, plain	1 oz.	111	0.9	0.1	248	0	0.0
Rye wafers	1 oz.	104	0.4	0.0	117	0	0.0
Saltines	5 crackers	66	2.0	0.0	105	0	1.0
Stacy's Pita Chips	1 package	200	8	0.5	400	0	0.0
Wheat Thins	16 crackers	136	5.8	0.9	180	0	0.0
Whole wheat wafers	5 crackers	50	1.3	0.0	135	0	0.0
Pastry:							
Croissant, butter	1	231	12.0	6.7	384	47	1.0
Danish, apple	1 piece	263	13.1	3.5	333	19	N/A
Cheese, Entenmann's	2 oz.	220	12.0	5.0	319	20	0.0
Donut:							
cake-type, plain	1	310	19.0	4.0	200	24	5.0
glazed	1	160	7.0	2.0	200	0	5.0
English muffin, plain	1	132	0.9	0.2	264	0	0.0

TR = nutrient present in trace amount
N/A = not available

	PORTION	K CAL (CALORIES)	FAT (GM.)	SATU-RATED FAT (GM.)	SODIUM (MG.)	CHOLES-TEROL (MG.)	TRANS FAT (MG.)
Flours							
All-purpose, unsifted	1 cup	400	0.0	0.0	3	0	0.0
Cake or pastry, sifted	1 cup	496	1.2	0.2	2	0	0.0
Self-rising, wheat	1 cup	443	1.2	0.2	1,588	0	0.0
Whole wheat	1 cup	407	2.2	0.4	6	0	0.0
French toast, frozen	2 slices	166	4.4	0.0	112	257	0.0
Macaroni, cooked:							
firm	1 cup	197	0.9	0.1	1	0	0.0
al dente	1 cup	155	0.6	N/A	0	0	0.0
Muffins, Dunkin' Donuts:							
blueberry	1	470	17.0	3.0	440	0	0.0
bran	1	140	4	1.3	385	28	0.0
corn	1	510	18.0	3.5	200	40	0.0
Noodles:							
chow mein, canned, La Choy	½ cup	130	5.0	1.5	198	0	1.5
egg, cooked	1 cup	213	2.4	0.5	11	53	0.0
Pancakes, from mix:							
buckwheat, Krusteaz	2	227	3.3	0.7	85	123	0.0
plain, Krusteaz	3	280	4.0	5.0	680	0	0.0
Popcorn:							
air-popped, unsalted	1 cup	31	0.3	0.1	0	0	0.0
popped in vegetable oil, salted	1 cup	55	3.1	0.5	97	0	0.0
Pretzels:							
sticks, fat-free	1 oz.	110	0.0	0.0	520	0	0.0
twisted, Olde Tyme, Snyder's	1 oz.	120	1.0	0.0	120	0	N/A

	PORTION	K CAL (CALORIES)	FAT (GM.)	SATU-RATED FAT (GM.)	SODIUM (MG.)	CHOLES-TEROL (MG.)	TRANS FAT (MG.)
Pretzels (cont.)							
twisted, thin, Rold Gold	9 pieces	110	1.0	0.0	420	0	0.0
Rice:							
brown, cooked	1 cup	218	1.6	0.3	10	0	0.0
white, cooked	1 cup	242	0.4	0.1	2	0	0.0
Rolls (commercial):							
dinner, whole wheat	1	96	1.7	0.3	155	TR	0.0
frankfurter or hamburger	1	120	1.9	0.5	220	0	0.0
hard	1	150	0.5	0.0	313	2	0.0
hoagie or submarine	1	400	8	1.8	683	TR	0.0
Soba pasta, cooked	1 cup	113	0.1	0.0	0	0	0.0
Spaghetti, cooked:							
firm (al dente)	1 cup	155	0.6	N/A	0	0	0.0
tender	1 cup	197	0.9	0.1	1	0	0.0
Tortilla, corn 6"	1 tortilla	70	1.0	0.0	40	0	0.0
Waffles, oat bran, homemade	½ piece	174	4.1	1.0	212	3	0.0
Dairy Products							
Butter, see *Fats & Oils*							
Cheese, natural:							
Blue	1 oz.	100	8.2	5.3	396	21	0.0
Camembert	1 oz.	85	6.9	4.3	239	20	0.0
Cheddar	1 oz.	114	9.4	6.0	176	30	0.0
Cottage cheese low fat, low sodium	½ cup	81	1.1	0.7	495	9	0.0
Cottage cheese, nonfat	½ cup	80	0.0	0.0	370	10	0.0

TR = nutrient present in trace amount
N/A = not available

	PORTION	K CAL (CALORIES)	FAT (GM.)	SATU-RATED FAT (GM.)	SODIUM (MG.)	CHOLES-TEROL (MG.)	TRANS FAT (MG.)
Cream cheese, brick, whipped, nonfat	1 oz.	100	10.0	6.0	90	30	0.0
Feta cheese, goat cheese	1 oz.	60	4.5	3.0	316	25	0.0
Mozzarella:							
nonfat	¼ cup	45	0.0	0.0	0	0	0.0
part skim	1 oz.	70	4.0	3.0	132	16	2.0
whole milk	1 oz.	80	6	3.7	106	22	N/A
Muenster	1 oz.	104	8.5	5.4	178	27	0.0
Parmesan, grated	2 tbsp.	14	1.0	0.6	85	5	0.0
Provolone	1 oz.	100	8.0	4.5	248	20	0.0
Ricotta:							
part skim	¼ cup	60	2.5	1.5	307	76	0.0
whole milk	¼ cup	108	8.1	5.1	74	26	0.0
Swiss	1 oz.	108	7.9	5.0	74	26	0.0
Cheese, pasteurized process:							
American	1 oz.	80	6.0	4.0	337	18	0.0
American, Alpine Lace, 33% less fat, 50% less salt	1 oz.	80	6.0	4.0	337	18	0.0
Swiss	1 oz.	108	7.9	5.0	388	24	0.0
Tofu cheddar	1 slice	40	2.5	0.0	220	0	0.0
Cream, sour:	2 tbsp.	62	6.0	3.8	15	13	0.2
Fat free	2 tbsp.	35	0.0	0.0	25	5	0.0
Cream substitutes, imitation (made with vegetable fat):							
Sweet Creamers:							
liquid (frozen)	1 tbsp.	20	1.5	1.4	12	0	N/A
powdered	1 tsp.	10	1	0.7	4	0	N/A
whipped topping, frozen	1 cup	240	19	16.3	19	0	N/A
	1 tbsp.	15	1	0.9	1	0	N/A

	PORTION	K CAL (CALORIES)	FAT (GM.)	SATU-RATED FAT (GM.)	SODIUM (MG.)	CHOLES-TEROL (MG.)	TRANS FAT (MG.)
Cream substitutes, imitation (made with vegetable fat) (cont.)							
powdered, whole milk	1 cup	150	10	8.5	53	8	N/A
pressurized	1 cup	185	16	13.2	43	0	N/A
	1 tbsp.	10	1	0.8	2	0	N/A
Cream, sweet:							
Half & half	2 tbsp.	39	3.5	2.2	12	11	0.1
Half & half, nonfat	2 tbsp.	20	0.0	0.0	25	0	0.0
Coffee creamer, nondairy	1 tbsp.	10	0.5	0.5	0	0	0.0
Heavy cream (volume double when whipped):							
unwhipped	2 tbsp.	103	11.0	6.9	11	41	0.3
whipped	2 tbsp.	52	5.5	3.4	6	20	0.2
Whipped topping: fat free, ReddiWhip	½ oz.	21	0.7	0.4	0	0	0.0
nondairy from can	2 tbsp.	23	2.0	1.7	5	0	0.0
Ice cream, See *Milk desserts, frozen*							
Ice milk, see *Milk desserts, frozen*							
Milk, fluid:							
Buttermilk, skim	1 cup	90	0.0	0.0	257	8.5	0.0
Lowfat: 2%, no milk solids added	1 cup	122	4.8	3.1	122	20	0.2
1%, no milk solids added	1 cup	102	2.4	1.5	122	10	0.1
Nonfat (skim), no milk solids added	1 cup	90	0.0	0.0	126	4	0.0

TR = nutrient present in trace amount
N/A = not available

	PORTION	K CAL (CALORIES)	FAT (GM.)	SATU-RATED FAT (GM.)	SODIUM (MG.)	CHOLES-TEROL (MG.)	TRANS FAT (MG.)
Whole, 3.3% fat	1 cup	146	7.9	4.6	120	34	0.2
Milk, canned:							
Condensed, sweetened	2 tbsp.	120	1.5	1.0	49	13	0.0
Evaporated:							
whole	1 cup	320	18.0	10.0	267	73	0.0
skim	1 cup	200	0.0	0.0	294	10	0.0
Milk, dried							
Buttermilk, water added	1 cup	98	2.2	1.3	620	83	0.1
Nonfat skim	1 cup	200	0.0	0.0	294	10	0.0
Milk Beverages:							
Chocolate (commercial)							
regular	1 cup	208	8.5	5.3	136	27	0.3
lowfat (1%)	8 oz.	150	2.5	1.5	153	8	0.0
Eggnog (commercial)	1 cup	400	18.0	10.0	137	150	0.0
Milk shakes, thick:							
chocolate	1 cup	211	6.2	3.9	263	24	0.0
vanilla	1 cup	185	5.0	3.1	225	28	0.0
Milk Desserts, frozen:							
Ice cream, vanilla (16% fat)	½ cup	260	16.0	10.0	108	88	0.0
Ice milk, vanilla (4% fat)	½ cup	130	4.5	3.0	105	18	N/A
Sherbet (orange)	½ cup	120	1.0	0.5	88	14	0.0
Frozen yogurt, nonfat (vanilla)	½ cup	90	0.0	0.0	64	4.8	0.0
Yogurt:							
whole milk	8 oz.	138	7.4	4.8	150	30	0.0
lowfat milk:							
fruit flavored	8 oz.	225	2.6	1.7	120	9	0.0
plain	8 oz.	143	3.5	2.3	170	20	0.0
nonfat milk	8 oz.	110	0.0	0.0	150	5	0.0

	PORTION	K CAL (CALORIES)	FAT (GM.)	SATU-RATED FAT (GM.)	SODIUM (MG.)	CHOLES-TEROL (MG.)	TRANS FAT (MG.)
Eggs:							
Cooked:							
fried in butter	1 egg	92	7.0	2.0	159	207	N/A
poached	1 egg	74	5.0	1.5	140	212	0.0
scrambled (milk added, in butter);							
also omelettes	1 egg	101	7.5	2.2	174	218	N/A
Raw, large:							
whole without shell	1	78	5.3	1.6	62	213	0.0
white	1	17	0.1	0.0	52	0	0.0
yolk	1	53	4.4	1.6	7	218	0.0
Substitute							
(Eggbeaters)	¼ cup	30	0.0	0.0	110	0	0.0
Fats and Oils							
Butter (4 sticks per pound):							
1 stick, salted	1 tbsp.	100	11.4	7.2	117	31	0.3
1 stick, unsalted	1 tbsp.	100	11.4	7.2	2	31	0.3
whipped	1 tbsp.	68	7.7	4.8	78	21	0.2
Lard	1 tbsp.	120	130	5.0	0	12	0.0
Margarine:							
Regular (about 80% fat):							
Hard (4 sticks/lb.), 1 tbsp.	1 tbsp.	90	10.0	2.0	132	0	2.5
Soft	1 tbsp.	80	8.0	2.0	151	0	0.0
Take Control Lite, no trans fat	1 tbsp.	45	5.0	0.5	134	0	0.0
Oils, salad or cooking (see chart p. 23)							
Shortening, Crisco	1 tbsp.	110	12.0	3.0	0	0	1.5
Salad dressings, commercial:							
Bleu Cheese, Kraft Free	2 tbsp.	45	0.0	0.0	360	0	0.0
French, Kraft	2 tbsp.	160	15.0	2.6	270	0	0.0

TR = nutrient present in trace amount
N/A = not available

	PORTION	K CAL (CALORIES)	FAT (GM.)	SATU-RATED FAT (GM.)	SODIUM (MG.)	CHOLES-TEROL (MG.)	TRANS FAT (MG.)
Kraft Free	2 tbsp.	45	0.0	0.0	300	0	0.0
Italian:							
Kraft Zesty	2 tbsp.	109	11.1	1.2	310	0	0.0
Kraft Free	2 tbsp.	20	0.3	0.2	430	0	0.0
Mayonnaise:							
Miracle Whip	1 tbsp.	70	7.0	1.0	78	8	0.0
Fat Free	1 tbsp.	13	0.4	0.1	120	0	0.0
Tartar sauce	2 tbsp.	90	9.0	1.5	170	10	N/A
Thousand Island:							
Kraft	2 tbsp.	110	10.0	1.5	310	10	N/A
Kraft Free	2 tbsp.	40	0.0	0.0	280	0	0.0
Finfish							
Anchovies, canned in oil, drained	1 oz.	60	2.8	0.6	1040	NA	0.0
Bass, striped, cooked	3.5 oz.	123	3.0	0.6	87	102	0.0
Bluefish, cooked	3.5 oz.	158	5.4	1.2	76	75	0.0
Carp, cooked	3.5 oz.	161	7.1	14	63	83	0.0
Catfish, cooked	3 oz.	129	6.8	1.5	68	54	0.0
breaded & fried	3 oz.	194	11.3	2.79	289	69	N/A
Caviar, black & red granular	1 tbsp.	40	2.9	0.7	240	94	0.0
Cod, Atlantic, cooked	3.5 oz.	104	0.9	0.17	77	55	0.0
Croaker, fried	3 oz.	187	10.8	3.0	296	71.4	0.0
Dolphin fish, cooked	3.5 oz.	108	0.9	0.2	96	80	0
Eel, cooked	3.5 oz.	231	14.0	3.0	55	137	0.0
Fish portions & sticks, frozen & reheated	1 stick (28 gm)	76	3.4	0.9	163	31	0.0
Gefilte fish: commercial, sweet recipe	1 piece (42 gm)	40	1.5	0.5	40	20	N/A

PORTION	K CAL (CALORIES)	FAT (GM.)	SATU-RATED FAT (GM.)	SODIUM (MG.)	CHOLES-TEROL (MG.)	TRANS FAT (MG.)
Grouper, cooked 3.5 oz.	117	1.3	0.3	53	47	0.0
Haddock, cooked 3.5 oz.	111	0.9	0.2	86	73	0.0
Halibut, cooked (dry heat) 3.5 oz.	139	2.9	0.4	68	41	0.0
Herring, Atlantic:						
pickled 3.5 oz.	262	15.3	2.4	870	51	0.0
kippered (40 gm.) 3.5 oz	217	12.4	12.8	918	82	N/A
Ling cod, cooked 3.5 oz.	108	1.3	0.25	75	66	0.0
Mackerel, Atlantic, cooked 3.5 oz.	260	17.7	4.1	82	74	0.0
Monkfish, cooked 3.5 oz.	96	1.9	0.5	23	32	0.0
Mullet, cooked 3.5 oz.	149	3.8	.7	70	63	0.0
Ocean perch, Atlantic, cooked 3.5 oz.	120	2.1	0.3	95	54	0.0
Pike, Walleye, cooked 3.5 oz.	118	1.6	0.3	64	109	0.0
Pollock, Atlantic, cooked 3.5 oz.	117	1.3	0.2	109	90	0.0
Pompano, cooked 3.5 oz.	209	12.1	4.5	75	64	0.0
Rockfish, cooked 3.5 oz.	120	2.0	0.5	76	44	0.0
Roughy, orange, raw 3 oz.	107	5.95	0.11	54	17	0.0
Sablefish, smoked 3.5 oz.	255	20.0	4.2	737	64	0.0
Salmon, Chinook:						
pink, canned 3.5 oz.	138	6.0	1.5	550	N/A	0.0
raw 3 oz.	153	8.88	2.13	40	56	0.0
smoked 3 oz.	99	3.67	.79	666	20	0.0
sockeye, canned 3.5 oz.	152	7.3	1.6	534	44	0.0

TR = nutrient present in trace amount
N/A = not available

	PORTION	K CAL (CALORIES)	FAT (GM.)	SATU- RATED FAT (GM.)	SODIUM (MG.)	CHOLES- TEROL (MG.)	TRANS FAT (MG.)
Sardines:							
Atlantic (canned in oil, drained solids with bone)	3.5 oz.	206	11.4	1.5	501	141	0.0
Pacific (canned in tomato sauce, drained solids with bone)	3.5 oz.	185	10.4	2.7	411	61	0.0
Sea bass, cooked	3.5 oz.	123	2.5	0.7	74	45	0.0
Shark, raw	3 oz.	111	3.83	0.78	67	43	0.0
Smelts, rainbow, cooked	3.5 oz.	123	3.1	0.6	76	89	0.0
Snapper, cooked	3.5 oz.	127	1.7	0.4	57	47	0.0
Sturgeon, cooked	3.5 oz.	134	5.1	1.2	N/A	N/A	0.0
Sucker, carp, cooked	3.5 oz.	161	7.1	1.4	63	83	0.0
Surimi (from pollock)	3 oz.	84	0.77	0.0	95	8	0.0
Swordfish, cooked	3.5 oz.	154	5.1	1.4	114	50	0.0
Trout, rainbow, cooked	3.5 oz.	149	5.8	1.6	56	69	0.0
Tuna:							
bluefin, raw	3 oz.	143	4.9	1.3	39	38	0.0
light (canned in oil, drained)	3 oz.	168	7.0	1.3	301	15	0.0
light (canned in water, drained)	3 oz.	99	0.7	0.2	287	26	0.0
white (canned in oil, drained)	3 oz.	158	6.9	1.1	337	26	0.0
white (canned in water, drained)	3 oz.	109	2.5	0.7	333	36	0.0

	PORTION	K CAL (CALORIES)	FAT (GM.)	SATU-RATED FAT (GM.)	SODIUM (MG.)	CHOLES-TEROL (MG.)	TRANS FAT (MG.)
Finfish:							
Turbot, cooked	3 oz.	104	13.2	N/A	163	52.7	0.0
Whitefish, cooked	3 oz.	146	6.4	1.0	64	76	0.0
smoked	3 oz.	92	0.8	0.2	1019	33	0.0
Whiting, cooked	3 oz.	99	1.4	0.3	112	71.4	0.0
Yellowtail, cooked	3 oz.	159	5.7	N/A	33	46.8	0.0
Shellfish—Crustaceans							
Crab:							
Alaska king, raw	3 oz.	83	1.3	0.1	912	45	0.0
blue, canned	3 oz.	84	1.1	0.2	283	76	0.0
Dungeness, cooked	3 oz.	94	1.1	0.1	321	65	0.0
Crayfish, cooked	3.5 oz.	81	1.2	0.2	67	177	0.0
Lobster northern, steamed	3.5 oz.	97	.60	0.1	377	71	0.0
Shrimp, canned:	3 oz.	102	1.67	0.31	143	147	N/A
breaded and fried	3 oz.	206	10.4	1.8	293	151	N/A
steamed	3 oz.	84	0.9	0.3	191	166	0.0
Spiny lobster, raw	3 oz.	95	1.29	0.2	150	60	N/A
Shellfish—Mollusks							
Abalone, raw	3 oz.	89	0.7	0.1	256	72	0.0
Clams:							
canned, drained	3 oz.	35	0.0	0.0	485	27	0.0
raw	3 oz.	63	0.8	0.1	48	29	0.0
Mussels, cooked	3 oz.	146	3.8	0.7	314	48	0.0
Oysters:							
fried	6 oz.	173	11.07	2.81	355	69	N/A
raw	3 oz.	50	1.3	0.4	95	47	0.0
Scallops:							
bay, raw	3.5 oz.	87	0.8	0.1	170	37	0.0

TR = nutrient present in trace amount
N/A = not available

	PORTION	K CAL (CALORIES)	FAT (GM.)	SATU-RATED FAT (GM.)	SODIUM (MG.)	CHOLES-TEROL (MG.)	TRANS FAT (MG.)
Squid, raw	3 oz.	78	1.2	0.0	37	198	0.0

Fruits and Fruit Juices

Apples, raw:

unpeeled, cored (2¾" diam.)	1 apple	72	0.2	0.0	0	0	0.0
peeled, sliced	1 cup	65	TR	0.1	TR	0	0.0
Apple juice	½ cup	55	0.0	0.0	4	0	0.0

Applesauce, canned:

sweetened	½ cup	97	0.2	0.0	4	0	0.0
unsweetened	½ cup	52	0.1	0.0	2	0	0.0

Apricots:

raw:

pitted	1	17	0.1	0.0	0	0	0.0
canned in heavy syrup	½ cup	107	0.1	0.0	5	0	0.0
juice pack	½ cup	59	0.1	0.0	5	0	0.0

dried:

uncooked	1	8	0.0	0.0	1	0	0.0
cooked, unsweetened	1 cup	210	TR	TR	8	0	0.0

Apricot nectar,

canned	½ cup	70	0.1	0.0	4	0	0.0

Avocado, raw, with skin & seed:

California (8 oz.)	1	289	26.7	3.7	21	0	0.0
Florida (8 oz.)	1	365	30.6	6.0	8	0	0.0

Banana:

whole	1 6-inch	105	0.4	0.1	1	0	0.0
sliced	1 cup	140	1	0.3	2	0	0.0
Blackberries	½ cup	31	0.4	0.0	0	0	0.0
Blueberries, raw	½ cup	41	0.2	0.0	4	0	0.0
Cantaloupe	¼ melon (5" diam)	47	0.3	0.1	12	0	0.0

Cherries, sweet,

raw	½ cup	46	0.1	0.0	TR	0	0.0

	PORTION	K CAL (CALORIES)	FAT (GM.)	SATU- RATED FAT (GM.)	SODIUM (MG.)	CHOLES- TEROL (MG.)	TRANS FAT (MG.)
Fruits and Fruit Juices (cont.)							
Cranberry juice cocktail, sweetened	8 oz. cup	130	0.0	0.0	5	0	0.0
Cranberry sauce, sweetened	½ cup	200	0.0	0.0	80	0	0.0
Dates, domestic	1	23	0.0	0.0	0	0	0.0
chopped	1 cup	490	TR	0.3	21	0	0.0
Figs, dried	1	47	0.2	0.0	2	0	0.0
Fruit cocktail:							
canned in heavy syrup	½ cup	90	0.0	0.0	8	0	0.0
juice pack	½ cup	60	0.0	0.0	5	0	0.0
Grapefruit:							
fresh	1	120	0.0	0.0	0	0	0.0
canned sections, with syrup	½ cup	76	0.1	0.0	9	0	0.0
Grapefruit juice:							
fresh	½ cup	95	TR	TR	2	0	0.0
canned, unsweetened	½ cup	47	0.1	0.0	1	0	0.0
canned, sweetened	1 cup	58	0.1	0.0	3	0	0.0
Grapes:							
Thompson seedless	½ cup	55	0.1	0.0	2	0	0.0
Emperor seeded	½ cup	55	0.1	0.0	2	0	0.0
Grape juice, canned or bottled	8 oz.	170	0.0	0.0	4	0	0.0
Honeydew melon	½ cup	31	0.1	0.0	8	0	0.0
Kiwi, raw	1	46	0.4	0.0	0	0	0.0

TR = nutrient present in trace amount
N/A = not available

	PORTION	K CAL (CALORIES)	FAT (GM.)	SATU-RATED FAT (GM.)	SODIUM (MG.)	CHOLES-TEROL (MG.)	TRANS FAT (MG.)
Lemon juice, fresh	1 cup	60	0.0	0.0	51	0	0.0
Mango, raw	½	67	0.3	0.1	4	0	0.0
Nectarine, fresh	1	70	0.5	0.0	0	0	0.0
Orange:							
whole fresh	1	62	0.2	0.0	0	0	0.0
sections, no							
membrane	1 cup	85	0.0	0.0	0.0	0	0.0
Orange juice, fresh	½ cup	56	0.3	0.0	1	0	0.0
Papaya, fresh	½	59	0.2	0.1	7	0	0.0
Peaches:							
fresh, whole	1	38	0.2	0.0	0.0	0	0.0
fresh, sliced	1 cup	75	0.2	0.0	0.0	0	0.0
canned, heavy							
syrup	½ cup	60	TR	TR	10	0	N/A
canned, juice							
pack	½ cup	35	TR	TR	3	0	N/A
Pears:							
fresh:							
Bartlett, cored	1	100	1	TR	TR	0	0.0
Bosc, cored	1	85	1	TR	TR	0	0.0
D'Anjou, cored	1	85	1	TR	TR	0	0.0
canned:							
in heavy syrup	½ cup	60	TR	TR	4	0	N/A
juice pack	½ cup	80	0.0	0.0	5	0	0.0
Pineapple:							
fresh, diced	½ cup	32	0.1	N/A	1	0	0.0
canned, heavy							
syrup	1 cup	200	TR	TR	1	0	0.0
canned, juice							
pack	½ cup	70	0.0	0.0	1	0	0.0
Pineapple juice,							
unsweetened	½ cup	70	0.1	0.0	1	0	0.0
Plantains, cooked	½ cup	89	0.1	0.1	4	0	0.0
Plums:							
fresh pitted	1(2⅛" diam.)	40	0.5	N/A	0	0	0.0

	PORTION	K CAL (CALORIES)	FAT (GM.)	SATU-RATED FAT (GM.)	SODIUM (MG.)	CHOLES-TEROL (MG.)	TRANS FAT (MG.)
Plums (cont.)							
canned, heavy syrup	½ cup	115	0.1	0.0	25	0	0.0
canned, juice pack	3	55	TR	TR	1	0	N/A
Pomegranate juice	1 cup	160	0.0	0.0	10	0	0.0
Prunes:							
dried, uncooked	1	20	0.0	0.0	0	0	0.0
cooked: unsweetened, fruit & liquid	½ cup	158	0.3	0.0	2	0	0.0
Prune juice, canned	½ cup	85	0.0	0.0	5	0	0.0
Raisins, seedless:							
not packed	½ cup	260	0.0	0.0	9	0	0.0
1 packet	½ oz.	40	0.0	0.0	2	0	0.0
Raspberries, fresh	½ cup	25	0.0	0.0	0	0	0.0
Rhubarb, cooked, sweetened	½ cup	139	0.1	0.0	1	0	0.0
Strawberries, raw, sliced	½ cup	27	0.3	0.0	1	0	0.0
Tangerine, fresh	1	45	0.3	0.0	1	0	0.0
Watermelon:							
fresh	1 slice (4"×8")	155	2	0.3	10	0	0.0
diced	½ cup	23	0.1	0.0	2	0	0.0
Legumes							
Beans, dry, cooked, & drained:							
Black beans	½ cup	114	0.5	0.1	1	0	0.0
Black-eyed peas	1 cup	190	1	0.2	20	0	0.0
Chickpeas (garbanzo beans)	½ cup	134	2.1	0.2	6	0	0.0

TR = nutrient present in trace amount
N/A = not available

	PORTION	K CAL (CALORIES)	FAT (GM.)	SATU-RATED FAT (GM.)	SODIUM (MG.)	CHOLES-TEROL (MG.)	TRANS FAT (MG.)
Great Northern beans	½ cup	104	0.4	0.1	5	0	0.0
Lima beans	½ cup	108	0.4	0.1	3	0	0.0
Navy beans	1 cup	225	1	0.1	13	0	0.0
Pinto beans	½ cup	122	0.6	0.0	2	0	0.0
Soy beans, edamame	½ cup	100	2.5	1.3	1	0	0.0
Beans, canned, solids & liquids:							
Lentils, dry, cooked	½ cup	115	0.4	0.1	2	0	0.0
Peas, split, dry, cooked	½ cup	116	0.4	0.1	2	0	0.0
Red kidney beans	½ cup	100	0.0	0.0	444	0	0.0
Refried beans:							
canned	½ cup	150	3.0	1.0	515	1	0.0
fat free	½ cup	110	0.0	0.0	560	0	0.0
Meat and Meat Products							
Beef (all grades, lean, trimmed):							
Brisket, flat cut, braised	3 oz.	185	8.6	3.1	66	77	0.7
Chuck:							
arm pot roast, braised	3 oz.	173	5.7	2.2	56	185	0.4
blade pot roast, braised	3 oz.	215	11.3	4.4	60	90	0.4
Flank steak, broiled	3 oz.	165	6.7	2.6	70	60	0.5
Ground beef:							
lean, broiled	3 oz.	213	13.2	5.0	65	74	0.6
extra lean, broiled	3 oz.	151	6.2	2.5	59	71	0.1
Rib:							
roast, lean, trimmed	3 oz.	201	11.48	4.87	64	68	N/A

	PORTION	K CAL (CALORIES)	FAT (GM.)	SATU-RATED FAT (GM.)	SODIUM (MG.)	CHOLES-TEROL (MG.)	TRANS FAT (MG.)
Beef (all grades, lean, trimmed) (cont.)							
steak, trimmed and broiled	3 oz.	188	9.53	4.03	58	68	N/A
Round:							
bottom round, braised	3 oz.	173	6.5	2.2	44	81	0.2
eye of round, roasted	3 oz.	138	35	1.2	52	59	0.0
top of round, broiled	3 oz.	169	4.3	1.5	51	72	N/A
round tip, roasted	3 oz.	148	5.3	1.9	55	69	0.2
Short ribs, braised	3 oz.	251	15.41	6.6	50	79	N/A
Sirloin steak, broiled	3 oz.	155	5.4	2.1	53	77	0.6
Tenderloin steak, broiled	3 oz.	164	6.7	2.6	54	72	0.5
Lamb (lean, trimmed):							
Chops (3 per lb. with bone):							
Arm, braised							
lean only	1.7 oz.	135	7	2.9	36	59	N/A
Leg, roasted:							
lean only	3 oz.	153	5.7	2.0	50	65	N/A
Loin, broiled:							
lean and fat	3 oz.	296	19.6	8.4	62	78	N/A
lean only	3 oz.	184	8.3	3.0	54	60	N/A
Rib rack, roasted:							
lean only	3 oz.	200	11.0	4.0	46	50	N/A
lean & fat	3 oz.	307	25.2	10.8	60	77	N/A
Pork, cured, cooked:							
Bacon:							
regular	3 slices	103	7.9	2.6	303	16	0.0
Canadian style	2 slices	86	3.9	1.3	711	27	0.0

TR = nutrient present in trace amount
N/A = not available

PORTION	K CAL (CALORIES)	FAT (GM.)	SATU-RATED FAT (GM.)	SODIUM (MG.)	CHOLES-TEROL (MG.)	TRANS FAT (MG.)
Ham:						
lean & fat,						
roasted	3 oz.	205	14	5.1	1,009	53	N/A
lean only	2.4 oz.	105	4	1.3	902	37	N/A
canned, roasted	1 oz.	68	5.3	1.8	908	35	N/A
Luncheon meat:						
Chopped ham,						
canned	1 oz.	68	5.3	1.8	576	21	N/A
Cooked ham (2 slices):						
regular	2 oz.	105	6	1.9	751	32	N/A
extra lean	2 slices	75	3	0.9	815	27	N/A
Pork, fresh, cooked:						
Chopped loin						
(3 per lb. with bone):						
broiled, lean						
only	3 oz.	199	11.8	4.3	56	84	0.0
pan fried, lean						
only	2.4 oz.	180	11	3.7	57	72	N/A
Leg roasted, lean						
only	2.5 oz.	160	8	2.7	46	68	N/A
Rib roasted, lean						
only	2.5 oz.	175	10	3.4	33	56	N/A
Shoulder cut,						
braised,						
lean only	2.4 oz.	165	8	2.8	68	76	N/A
Sausages:						
brown and						
serve	2 pieces	190	18.0	6.0	105	9	0.0
pork link						
(16 per lb)	1 piece	134	11.6	4.9	168	11	0.0
pork, fresh	1 patty (1 oz.)	76	5.7	1.6	349	22	0.0
Spare ribs, roasted	3 oz.	338	25.8	9.5	N/A	N/A	N/A
Tenderloin, lean						
roasted	3 oz.	130	4.0	1.5	50	79	0.0
Sausages, Franks, and Luncheon Meats:						
Blood sausage	1 slice (1 oz.)	95	8.6	3.3	N/A	30	N/A

	PORTION	K CAL (CALORIES)	FAT (GM.)	SATU-RATED FAT (GM.)	SODIUM (MG.)	CHOLES-TEROL (MG.)	TRANS FAT (MG.)

Sausages, Franks, and Luncheon Meats (cont.)

	PORTION	K CAL (CALORIES)	FAT (GM.)	SATU-RATED FAT (GM.)	SODIUM (MG.)	CHOLES-TEROL (MG.)	TRANS FAT (MG.)
Bockwurst (raw pork, veal, etc.)	2 oz.	158	14.6	5.8	N/A	N/A	0.0
Bologna:							
beef, 1 slice	1 slice	59	6.4	2.0	230	13	0.0
beef & pork, 1 slice	1 slice	87	7.0	2.6	234	13	0.0
turkey	1 slice	52	3.7	1.1	222	20	0.0
Bratwurst (cooked pork)	1 link	281	24.8	8.6	473	51	0.0
Braunschweiger (pork)	2 oz.	185	16.2	5.3	206	28	0.0
Bratwurst (pork, beef)	1 link	281	248	8.6	778	44	0.0
Chorizo (pork, beef)	1 link	273	23.0	8.6	N/A	N/A	N/A
Frankfurter:							
beef	1 frank	147	13.6	5.6	461	22	1.0
beef & pork (1¾ oz.)	1 frank	90	6.0	2.0	75	22	0.0
chicken	1 frank	116	8.8	2.5	617	45	0.0
pork & beef, battered & fried (corn dog)	1 frank	330	20	8.4	1,252	37	N/A
turkey	1 frank	90	6.0	1.5	472	39	0.0
Ham (See chart page 369)							
Italian sausage, pork, cooked	1 link	216	17.2	6.1	618	52	N/A
Kielbasa—Kolbassy (pork & beef)	1 link	81	7.0	2.6	280	17	0.0
Knockwurst (pork & beef)	1 link	209	18.8	6.9	687	39	1.0

TR = nutrient present in trace amount
N/A = not available

	PORTION	K CAL (CALORIES)	FAT (GM.)	SATU-RATED FAT (GM.)	SODIUM (MG.)	CHOLES-TEROL (MG.)	TRANS FAT (MG.)
Liver cheese (pork liver)	1 slice	115	9.7	3.4	465	66	N/A
Mortadella (beef & pork)	1 oz.	88	7.2	2.7	187	8	N/A
Pepperoni	1 oz.	132	11.4	4.6	112	N/A	N/A
Salami:							
cooked beef	1 slice	75	6.5	3.0	607	37	N/A
cooked turkey	1 slice	43	2.7	0.8	251	20	0.0
dried/hard (Italian, pork & beef)	1 slice (⅓ oz.)	42	3.4	1.2	186	8	N/A
Turkey, breast meat loaf (8 slices per 6 oz.)	1 oz.	41	0.3	0.0	608	17	0.0
Veal:							
Breast, lean, braised	3 oz.	443	45.4	18.2	64	N/A	N/A
Cutlet, braised or broiled	3 oz.	160	3.7	1.1	56	109	N/A
Loin chop, lean only, broiled	3 oz.	149	5.9	2.2	80	90	N/A
Rib, roasted, lean	3 oz.	151	6.3	1.8	57	109	N/A
Venison, roasted	3 oz.	134	2.7	1.1	70	79	0.0
Miscellaneous							
Baking powder:							
regular	1 tsp.	5	0	0	329	0	0.0
low sodium	1 tsp.	5	0	0	TR	0	0.0
Black pepper	1 tsp.	5	0.0	0.0	1	0	0.0
Celery seed	1 tsp.	10	1	0.0	3	0	0.0
Chili powder	1 tsp.	10	0.0	0.0	26	0	0.0
Chocolate							
bitter or baking	1 oz.	158	9.6	5.9	1	0	0.0
semisweet (see Sugars & Sweets, Candy)							

	PORTION	K CAL (CALORIES)	FAT (GM.)	SATU-RATED FAT (GM.)	SODIUM (MG.)	CHOLES-TEROL (MG.)	TRANS FAT (MG.)
Miscellaneous (cont.)							
Cinnamon	1 tsp.	5	0.0	0.0	1	0	0.0
Curry powder	1 tsp.	7	0.3	0.0	1	0	0.0
Dried chipped beef	2.5 oz.	145	4	1.8	3,053	46	N/A
Garlic powder	1 tsp.	9	0.0	0.0	1	0	0.0
Gelatin, dry	1 envelope	25	0.0	0.0	6	0	0.0
Ketchup	1 tbsp.	15	0.0	0.0	156	0	0.0
reduced sodium and reduced calorie	1 tbsp.	15	0.0	0.0	110	0	0.0
Mustard, prepared, yellow	1 tsp. (or 1 packet)	5	0.0	0.0	63	0	0.0
Olives, canned:							
green, stuffed	2 each	8	0.9	0.1	312	0	0.0
black, ripe, pitted	2 each	10	0.9	0.1	68	0	0.0
Onion powder	1 tsp.	5	0.0	0.0	1	0	0.0
Oregano	1 tsp.	5	0.0	0.0	TR	0	0.0
Paprika	1 tsp.	5	0.0	0.0	1	0	0.0
Pickles, cucumber:							
dill	1 (3¾" long)	23	0.0	0.0	928	0	0.0
sweet gherkin, 1 small whole	1 (2½" long)	29	0.1	0.0	107	0	0.0
Popcorn (see Grains & Grain Products)							
Relish, chopped sweet	1 tbsp.	20	0.1	0.0	107	0	0.0
Salt	1 tsp.	0	0.0	0.0	2,132	0	0.0
Soy products:							
Miso	1 cup	470	13	1.8	8,142	0	0.0

TR = nutrient present in trace amount
N/A = not available

	PORTION	K CAL (CALORIES)	FAT (GM.)	SATU-RATED FAT (GM.)	SODIUM (MG.)	CHOLES-TEROL (MG.)	TRANS FAT (MG.)
Tofu (1 2½" × 2¾" × 1")	1 piece	85	5	0.7	8	0	0.0
Tahini (sesame)	1 tbsp.	90	8	1.1	5	0	N/A
Vinegar, cider	1 tbsp.	0.0	0	0	TR	0	0.0
Yeast:							
baker's, dry, active	1 package	20	0.0	0.0	4	0	0.0
brewer's, dry	1 tbsp.	25	0.0	0.0	10	0	0.0

Mixed Dishes and Fast Foods

	PORTION	K CAL (CALORIES)	FAT (GM.)	SATU-RATED FAT (GM.)	SODIUM (MG.)	CHOLES-TEROL (MG.)	TRANS FAT (MG.)
Beef & vegetable stew	1 cup	220	11	4.4	292	71	N/A
Beef pot pie, 9" diam.	⅓ pie	515	30	7.9	596	42	N/A
Chicken à la king	1 cup	470	34	12.9	760	221	N/A
Chicken & noodles	1 cup	365	18	5.1	600	103	N/A
Chicken chow mein:							
canned	1 cup	95	TR	0.11	725	8	N/A
home recipe	1 cup	255	10	4.1	473	75	N/A
Chicken pot pie, 9" diam.	½ pie	750	46.0	14.0	594	56	N/A
Chili con carne, canned with beans	1 cup	340	16	5.8	1,354	28	N/A
Chop suey, with stir fried vegetables	1 cup	135	7.5	0.0	505	0	0.0
Fast-food entrées:							
Cheeseburger, 4-oz. patty	1 sand.	490	29.0	12.0	770	65	1.5
Chicken, fried, with skin:							
breast	1 piece	460	28.0	8.0	1,116	135	4.5
drumstick (3.4 oz. with bones)	1 piece	160	10.0	2.5	422	75	1.5

	PORTION	K CAL (CALORIES)	FAT (GM.)	SATU-RATED FAT (GM.)	SODIUM (MG.)	CHOLES-TEROL (MG.)	TRANS FAT (MG.)
Fast-food entrées *(cont.)*							
Enchilada, chicken	1	399	18.2	5.5	1,319	40	N/A
English muffin with egg & cheese	1 sand.	290	11.0	4.5	826	71	0.0
Fish sandwich, large (fried)	1 sand.	470	27	6.3	621	91	N/A
Hamburger:							
regular	1 sand.	700	42.0	13.0	463	32	1.0
4-oz. patty	1 sand.	390	22.0	7.0	763	71	0.5
Pizza, cheese, 15" diam.	1 slice (⅛ pie)	280	12.0	6.0	699	56	0.5
Roast beef sandwich	1 sand.	320	13.0	6.0	757	55	1.0
Taco, fish	1 taco	290	16.0	3.0	226	21	N/A
Macaroni & cheese	1 serving	400	18.0	5.0	730	24	2.5
Quiche Lorraine, 8" diam.	1 slice	600	48	23.2	653	285	N/A
Spaghetti and tomato sauce:							
with cheese	1 cup	383	10.1	0.4	477	0	N/A
with meatballs: canned	½ cup	260	10	2.4	1,220	23	N/A

Nuts and Seeds *(See chart page 20)*

Poultry
Capon:

	PORTION	K CAL (CALORIES)	FAT (GM.)	SATU-RATED FAT (GM.)	SODIUM (MG.)	CHOLES-TEROL (MG.)	TRANS FAT (MG.)
with skin, roasted	3½ oz.	227	11.6	3.2	49	86	0.1

TR = nutrient present in trace amount
N/A = not available

	PORTION	K CAL (CALORIES)	FAT (GM.)	SATU-RATED FAT (GM.)	SODIUM (MG.)	CHOLES-TEROL (MG.)	TRANS FAT (MG.)
Chicken:							
Broilers/Fryers, light meat:							
with skin, fried	3½ oz.	220	8.8	2.4	77	87	0.0
without skin, fried	3½ oz.	186	4.7	1.6	81	90	0.0
with skin, baked or broiled	3½ oz.	195	7.7	2.2	63	74	0.1
without skin, baked or broiled	3½ oz.	164	3.5	1.0	65	77	0.0
Broilers/Fryers, dark meat							
with skin, fried	3½ oz.	238	14.2	3.8	89	92	N/A
with skin, roasted	3½ oz.	153	9.6	2.7	87	91	0.2
without skin, roasted	3½ oz.	109	5.7	1.6	93	93	0.2
Broilers/Fryers, wings:							
with skin, fried	1 wing	159	10.7	2.9	25	26	N/A
with skin, roasted	1 wing	99	6.6	1.9	28	29	0.1
Duck:							
with skin, roasted	3½ oz.	334	28.1	9.6	59	84	N/A
without skin, roasted	3½ oz.	199	1.1	4.1	65	89	N/A
Turkey:							
Light meat, roasted:							
with skin	3½ oz.	195	8.3	2.3	63	76	0.0
without skin	3½ oz.	156	3.2	1.0	64	69	0.0
Dark meat, roasted:							
with skin	3½ oz.	219	11.5	3.5	76	89	0.0
without skin	3½ oz.	186	7.2	2.4	79	85	0.0
Breast, roasted, no skin	3½ oz.	134	0.7	0.2	959	31	0.0

	PORTION	K CAL (CALORIES)	FAT (GM.)	SATU-RATED FAT (GM.)	SODIUM (MG.)	CHOLES-TEROL (MG.)	TRANS FAT (MG.)
Soups							
Canned, condensed:							
Asparagus, cream of:							
made with milk	1 cup	161	8.2	3.3	1,041	22	0.0
made with							
water	½ cup	110	7.0	2.0	981	5	0.0
Bean with bacon,							
made with water	1 cup	172	6.0	1.5	952	3	0.0
Bean, black,							
Health Valley	1 cup	120	0.0	0.0	1,198	0	0.0
Beans with franks,							
made with water	1 cup	187	7.0	2.1	1,092	12	N/A
Beef broth							
bouillon	1 cup	19	0.7	0.3	782	TR	0.0
Celery, cream of,							
condensed	½ cup	90	6.0	1.0	1,010	32	0.0
Cheese:							
made with milk	1 cup	230	14.6	9.1	1,020	48	N/A
made with water	1 cup	155	10.5	6.7	950	30	N/A
Chicken broth,							
made with water	1 cup	34	0.0	0.0	776	1	0.0
Chicken, cream of:							
condensed	½ cup	120	8.0	0.0	1,046	27	0.0
low sodium	½ cup	80	2.5	1.0	986	10	0.0
Chicken gumbo,							
Campbell's	1 cup	60	1.0	0.5	955	5	N/A
Chicken noodle	1 cup	100	2.0	0.5	1,107	7	0.0
Chicken noodle							
with dumplings	1 cup	70	2.0	0.0	1,039	10	0.0
Chicken rice	1 cup	130	2.0	0.0	814	7	N/A
Chicken vegetable,							
Progresso	1 cup	90	1.5	0.0	944	10	0.0

TR = nutrient present in trace amount
N/A = not available

	PORTION	K CAL (CALORIES)	FAT (GM.)	SATU- RATED FAT (GM.)	SODIUM (MG.)	CHOLES- TEROL (MG.)	TRANS FAT (MG.)
Chili beef, made with water	1 cup	169	6.6	3.3	1,035	12	N/A
Clam chowder:							
Manhattan, chunky, ready to serve	1 cup	134	3.4	2.1	1,000	14	N/A
New England, made with milk	1 cup	190	10.0	2.5	992	22	0.0
Consommé beef, made with water	1 cup	29	0	0.0	637	0	0.0
Green pea, made with water	½ cup	164	2.9	1.4	987	0	0.0
Minestrone, made with water	1 cup	100	0.0	0.0	911	0.0	0.0
Mushroom, cream of	½ cup	100	6.0	1.5	1,076	20	0.0
Oyster stew	1 cup	80	6.0	3.5	1,040	32	N/A
Potato, cream of	½ cup	90	2.0	1.0	1,060	22	0.0
Shrimp, cream of	1 cup	90	6.0	2.0	1,036	35	N/A
Split pea with ham, ready to serve	1 cup	170	7.0	0.5	965	7	0.0
Tomato bisque	½ cup	130	3.5	1.5	1,108	22	0.0
Turkey noodle	1 cup	100	0.5	0.0	815	5	0.0
Turkey vegetable	1 cup	90	2.0	0.0	905	2	0.0
Vegetable:							
with beef	1 cup	120	1.0	0.0	957	5	0.0
chunky	1 cup	110	1.0	0.0	1,010	0	0.0
vegetarian	½ cup	90	5.0	0.0	823	0	0.0
Dehydrated soups:							
Beef broth, cube	½ cube	20	1.0	0.5	864	TR	0.0
Chicken broth, cube	1 cube	9	0.2	0.1	1,152	1	N/A
Cup of Soups, prepared with water:							
Chicken noodle	6 oz.	40	1.0	0.2	957	2	N/A
Onion	6 oz.	20	TR	0.1	635	0	N/A

	PORTION	K CAL (CALORIES)	FAT (GM.)	SATU- RATED FAT (GM.)	SODIUM (MG.)	CHOLES- TEROL (MG.)	TRANS FAT (MG.)
Soups (cont.)							
Tomato							
vegetable	6 oz.	40	1.0	0.3	856	0	N/A
Onion soup mix	1 packet	115	2.3	0.5	3,493	2	N/A
Reconstituted with water:							
Celery, cream							
of	1 cup	63	1.6	0.2	839	1	N/A
Chicken noodle	1 cup	53	1.2	0.3	1,284	3	N/A
Leek	1 cup	71	2.1	1.0	966	3	0.0
Onion	1 cup	28	0.6	0.1	848	0	N/A
Oxtail	1 cup	71	2.6	1.3	1,210	3	N/A
Pea, green/split	1 cup	133	1.6	0.4	1,220	3	0.0
Sugars:							
Brown, packed	1 cup	829	0.0	0.0	97	0	0.0
White:							
granulated	1 cup	774	0.0	0.0	5	0	0.0
powdered, sifted	1 cup	467	0.1	0.0	02	0	0.0
Sugars and Sweets							
Candy:							
Caramels	1 piece	39	0.8	0.7	64	1	0.0
Chocolate:							
milk, plain	1 oz.	90	5.0	3.5	23	6	0.0
milk, with							
almonds	1 oz.	100	6.0	3.0	23	6	0.0
milk, with							
peanuts	1 oz.	147	9.5	4.1	19	5	N/A
milk, with rice							
cereal	1 oz.	140	7	4.4	46	6	N/A
semi-sweet,	6 oz.						
chips	(or 1 cup)	860	61	36.2	24	0	N/A
sweet, dark	1 oz.	150	10	5.9	5	0	N/A
Fondant (uncoated							
mints, creme							
filling, etc.)	1 oz.	105	0	0	57	0	0.0

TR = nutrient present in trace amount
N/A = not available

	PORTION	K CAL (CALORIES)	FAT (GM.)	SATU-RATED FAT (GM.)	SODIUM (MG.)	CHOLES-TEROL (MG.)	TRANS FAT (MG.)
Fudge, chocolate, plain	1 oz.	124	5.3	3.3	57	0	0.0
Gumdrops	1 oz.	112	0.0	0.0	10	0	0.0
Hard candy	1 oz.	112	0.1	0.0	7	0	0.0
Jelly beans	1 oz.	106	0.0	0.0	7	0	0.0
Marshmallows	1 oz.	90	0.1	0.0	25	0	0.0
Custard, baked	1 cup	305	15	6.8	209	278	N/A
Gelatin dessert	½ cup	70	0	0.0	55	0	N/A
Honey	1 cup	1021	0.0	0.0	17	0	0.0
Jams & Preserves	1 tbsp.	50	0.0	0.0	2	0	0.0
Jelly	1 tbsp.	50	0.0	0.0	4	0	0.0
Popsicle	1 (3 oz.)	45	0.0	0.0	11	0	0.0
Puddings, canned:							
Chocolate	5 oz. can	205	11	9.5	285	1	N/A
Tapioca	5 oz. can	160	5	4.8	252	TR	N/A
Vanilla	5 oz. can	220	10	9.5	305	1	N/A
Puddings, dry mix, made with whole milk:							
Chocolate:							
instant	½ cup	155	4	2.3	440	14	N/A
cooked	½ cup	150	4	2.4	167	15	N/A
Tapioca	½ cup	145	4	2.3	152	15	N/A
Vanilla:							
instant	½ cup	150	4	2.2	375	15	N/A
cooked	½ cup	145	4	2.3	178	15	N/A
Syrups:							
Chocolate flavored syrup or topping:							
thin type	2 tbsp.	85	TR	0.2	36	0	N/A
fudge type	2 tbsp.	125	5	3.1	42	0	N/A
Molasses	1 cup	951	0.3	0.1	38	0	0.0
Table syrup, corn or maple	2 tbsp.	122	0	0.0	19	0	0.0

	PORTION	K CAL (CALORIES)	FAT (GM.)	SATU-RATED FAT (GM.)	SODIUM (MG.)	CHOLES-TEROL (MG.)	TRANS FAT (MG.)

Vegetables and Vegetable Products

Alfalfa seeds,

sprouted, raw	½ cup	5	0.1	0.0	2	0	0.0

Artichokes, globe or French,
cooked &

drained	1	60	0.2	0.0	79	0	0.0

Asparagus, green,
cooked from raw:

cuts and tips	½ cup	3	0.0	0.0	7	0	0.0
spears	½ cup	15	0.0	0.0	2	0	0.0

Bamboo shoots,

canned, drained	½ cup	20	0.2	0.1	9	0	0.0

Beans:

Lima, frozen, cooked:

Fordhook	1 cup	170	1	0.1	90	0	N/A
Baby limas	1 cup	190	1	0.1	52	0	N/A

Snap beans:

cooked	½ cup	22	0.2	0.0	4	0	0.0
frozen	½ cup	19	0.1	0.0	18	0	0.0
canned, drained	½ cup	14	0.1	0.0	339	0	0.0

Bean sprouts:

raw	1 cup	30	TR	TR	6	0	0.0
cooked, drained	1 cup	25	TR	TR	12	0	0.0

Beets:

cooked:

fresh	½ cup	22	0.1	0.0	83	0	0.0
pickled	½ cup	65	0.0	0.0	49	0	0.0
canned	½ cup	26	0.1	0.0	466	0	0.0

Beet greens,
leaves and stems,

cooked	1 cup	40	TR	TR	347	0	0.0

Black-eyed peas:
cooked and drained:

from raw	1 cup	180	1	0.3	7	0	0.0

TR = nutrient present in trace amount
N/A = not available

	PORTION	K CAL (CALORIES)	FAT (GM.)	SATU- RATED FAT (GM.)	SODIUM (MG.)	CHOLES- TEROL (MG.)	TRANS FAT (MG.)
from frozen	1 cup	225	1	0.3	9	0	0.0
Broccoli:							
raw	½ cup	10	0.1	0.0	41	0	0.0
cooked, from							
raw	½ cup	22	0.3	0.0	17	0	0.0
cooked, from							
frozen	½ cup	20	0.2	0.0	7	0	0.0
Brussels sprouts,							
cooked, drained	½ cup	28	0.4	0.1	33	0	0.0
Cabbage:							
Chinese,							
cooked, drained	½ cup	10	0.1	0.0	58	0	0.0
red, raw	½ cup	11	0.1	0.0	8	0	0.0
Savoy	1 cup	20	TR	TR	20	0	0.0
Cabbage:							
green, raw	½ cup	8	0.0	0.0	13	0	0.0
cooked, drained	½ cup	17	0.3	0.0	29	0	0.0
Carrots:							
raw	½ cup	25	0.2	0.0	25	0	0.0
cooked	½ cup	27	0.1	0.0	39	0	0.0
Cauliflower:							
raw	½ cup	13	0.1	0.0	15	0	0.0
cooked	½ cup	14	0.3	0.0	8	0	0.0
Celery, raw	1 stalk	10	0.0	0.0	35	0	0.0
	½ cup	8	0.1	0.0	106	0	0.0
Collards, cooked	½ cup	25	0.3	0.0	36	0	0.0
Corn, sweet, cooked:							
from raw	1 ear	85	1	0.2	13	0	0.0
kernels, from							
frozen	1 cup	135	0.0	0.0	8	0	0.0
cream style	½ cup	100	0.5	0.0	730	0	0.0
whole kernel	1 cup	165	1	0.2	571	0	0.0
Cucumber, fresh	½ cup	24	0.3	0.0	1	0	0.0
Dandelion greens,							
cooked, drained	½ cup	17	0.3	0.1	46	0	0.0

	PORTION	K CAL (CALORIES)	FAT (GM.)	SATU-RATED FAT (GM.)	SODIUM (MG.)	CHOLES-TEROL (MG.)	TRANS FAT (MG.)
Vegetables and Vegetable Products (cont.)							
Eggplant, cooked, steamed	½ cup	17	0.1	0.0	3	0	0.0
Endive, Belgian, fresh	½ cup	8	0.0	0.0	11	0	0.0
Ginger root, raw	1 tsp.	2	0.0	0.0	6	0	0.0
Hominy, canned, white	1 cup	140	0.0	0.0	710	0	0.0
Jerusalem artichoke, raw	½ cup	57	0.0	0.0	6	0	0.0
Kale, cooked, drained	1 cup	40	1	0.1	30	0	0.0
Kohlrabi cooked, drained	½ cup	24	0.1	0.0	35	0	0.0
Lettuce raw:							
butterhead	½ cup	4	0.1	0.0	8	0	0.0
iceberg	½ cup	4	0.0	0.0	49	0	0.0
loose leaf (as romaine), shredded	½ cup	4	0.0	0.0	5	0	0.0
Mushrooms:							
raw, button	½ cup	8	0.1	0.0	3	0	0.0
cooked, drained	1 cup	40	1	0.1	3	0	0.0
canned, drained	½ cup	20	0.2	0.0	663	0	0.0
Mustard greens, cooked	½ cup	11	0.2	0.0	22	0	0.0
Okra, cooked	½ cup	18	0.1	0.0	4	0	0.0
Onions, raw	½ cup	34	0.1	0.0	3	0	0.0
onion rings	1 serving	320	16.0	4.0	17	0	N/A
Onions (scallions) white portion only	6	10	0.0	0.0	1	0	0.0

TR = nutrient present in trace amount
N/A = not available

	PORTION	K CAL (CALORIES)	FAT (GM.)	SATU-RATED FAT (GM.)	SODIUM (MG.)	CHOLES-TEROL (MG.)	TRANS FAT (MG.)
Parsley, raw	½ cup	11	0.2	0.0	2	0	0.0
Parsnips, cooked	½ cup	55	0.2	0.0	6	0	0.0
Peas, snow, cooked	½ cup	35	0.2	0.0	6	0	0.0
Peas, green, cooked	½ cup	67	0.2	0.0	2	0	0.0
sugar snap	½ cup	38	0.0	0.0	139	0	0.0
Peppers, bell, raw	½ cup	15	0.1	0.0	2	0	0.0
Peppers, hot chili, raw	½ cup	14	0.3	0.0	3	0	0.0
Potatoes:							
baked with skin	6 oz.	128	0.2	0.1	16	0	0.0
boiled	½ cup	67	0.1	0.0	5	0	0.0
French fried, frozen, fried in vegetable oil	10 strips	160	8	2.5	108	0	N/A
oven heated	10 strips	110	4	2.1	16	0	N/A
Potato products, prepared:							
Au gratin:							
dry mix	1 packet	230	10	6.3	1,076	12	N/A
home recipe	1 cup	325	19	11.6	1,061	56	N/A
Hash browns, from frozen	½ cup	62	4.8	1.9	53	0	0.0
Mashed, home recipe:							
milk added	1 cup	160	1	0.7	636	4	N/A
milk & margarine added	½ cup	119	4.4	1.8	620	4	0.1
from dehydrated flakes	1 cup	235	12	7.2	697	29	N/A
Potato salad, made with mayonnaise	1 cup	360	21	3.6	1,323	170	N/A
Scalloped potatoes:							
home recipe	1 serving	30	0.7	N/A	821	29	N/A
cheesy	½ cup	110	1.5	0.0	94	0	N/A

PORTION	K CAL (CALORIES)	FAT (GM.)	SATU-RATED FAT (GM.)	SODIUM (MG.)	CHOLES-TEROL (MG.)	TRANS FAT (MG.)
Vegetables and Vegetable Products (cont.)						
Pumpkin, canned ½ cup	42	0.3	0.2	12	0	0.0
Radishes ½ cup	9	0.1	0.0	4	0	0.0
Rutabaga, cooked ½ cup	33	0.2	0.0	4	0	0.0
Sauerkraut, canned ½ cup	16	0.0	0.0	1,560	0	0.0
Seaweed (kelp), raw ½ cup	17	0.2	0.1	66	0	0.0
Spinach:						
raw, chopped ½ cup	3	0.1	0.0	43	0	0.0
cooked ½ cup	21	0.2	0.0	126	0	0.0
creamed ½ cup	111	8.0	4.6	163	0	0.0
Spinach soufflé 1 cup	220	18	7.1	763	184	N/A
Squash, summer ½ cup	18	0.3	0.1	2	TR	0.0
Sweet potato, cooked: baked in skin,						
peeled 6 oz.	93	0.2	0.1	20	0	0.0
mashed ½ cup	125	0.2	0.1	20	0	0.0
candied ½ cup	276	0.8	0.4	74	8	0.0
Tomato:						
raw 1	35	0.5	0.0	10	0	0.0
canned, Del Monte ½ cup	25	0.0	0.0	391	0	0.0
Tomato juice, canned ½ cup	25	0.0	0.0	881	0	0.0
Tomato products, canned: paste,						
Contadina 2 tbsp.	30	0.0	0.0	170	0	0.0
puree, Progresso ½ cup	50	0.0	0.0	50	0	0.0
Turnips, cooked ½ cup	17	0.1	0.0	78	0	0.0

TR = nutrient present in trace amount
N/A = not available

PORTION	K CAL (CALORIES)	FAT (GM.)	SATU- RATED FAT (GM.)	SODIUM (MG.)	CHOLES- TEROL (MG.)	TRANS FAT (MG.)
Turnip greens, cooked 1 cup	14	0.2	0.0	42	0	0.0
Vegetable juice, V-8 Low Sodium, canned 5.5 oz.	30	0.0	0.0	80	0	0.0
Water chestnuts, ½ cup	60	0.1	0.0	11	0	0.0
Watercress ½ cup	2	0.0	0.0	1	0	0.0
Zucchini, cooked ½ cup	13	0.1	0.0	2	0	0.0

The average person should try to consume between 25 and 30 grams of fiber daily. This expedites the passage of food through the gastrointestinal tract and helps to lessen the absorption of cholesterol. Fiber consumption is also helpful in weight-loss management.

The Dietary Fiber Content of Selected Foods

There are two types of fiber—soluble helps lower cholesterol and insoluble helps prevent constipation.

FOOD ITEM	TOTAL DIETARY FIBER
	gm. per 100 gm. *(about 3½ ounces)* edible portion
Baked Products	
Bagels, plain	2.1
Bread:	
Boston brown	4.7
Bran	8.5
Cornbread mix, baked	2.6
Cracked wheat	5.3
French	2.3
Hollywood-type, light	4.8
Italian	2.7
Mixed-grain	6.3
Oatmeal	3.9
Pita:	
White	1.6
Whole wheat	7.4
Pumpernickel	5.9
Reduced-calorie, high-fiber	
Wheat	11.3
White	7.9
Rye	6.2
Wheat	3.5
Toasted	5.2
White	1.9
Toasted	2.5
Whole Grain	3.2

The Dietary Fiber Content of Selected Foods

*Foods high in fiber are filling and thus
are appetite suppressants.*

FOOD ITEM	TOTAL DIETARY FIBER
	gm. per 100 gm. *(about 3½ ounces)* *edible portion*
Whole wheat	7.4
Toasted	8.9
Bread crumbs, plain or seasoned	4.2
Bread stuffing, flavored, from dry mix	2.9
Cookies:	
Brownies	2.2
With nuts	2.6
Butter	2.4
Chocolate chip	2.7
Chocolate sandwich	2.9
Fig bars	4.6
Fortune	1.6
Oatmeal	2.9
Oatmeal, soft-type	2.7
Peanut butter	1.8
Shortbread with pecans	1.8
Crackers:	
Crisp bread, rye	16.2
Graham cracker	3.2
Honey	1.7
Matzo:	
Plain	2.9
Egg/onion	5.0
Whole wheat	11.8
Melba toast:	
Plain	6.3
Rye	7.9
Wheat	7.4
Rye	15.8

The Dietary Fiber Content of Selected Foods

*In cultures where natural fiber consumption
is high, obesity is low!*

FOOD ITEM	TOTAL DIETARY FIBER
	gm. per 100 gm. *(about 3½ ounces)* *edible portion*

Baked Products (cont.)

Saltines	2.6
Snack-type	1.2
Wheat	5.5
Whole wheat	10.4
English muffin, whole wheat	6.7
French toast, commercial, ready-to-eat	3.1
Muffins, commercial, oat bran	7.5

Pancake/waffle mix:

regular, prepared	1.4
Buckwheat, dry	2.3
Taco shells	8.0

Tortillas:

Corn	5.2
Flour, wheat	2.9
Waffles, commercial, frozen, ready-to-eat	2.4

Breakfast Cereals, Ready-to-Eat

Bran:

extra fiber	45.9
high fiber	35.3
Bran flakes	18.8
Bran flakes with raisins	13.4

Corn flakes:

Plain	2.0
Frosted or sugar-sparkled	2.2
Fiber cereal with fruit	14.8
Granola	10.5
Oat cereal	10.6
Oat flakes, fortified	3.0

The Dietary Fiber Content of Selected Foods

*Fiber helps you limit calories, lose weight,
and promotes bowel regularity.*

FOOD ITEM	TOTAL DIETARY FIBER
	gm. per 100 gm. *(about 3½ ounces)* edible portion

Wheat and malted barley:

Flakes	6.8
Nuggets	6.5
With raisins	6.0
Wheat flakes	9.0

Cereal Grains

Amaranth	15.2
Amaranth flour, whole grain	10.2
Arrowroot flour	3.4
Barley	17.3
Barley, pearled, raw	15.6
Bulgur, dry	18.3
Corn bran, crude	84.6
Corn flour, whole grain	13.4

Cornmeal:

Whole grain	11.0
Degermed	5.2

Farina:

Dry	2.7
Cooked	1.4
Millet, hulled, raw	8.5
Oat bran, raw	15.9
Oat flour	9.6
Oats, rolled or oatmeal, dry	10.3

Rice, brown, long grain:

Raw	3.5
Cooked	1.7

The Dietary Fiber Content of Selected Foods

*Fiber results in better blood-sugar balance and
reduces the risk of developing and helps control Type 2 diabetes.*

FOOD ITEM	TOTAL DIETARY FIBER
	gm. per 100 gm. *(about 3½ ounces)* edible portion

Rice, brown, long grain (cont.)

Rice, white:

Long grain:	
Cooked	0.5
Precooked or instant:	
Dry	1.6
Cooked	0.8
Medium grain, raw	1.4

Rice flour:

Brown	4.6
White	2.4
Rye flour, medium or light	14.6
Semolina	3.9
Tapioca, pearl, dry	1.1
Triticale	18.1
Triticale flour, whole grain	14.6
Wheat bran, crude	42.4

Wheat flour:

White, all-purpose	2.7
Whole grain	12.6

Wheat germ:

Crude	15.0
Toasted	12.9
Wild rice, raw	5.2

Fruits and Fruit Products

Apples, raw:

With skin	2.2
Without skin	1.9
Apple juice, unsweetened	0.1

The Dietary Fiber Content of Selected Foods

*Foods high in fiber are high in volume
and low in calories.*

FOOD ITEM	TOTAL DIETARY FIBER
	gm. per 100 gm. (about 3½ ounces) edible portion
Applesauce, unsweetened	1.5
Apricots, dried	7.8
Apricot nectar	0.6
Bananas, raw	1.6
Blueberries, raw	2.3
Cantaloupe, raw	0.8
Figs, dried	9.3
Grapefruit, raw	0.6
Grapes, Thompson seedless, raw	0.7
Kiwi fruit, raw	3.4
Nectarines, raw	1.6
Oranges, raw	2.4
Orange juice, frozen concentrate, prepared	0.2
Peaches:	
Canned in juice, drained	1.0
Dried	8.2
Raw	1.6
Pears, raw	2.6
Pineapple:	
Canned in heavy syrup, chunks, drained	1.1
Raw	1.2
Prunes:	
Dried	7.2
Stewed	6.6
Prune juice	1.0
Raisins	5.3
Strawberries	2.6
Watermelon	0.4
Legumes, Nuts, and Seeds	
Almonds, oil-roasted	11.2

The Dietary Fiber Content of Selected Foods

*We should try to consume 25 to 30 grams
of dietary fiber each day.*

FOOD ITEM	TOTAL DIETARY FIBER
	gm. per 100 gm. (about 3½ ounces) edible portion

Legumes, Nuts, and Seeds (cont.)

Baked beans, canned:

Sweet or tomato sauce	7.7
Plain	7.7
Beans, Great Northern, canned, drained	5.4
Chickpeas, canned, drained	5.8
Cowpeas (black-eyed peas), cooked, drained	9.6
Hazelnuts, oil-roasted	6.4
Lima beans, cooked, drained	7.2
Pecans, dried	6.5
Pistachio nuts	10.8
Tahini	9.3
Tofu	1.2

Walnuts, dried:

Black	5.0
English	4.8

Pasta

Macaroni (see Spaghetti)	
Macaroni, protein-fortified, dry	4.3
Macaroni, tricolor, dry	4.3

Noodles, Japanese, dry:

Somen	4.3
Udon	5.4
Noodles, spinach, dry	6.8

Spaghetti and macaroni:

Dry	2.4
Cooked	1.6

Spaghetti, dry:

Spinach	10.6
Whole wheat	11.8

The Dietary Fiber Content of Selected Foods

FOOD ITEM	TOTAL DIETARY FIBER
	gm. per 100 gm.
	(about 3½ ounces)
	edible portion

Popcorn:
Air-popped — 15.1

Vegetables and Vegetable Products
Artichokes, raw — 5.2
Beans, snap, raw — 1.8
Beets, canned, drained solids, sliced — 1.7

Broccoli:
Raw — 2.8
Cooked — 2.6
Brussels sprouts, boiled — 4.3

Cabbage, red:
Raw — 2.0
Cooked — 2.0
Cabbage, white, raw — 2.4
Carrots, raw — 3.2

Cauliflower:
Raw — 2.4
Cooked — 2.2

Celery:
Raw — 1.6
Cooked — 3.7

Canned corn:
Cream-style — 1.2
Cucumbers, raw — 1.0

Lettuce:
Butterhead or iceberg — 1.0
Romaine — 1.7

Mushrooms:
Raw — 1.3
Broiled — 2.2
Onions, raw — 1.6
Onions, spring, raw — 2.4

The Dietary Fiber Content of Selected Foods

FOOD ITEM	TOTAL DIETARY FIBER
	gm. per 100 gm. *(about 3½ ounces)* *edible portion*
Vegetables and Vegetable Products (cont.)	
Parsley, raw	4.4
Peas, edible-podded, cooked	2.8
Peppers, sweet, raw	1.6
Potatoes:	
Baked:	
Flesh	1.5
Skin	4.0
Boiled	1.5
Spinach, raw	2.6
Squash:	
Summer:	
Raw	1.2
Cooked	1.4
Winter:	
Raw	1.8
Cooked	2.8
Sweet potatoes:	
Raw	3.0
Cooked	3.0
Tomatoes, raw	1.3
sauce	1.5
Turnip greens, boiled	3.1
Turnips:	
Raw	1.8
Boiled	2.0
Vegetables, mixed, frozen, cooked	3.8
Watercress	2.3

Anderson, James W., and Susan R. Bridges, "The Dietary Fiber of Selected Foods," *American Journal of Clinical Nutrition*, 47:440–7, 1988.

Bibliography

BOOKS

Farquhar, John W., *How to Reduce Your Risk of Heart Disease.* Stanford Center for Research, 1996.

———*The American Way of Life Need Not Be Hazardous to Your Health.* Norton, 1989.

Jacobson, Michael, and Bruce Marder, *What Are We Feeding Our Kids?* Workman, 1994.

Ornish, Dean, M.D., *Stress, Diet, and Your Heart.* Signet, 1984.

Pennington, Jean A. T., and Judith S. Douglass, *Bowes and Church's Food Values of Portions Commonly Used,* 18th Edition. Lippincott and Wilkins, 2005.

Peters, Anne, M.D. *Conquering Diabetes.* Penguin Group USA, 2005.

Pritikin, Nathan, *The Pritikin Promise: 28 Days to a Longer, Healthier Life.* Simon & Schuster, 1983.

Roth, Harriet, *Harriet Roth's Fat Counter. Revised Edition.* Signet, 2007.

———*Harriet Roth's Fat Counter.* Signet, 1999.

———*Deliciously Healthy Jewish Cooking.* Dutton, 1996.

———*Complete Guide to Fats, Calories and Cholesterol.* New American Library, 1993.

———*Harriet Roth's Guide to Low-Cholesterol Dining Out.* Signet, 1990.

———*Cholesterol Control Cookbook.* Plume, 1991.

———*Cholesterol Control Cookbook.* New American Library, 1989.

———*Deliciously Simple.* New American Library, 1986.

———*Deliciously Low.* New American Library, 1983.

Saltsman, Amelia, *The Santa Monica Farmers' Market Cookbook.* Blenhaim Press, 2007.

Wansink, Brian, *Mindless Eating: Why We Eat More Than We Think.* Bantam, 2007.

BOOKLETS

American Heart Association, *Calories Do Count!* To learn more, call toll-free (800) AHA-USA1 or (800) 242-8721. For futher information, visit www.americanheart.org.

——*Understanding and Controlling Cholesterol.* To learn more, call toll-free (800) AHA-USA1 or (800) 242-8721. For further information visit www.americanheart.org.

National Cholesterol Education Program. *Live Healthier, Live Longer: Preventing Heart Disease.* Adult Treatment Panel III guidelines, available online at http://www.nhlbi.nih.gov/chd/.

National Heart, Lung and Blood Institute, *Exercise and Your Health.* U.S. Department of Health and Human Services; National Institutes of Health; National Heart, Lung and Blood Institute. NIH Publication No. 81-1677.

——*Your Guide to Lowering Your Cholesterol with Therapeutic Lifestyle Changes* (TLC). U.S. Department of Health and Human Services; National Institutes of Health; National Heart, Lung and Blood Institute. NIH Publication No. 06-5235.

National Institutes of Health, U.S. Department of Health and Human Services. *National Cholesterol Education Month Kit, 2006,* available online at hp2010. nhlbihin.net/cholmonth/chool_kit.htm. To contact a trained information specialist, phone (301) 592-8573 or write to NHLBI Health Information Center, P.O. Box 30105, Bethesda, MD 20824-0105. Also, for health information, visit www.nhlbi.hih.gov.

Office of the Surgeon General, U.S. Department of Health and Human Services. *The Health Consequences of Smoking, A Report of the Surgeon General,* 2004; *The Surgeon General's Call to Action to Prevent and Decrease Overweight and Obesity,* 2004. Available online at www.surgeongeneral.gov, or write to: 5600 Fishers Lane, Room 18-66, Rockville, MD 20857. Phone (301) 443-4000.

U.S. Department of Agriculture, Nutrition and Health Issues, Heart Health. *High Blood Cholesterol, What You Need to Know,* NIH Publication No. 05-3290. Available online at www.nutrition.gov. To contact a nutrition information specialist write to: National Agricultural Library, Food and Nutrition Information Center, Nutrition.gov Staff, 10301 Baltimore Ave., Beltsville, MD 20705-2351.

RECOMMENDED PERIODICALS AND NEWSLETTERS

Center for Science in the Public Interest, "Nutrition Action Health Letter." Nutrition Action Circulation Department, 1875 Connecticut Avenue, N.W., Suite 300, Washington, D.C. 20009-5728 (www.cspinet.org/nah/).

Cleveland Clinic Heart and Vascular Institute, "Health Extra" newsletter. Subscribe online at www.clevelandclinic.org/healthextra/.

"Environmental Nutrition," P.O. Box 5656, Norwalk, CT 06856-5656 (www.environmentalnutrition.com).

Harvard Medical School, "Harvard Health Letter." Subscribe online at www.health.harvard.edu/newsletters/Harvard_Health_Letter.htm.

Johns Hopkins Medical Letter, "Health After Fifty," P.O. Box 420178, Palm Coast, FL 32142-0178 (www.johnshopkinshealthalerts.com/health_after_50/).

Latino Nutrition Council (www.latinonutrition.org).

Loma Linda University Medical Center: "A Healthy Tomorrow." 11234 Anderson Street, Loma Linda, CA 92354-2804 (www.llu.edu/news/healthy/).

Mayo Clinic Health Letter, P.O. Box 53889, Boulder, CO 80322-3889.

Mt. Sinai School of Medicine, "Focus in Health Aging," P.O. Box 420235, Palm Coast, FL 32142-0235.

Tufts University, "Health & Nutrition Letter." P.O. Box 420235, Palm Coast, FL 32142-0235 (healthletter, tufts.edu/).

University of California, Berkeley, "Wellness Letter." P.O. Box 420148, Palm Coast, FL 32142-0235 (www.wellnessletter.com).

University of California, Los Angeles, "Healthy Years." P.O. Box 420235, Palm Coast, FL 32142-0235 (www.healthy-years,com/cs).

University of Texas, "Lifetime Health Letter," 7000 Tannen, DCT 12012, Houston, TX 77030.

Weil Medical College of Cornell University, "Women's Health Advisor," P.O. Box 420235, Palm Coast, FL 32142-0235.

ARTICLES

Anderson, James W., and Susan B. Bridges, "The Dietary Fiber Content of Selected Foods," *American Journal of Clinical Nutrition* 47:440–7, 1988.

RECOMMENDED PEDOMETERS

www.omronhealthcare.com   Pocket Pedometer HJ-112, costs about $35.
www.new-lifestyles.com, www.thepedometercompany.com/nl2000.html   NL-2000 Activity Monitor, $59.95.

Index